Head and Neck Surgery
Volume 2

Head and Neck Surgery

Indications · Techniques · Pitfalls

Edited by H. H. Naumann
With a Foreword by R. A. Buckingham

Volume 2
Face and Facial Skull
(Chapters 8 to 15)

With Contributions by

H. G. Boenninghaus, Heidelberg
C. A. Hamberger, Stockholm
J. Kinnman, Stockholm
G. Mårtensson, Stockholm
A. Miehlke, Göttingen
K. Mündnich, Münster
E. Nessel, Münster
R. M. Rankow, New York, N. Y.
B. Spiessl, Basel
G. Theissing, Erlangen
H. M. Tschopp, Basel

Translated by P. M. Stell

648 Illustrations
901 Individual Figures

W. B. Saunders Company Philadelphia · London · Toronto
Georg Thieme Publishers Stuttgart   1980

Original German Edition: Kopf- und Hals-Chirurgie
© 1974 by Georg Thieme Verlag, Stuttgart

Authorized English edition copublished 1980
by W. B. Saunders Company, Philadelphia, London, Toronto
and Georg Thieme Verlag, Stuttgart.

© 1980 Georg Thieme Verlag, Herdweg 63, P.O.B. 732, D-7000 Stuttgart 1, West Germany
Printed in Germany

Typesetting: Sulzberg-Druck GmbH, Sulzberg im Allgäu (Linotype VIP)
Printing: Bechtle-Druck, Esslingen

ISBN 3-13-546901-8 (Thieme)
ISBN 0-7216-6664-7 (Saunders)
LCCCN 79-3798 (Saunders)

Editor

Naumann, H. H., Prof Dr
Director, Universitäts-Hals-Nasen-Ohren-Klinik München
D-8000 Munich 2, FRG

Authors

Boenninghaus, H. G., Prof Dr
Director, Universitäts-Hals-Nasen-Ohren-Klinik Heidelberg
D-6900 Heidelberg FRG

Hamberger, C. A., Prof Dr
Chief, Clinic of Oto-Rhino-Laryngology, Karolinska Sjukhuset
S-10401 Stockholm 60, Sweden

Kinnman, J., Prof Dr
Karolinska Sjukhuset
S-10401 Stockholm 60, Sweden

Mårtensson, G., Prof Dr Dr
Chief, Department of Tooth and Jaw Diseases, Karolinska Sjukhuset
S-10401 Stockholm 60, Sweden

Miehlke, A., Prof Dr
Director, Universitäts-Hals-Nasen-Ohren-Klinik Göttingen
D-3400 Göttingen, FRG

Mündnich, K., Prof Dr
Director, Universitäts-Hals-Nasen-Ohren-Klinik Münster/Westfalen
D-4400 Münster, FRG

Nessel, E., Prof Dr
Wissenschaftlicher Rat and Professor, Universitäts-Hals-Nasen-Ohren-Klinik Münster/Westfalen
D-4400 Münster, FRG

Rankow, R. M., DDS, MD
Associate Professor of Clinical Otolaryngology (Surgery of the Head and Neck), College of Physicians and Surgeons, Columbia University, and the Head and Neck Surgical Service, Presbyterian Hospital, New York, NY, Attending Surgeon, Chief, Head and Neck Surgical Service, Bronx Lebanon Hospital Center, Attending Surgeon, Plastic and Maxillofacial Surgical Service, Doctors Hospital, New York, NY, USA

Spiessl, B., Prof Dr Dr
Chief, Klinik für Plastische und Wiederherstellende Chirurgie, Department für Chirurgie, Kantonsspital Basel, Universitätskliniken
CH-4004 Basel, Switzerland

Theissing, G., Prof Dr
em. Director, Universitäts-Hals-Nasen-Ohren-Klinik Erlangen-Nürnberg
D-8520 Erlangen, FRG

Tschopp, H. M., Dr
   Head, Klinik für Plastische und Wiederherstellende Chirurgie, Department für Chirurgie,
   Kantonsspital Basel, Universitätskliniken
   CH-4004 Basel, Switzerland

Translator

Stell, P. M., ChM, FRCS
   Professor of Otorhinolaryngology, The University of Liverpool, Department of Otorhinolaryngology, Royal Liverpool Hospital
   Liverpool L7, UK

Foreword

This volume should be of interest and practical value to all students of head and neck diseases and their surgical treatment. Since the physician is a student for as long as he practices his art, medical students, residents, and specialists, young and old, will find this book to be an excellent treatise of head and neck surgery.

Professor Naumann has enlisted surgeons from clinics and universities of Europe and America to write chapters on the procedures with which they are most familiar, ones which in many cases they have themselves originated. The result is this authoritative volume in which various surgical diseases and their treatments are detailed by international authorities.

Since the authors are experts and leaders in their respective fields, they describe the most modern treatment of head and neck disorders. But the book is not an encyclopedia of surgical procedures, because each author describes operations with which he has had most experience and which he knows to be the most effective for the particular disease described.

As Professor Naumann states in his Foreword, the primary aim of the book is to describe surgical procedures of the head and neck. He has done this by using drawings which illustrate the basic steps of the various surgical procedures. The textual descriptions of the procedures are concise and informative.

While the book is profusely illustrated, each author has followed an outline which completely describes the protocol for each operative procedure. Thus, a description of a surgical procedure is preceded by a brief statement of the rationale and purpose for which the procedure is recommended. The indications for surgery, the methods of establishing the preoperative diagnosis, the preoperative procedures and the type of anesthesia are described. When special instruments are required they are described and illustrated.

Following the description and illustration of the procedure, important modifications and alternative techniques are presented. Important surgical landmarks and sites where iatrogenic injury can occur are detailed. For each procedure a section on rules, hints and typical errors gives the kind of practical information that only an experienced and seasoned surgeon can give. Finally, the postoperative care is outlined as well as a discussion of the functional sequelae of the surgery.

This method of describing surgical procedures is so complete and yet so concise that the descriptions could almost be used verbatim as Pattern Criteria for Surgical Procedures that today are required by the Joint Commission on Hospital Accreditation in the USA.

In his Preface, Professor Naumann states that there are many different surgical disciplines involved in treatment of the head and neck. In some instances two or more specialists may be involved in treatment of the same region of the head or neck in the same patient, and they may be more or less unaware of what their colleagues are attempting to accomplish. By making this book available and convenient for these different specialists, Professor Naumann has increased interdisciplinary knowledge and understanding and contributed greatly to improved patient care, the goal of all physicians. The Chapter, Operations on the Eyelids, the Lacrimal Apparatus and the Orbit, for instance, written by an outstanding ophthalmologist from Germany, discusses clearly the relationship of the plastic surgeon and ophthalmologist in the treatment of lesions of the lids, orbits, and lacrimal apparatus. At the same time, surgeons trained in basic plastic procedures will be helped in the correct evaluation and treatment of lid injuries should they be in a position where no ophthalmological consultation is available. Similarly, the Chapter, Trauma of the Base of the Skull and Intracranial Complications of Nasal Disease, stresses the close cooperation between the neurosurgeon and the rhinologic surgeon required in the treatment of these often dread illnesses.

This book is in no way intended to enable an inexperienced surgeon to perform complex, difficult head and neck surgical procedures, but residents and fellows will find it invaluable for their study and preparation for surgery.

The mature surgeon will find this volume to be valuable for information about up-to-date surgical procedures and for review of operations which he may not have performed for several years. Whether he wishes or is forced by circumstances to perform a procedure that he has not done for a long time, this book presents a stepwise method for his review.

The pre- and postoperative management, anatomical landmarks and pitfalls to be avoided are clearly spelled out so that he can complete the procedure successfully.

For the physician who may be required to take a re-qualification examination on procedures which he has not done since his residency, perusal of this book should jog his memory sufficiently for him to be able to pass successfully.

Professor Naumann is to be congratulated for making the fruits of the labors of many outstanding surgeons available to the profession.

Park Ridge, Ill.,   *Richard A. Buckingham*
June 1979

Preface

This manual is organized practically: for the operating table. The illustrations therefore are central; the text provides additional information which the illustrations cannot supply.

This atlas is intended for physicians who are familiar with the principles of general surgery and the clinical aspects of diseases of the head and neck, but who require more detailed information concerning special surgical techniques for the head and neck region.

More surgical specializations are employed in the region of the head and neck than in any other part of the body. This close relationship necessarily results in a certain amount of overlapping. Increasing specialization, however, also means that the operator is no longer aware of all details of all procedures within his own field of specialization, and he knows less and less about the problems in related fields, even though these specializations are involved with the same region of the body and frequently even with the same patient. The manual, therefore, is intended to broaden the horizon of the operator. We do not intend to remove established borders for the respective operative specializations. Knowledge of methods and possibilities of related fields of specializations, however, should influence the therapeutic measures employed by the operator – usually for the good of the patient.

We have carefully selected the operative methods and their modifications for each indication so that the less experienced reader will not be forced to choose among many different methods. Basically we have presented a detailed description of only one method for each indication. If necessary, brief mention was also made of a few important alternative methods. In this way a selection of established procedures is presented which covers all possible eventualities.

Authors from various fields of specializations were asked to contribute chapters. Some overlapping, therefore, was unavoidable. The repetition was retained so that the style of the author and the balance of each chapter could be maintained.

Since this manual is intended for practical use, only limited bibliographic references are given so that the reader may consult the relevant literature for more detailed information.

The authors and the editors hope that this manual will become a useful aid for training young surgeons. We are aware that it is not perfect and, therefore, are grateful for any constructive criticism or helpful suggestions.

On behalf of all the contributors, I wish to render my sincere gratitude to Professor P. M. Stell who has fulfilled the difficult task to perform the translation from German in such an excellent manner. I also would like to thank Messrs. R. Brammer, H. Seeber, and P. Haller, the medical illustrators, for their collaboration; the book would not have been possible without their technical knowledge and artistic ability. Dr. K. R. Deck helped with the translation and the editing. I would like to express my gratitude to Dr. G. Hauff and his coworkers at Georg Thieme Publishers for their advice and assistance concerning the production and technical presentation of the manual.

Munich, June 1979   *H. H. Naumann*

Contents

8 Trauma of the Anterior Cranial Fossa and of the Base of the Skull and Intracranial Complications of Nasal Disease

By H. E. Boenninghaus

9 Surgery of Injuries of the Skeleton and the Soft Tissues of the Face

By G. Mårtensson

10 Transsphenoidal Surgery of the Pituitary Gland

By C.-A. Hamberger and J. Kinnman

11 Surgery of the Nasopharynx

By E. Nessel and K. Mündnich

12 Surgery of the Jaws

By B. Spiessl and H. M. Tschopp

13 Surgery of Malignant Tumors of the Tongue and the Floor of the Mouth

By R. M. Rankow

14 Surgery of the Oropharynx and of the Tonsils

By G. Theissing

15 Surgery of the Salivary Glands and the Extratemporal Portion of the Facial Nerve

By A. Miehlke

Contents of Volume 1

8 Trauma of the Anterior Cranial Fossa and Intracranial Complications of Nasal Disease

By H. G. Boenninghaus

Surgery of Frontobasal Injuries

The term frontobasal fracture (fracture of the rhinobasis; Wullstein and Wullstein 1970) indicates a fracture of the base of the skull which involves any wall of any of the accessory nasal sinuses forming part of the base of the skull. It, therefore, includes fractures of the posterior wall of the frontal sinus, the roof of the ethmoid sinus and the cribriform plate as well as the roof and lateral wall of the sphenoid sinus (Fig. 8.1). The roof of the orbit is also often involved. Operative intervention on the superior sinuses (frontal sinus, ethmoid sinuses and sphenoid sinuses) is often necessary in frontobasal fractures (Figs. 8.2, 8.3).

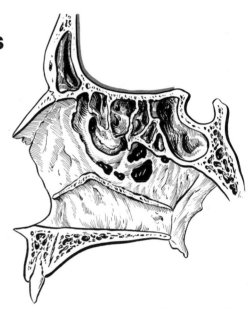

Fig. 8.1 The base of the skull (red) in the region of the nasal sinuses.

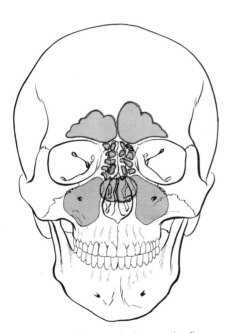

Fig. 8.2 The superior nasal sinuses (red).

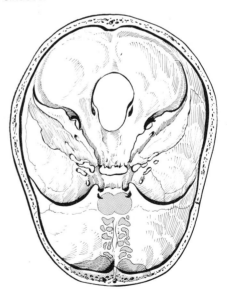

Fig. 8.3 The superior nasal sinuses projected on the base of the skull.

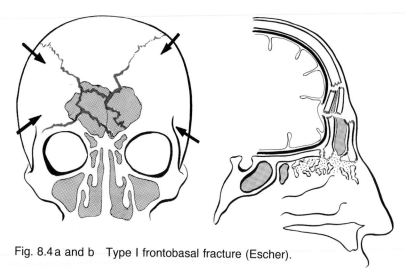

Fig. 8.4a and b   Type I frontobasal fracture (Escher).

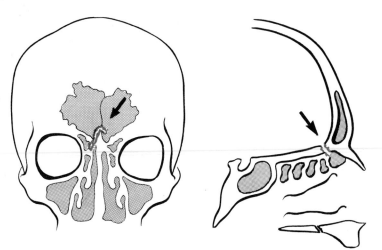

Fig. 8.5a and b   Type II frontobasal fracture (Escher).

Classification

These fractures were classified by Escher (1969) as follows:

Type I   Extensive, comminuted frontobasal fractures with comminution of the frontal bone (Figs. 8.4a, b).

Type II   Localized frontobasal fractures (Figs. 8.5a, b).

Type III   Avulsion of the central part of the face from the base of the skull (Fig. 8.6).

Type IV   Lateral orbital frontobasal fractures with involvement of the roof of the orbit (Fig. 8.7).

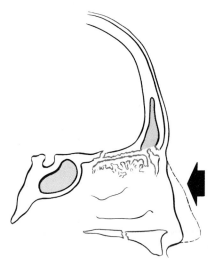

Fig. 8.6   Type III frontobasal fracture (Escher).

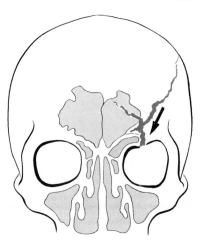

Fig. 8.7   Type IV frontobasal fracture (Escher).

Frequency: The posterior wall of the frontal sinus is most frequently involved, followed by the roof of the ethmoids; involvement of the roof of the sphenoid is the least frequent. The junction of the posterior wall of the frontal sinus and the roof of the ethmoid sinus is frequently affected since the bone here is thin and easily splintered. Most tears of the dura also occur at this point.

Dangers: Damage to the dura overlying the roof of the sinuses can at any time lead to an ascending infection and rhinogenic meningitis. The prognosis depends on the intracranial complications which may occur and on the extent of simultaneous brain damage. Surgery is indicated for frontobasal fractures and for damage to the dura in order to prevent or manage intracranial complications.

Cause: The most common cause of this injury is a traffic accident; occasionally the cause is an accident at work, during sport activities or from other causes. Injuries to the dura occur occasionally during operations on the ethmoid sinuses and in extensive tumor operations.

Diagnostic Preoperative Measures

Inspection. A *unilateral or bilateral orbital hematoma* and epistaxis are almost always present, but these symptoms can also occur in the absence of a fracture of the base of the skull, for example, following injuries to the nose or to the anterior wall of the frontal sinus. The more important sign pointing to a fracture of the base of the skull is bleeding into the medial side of the upper eyelid behind the tarsus, a point which can be verified by everting the upper lid.

Surgical *emphysema* of the lids indicates a fracture of the ethmoid sinuses where air is forced into the upper and lower lids on straining or sneezing. It is not, however, evidence of a fracture of the base of the skull communicating with the inside of the cranial cavity. Surgical emphysema in the orbital apex, which may be easily recognized by palpation, can exert pressure on the optic nerve.

Skin wounds are no indication of the extent of deeper injuries; they may even be absent. It is never sufficient to treat the skin wounds alone without checking for a fracture. Cerebrospinal fluid leakage

from the skin wound or a prolapse of brain tissue indicates that the cranial cavity has been breached and the dura torn.

Investigation of cerebrospinal fluid. In contrast to epistaxis cerebrospinal fluid rhinorrhea following an accident is a certain sign of a fracture of the base of the skull. The fracture is usually to be found in the anterior cranial fossa, but it can also occur in the lateral part of the base of the skull. In a transverse fracture of the petrous bone with an intact tympanic membrane, the cerebrospinal fluid can escape from the middle ear, pass down the eustachian tube and escape from the nose. In the differential diagnosis, deafness should draw attention to the aural origin of the C.S.F. leak (Boenninghaus 1960). The term *cerebrospinal fluid rhinorrhea* indicates an escape of fluid immediately after the injury; the term *cerebrospinal fluid fistula* indicates the escape of cerebrospinal fluid weeks or even months after the accident.

Several methods can be used to establish that the fluid escaping from the nose is cerebrospinal fluid. These methods can also be used in cases of spontaneous nontraumatic rhinorrhea:

● Bending the head forward, possibly accompanied by compression of the internal jugular vein, increases the rate of flow.

● Cerebrospinal fluid stains glucose reagent sticks, whereas a high concentration of protein indicates that the fluid is nasal secretion or tears (Rollin 1970).

● 1–2 ml of 5% fluorescein is injected intrathecally. In the presence of a cerebrospinal fluid leak, the fluorescein can be picked up 1 hour later on pledgets placed in different positions in the nose and its presence demonstrated by fluorescence (Simon 1970) in the nose or accessory sinuses, by endoscopy using ultraviolet light (Messerklinger 1972).

● The radioactive isotopes ^{169}Yb (1 mCi ^{169}Ytterbium, which has a half-life of 31 days) or human serum albumen tagged with ^{131}I (100 μCi ^{131}I, which has a half-life of 8.04 days) are particularly valuable. They are introduced into the cerebrospinal fluid and are collected on marked pledgets. The activity on the pledgets is then measured or it can be used to make a scintigram. The findings, however, can only be evaluated if profuse rhinorrhea is present. It usually suffices to produce simple evidence of rhinorrhea. On lateral views taken with the scanner or the scintillation camera, both sides are superimposed on each other; lateral localization, therefore, is difficult. This method of examination should only be used in a persistent rhinorrhea where there is some doubt as to whether a fistula is present.

● During the operation it is possible to demonstrate small localized or previously unrecognized tears of the dura by using the operating microscope to observe transport disturbances of the secretions (Messerklinger 1967).

Evidence of disturbances of smell. Disturbances of smell are certainly not evidence of a basal fracture, since they can also occur due to respiratory anosmia, nasal injuries with obstruction to nasal respiration or in central anosmia due to damage to the olfactory bulb and track. They are always present, however, in frontobasal fractures with tearing of the olfactory nerve. Unilateral anosmia indicates the side of the injury of the base of the skull.

Radiological investigation. Radiographs are taken of the base of the skull in three planes using postero-anterior views in the occipitofrontal, occipitonasal and occipitomental positions, lateral views of the skull and Welin's overextended axial view (Boenninghaus 1960). The posterior wall of the frontal sinus, which is of particular interest to the rhinologist, is well shown on Welin's view, but the roof of the ethmoids is well shown on the lateral view. If the radiological findings in the standard views are not clear cut, tomography with sagittal and frontal cuts is indicated. Depending on the availability of the apparatus, linear, cyclical or preferably paracyclical tomograms are used.

A collection of air, which is a certain sign of tearing of the dura, should be looked for on the radiographs. A pneumatocele can occur in the subdural, subarachnoid or intraventricular spaces (in a pre-existing space) or there may be an intracerebral *pneumatocele* (air in a cavity produced by damage to the brain substance). Both may occur relatively often together.

Neurological examination. In addition to a general neurological examination computerized tomography, echoencephalography or occasionally angiography should be carried out if there is the slightest suspicion of a space-occupying intracranial hematoma since the typical signs (a symptom free interval, homolateral dilation of the pupil, fixed pupil and contralateral neurological signs) only occur in 50% of acute hematomas.

Cooperation with other specialists. In patients with damage to the lacrimal apparatus, the orbit and the eyeball as well as those with disturbances of vision, an ophthalmologist should be consulted for help with the diagnosis and management of the injury. An oral surgeon should be consulted in injuries to the middle third of the face (Le Fort fractures, see Chapter 9) which require specialized repositioning and fixation. A neurosurgeon is required for intradural procedures (via a transfrontal craniotomy) in open injuries to the brain, disturbances of the cerebral substance, fresh intracranial bleeding and for late complications if an encapsulated abscess is present. If operative management by a neurosurgeon is indicated, care of the injured accessory sinuses by the rhinologist should not be neglected. The nasal operation should preferably be carried out *immediately* after intradural repair of the trauma to the brain and skull. Closure of the dura in such a staged procedure will then have already been carried out by the neurosurgeon at the first operation via the intradural route.

Therapeutic Preoperative Measures

Before operative procedures can be carried out in frontobasal fractures, the airway must be free, shock must have been treated and the circulation must have been stabilized. Before every operation for trauma, the vital signs must be normal (Schürmann 1967). Furthermore, intracranial hemorrhage and profuse hemorrhage from the nose or mouth take precedence in treatment.

a) If there is respiratory obstruction, intubation or tracheostomy is carried out. A tracheostomy is preferred if it is anticipated that the patient will be unconscious for more than 1 or 2 days. The tracheobronchial tree should also be aspirated.

b) If the patient is in shock, an intravenous infusion is set up with low molecular weight colloidal solutions.

c) If there is intracranial bleeding, the hematoma must be relieved immediately via a burr hole or an osteoplastic craniotomy. The craniotomy should preferably be carried out by a neurosurgeon, who will usually have had a C.A.T. scan and an echoencephalogram and an angiogram made first (see p. 4).

d) Severe nasal bleeding should be treated by packing (see Vol. 1, p. 342) or ligature of the vessels (see Vol. 1, p. 347).

e) In recent accidents with open wounds (for example, after traffic accidents or accidents at work), a prophylactic injection against tetanus is necessary.

Indications

Absolute indications:

● Tears of the dura with cerebrospinal fluid rhinorrhea or a pneumatocele due to an accident or occurring during an operation.

● Open injuries to the brain.

● Traumatic infectious meningitis.

● Penetrating foreign bodies (closed injury).

● Orbital complications.

● Late complications arising from the accessory sinuses such as a dural fistula communicating with the posterior wall of the frontal sinus or of the roof of the ethmoid or sphenoid with rhinorrhea, late meningitis, encephalitis, brain abscess or osteomyelitis of the frontal bone.

Relative indications:

● Fractures of the posterior wall of the frontal sinus, of the roof of the ethmoid sinus or of the roof of the sphenoid sinus with radiological evidence of bone displacement and the *possibility* of a dural tear.

● Comminuted fractures of the superior sinuses implicating the frontonasal duct or the orbit.

● Depressed fractures involving the frontal sinus.

● Stab wounds without penetrating foreign bodies and without tearing of the dura.

● Soft tissue injuries with exposure of the underlying sinuses.

● Infection of the sinuses originating at the time of the accident.

● Mucoceles and pyoceles.

Contraindications:

The decision not to operate involves great responsibility and should only be taken in the following circumstances:

● The fracture line involving the frontal sinus shows no bony displacement and no signs of involvement of the dura.

● No comminution of the base of the skull.

● In fractures of the vault of the skull, which do not reach the base of the skull.

● In fractures of the anterior wall of the frontal sinus without bony displacement or comminution.

● In fractures of the nasal bones, without comminution, in the region of the frontonasal duct; in this case, management of the nasal bones alone will suffice.

Timing of the Operation

After resolution of shock and carrying out the preoperative measures mentioned on page 4, surgery should not be delayed for any of the absolute indications. Patients with meningitis of late onset often present to an internist first rather than to the surgeon (in contrast to acute trauma) since the traumatic incident is no longer suspected. As soon as the meningitis begins to improve, the patient must be transferred and the operation carried out. In trauma due to surgery, immediate exploration of the base of the skull is indicated.

In the relative indications, a delay of 1 or 2 weeks under antibiotic cover is possible until the patient begins to recover, but *the operation should not be omitted for patients with relative indications.*

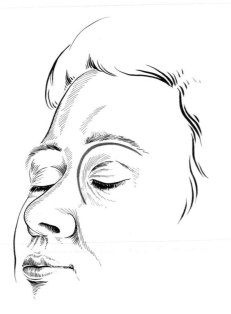

Fig. 8.8   Incision for exposure of the base of the skull over the roof of the sinuses (curved incision).

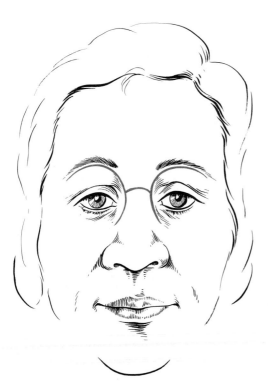

Fig. 8.9   Incision for a bilateral operation.

Principles of the Operation

Surgery is necessary to prevent or relieve a local or intracranial complication. The operation must achieve the following:

● Debridement of the sinus with maintenance of the lumen and restoration of normal relationships at the base of the skull as well as creation of a wide and permanent drainage from the sinus to the nose. If maintenance of the lumen of the frontal sinus is not possible, the sinus should be obliterated.

● In injuries to the dura, a watertight closure between the roof of the sinus and the cranial cavity should be achieved by repair of the dura, so that open injuries to the brain are walled off.

Preparation for Surgery and Anesthesia

Premedication, positioning, preparation, infiltration anesthesia, draping, placement of the surgical team and instruments are the same as described for operations on the frontal sinus (Vol. 1, Chap. 7). The following should also be available for operations on the base of the skull and for repair of the dura: an operating microscope, a drill, lyophilized dura and tissue adhesives.

The operation is carried out under endotracheal anesthesia.

Operative Technique

Fronto-orbital (Extracranial) Procedure

A curved incision is made from the lateral side of the nose terminating within or beneath the eyebrow (Fig. 8.8). For a bilateral frontobasal fracture, a bilateral curved incision is made with a connection over the bridge of the nose (Fig. 8.9). In soft tissue injuries in the region of the eyebrow or the root of the nose, the skin wounds can be included in the incision. The periosteum is divided and the soft tissues are retracted along with the trochlea. The periosteum of the frontal bone is preserved so that an osteoplastic procedure can be carried out if necessary. Furthermore, the periosteum can later be used as a free transplant to repair the dura. The bony floor of the frontal sinus, the lacrimal fossa and the nasal bone are exposed by careful elevation of the lacrimal sac.

The floor of the frontal sinus is removed as in Jansen-Ritter's operation (see Vol. 1, Chap. 7) beginning in the lacrimal fossa. The fossa is penetrated with Hajek's forceps (Fig. 8.10).

If the bone is very thick at this point, a hammer and chisel must be used.

If the posterior wall of the frontal sinus cannot be fully seen after removal of the floor of the sinus, an osteoplastic flap of the anterior wall of the sinus must be turned *upward* or be temporarily removed after division with a Stryker saw in order to reach a fracture of the posterior wall. A typical osteoplastic flap of the anterior wall of the frontal sinuses is described in Vol. 1, Chap. 7.

Loose fragments of the anterior wall are removed, but large bony fragments still attached by their periosteum can be preserved and replaced later or wired in place by intraosseous wires (Matzker 1961) (Fig. 8.11). Depressed fragments of bone are elevated if possible. If the anterior wall of the sinus is extensively comminuted, it must be removed to allow obliteration of the sinus (see p. 18).

More extensive procedures, such as the radical operations on the frontal sinus, the ethmoids and the sphenoids (see Vol. 1, Chap. 7, p. 399) include removal of torn mucosa with curettes or with the drill, clearance of the ethmoids including removal of the floor of the ethmoids, removal of the anterior wall of the sphenoid and, in fractures affecting the sphenoid, removal of the mucosa of this sinus.

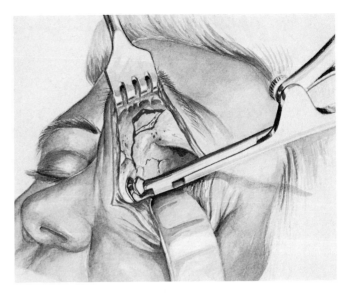

Fig. 8.10

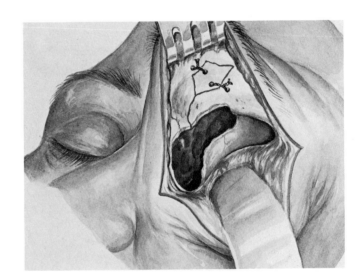

Fig. 8.11

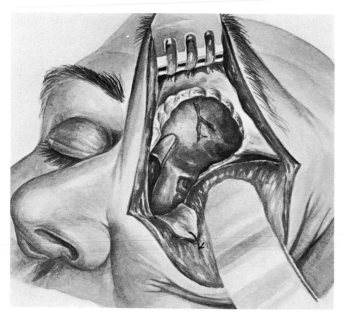

Fig. 8.12

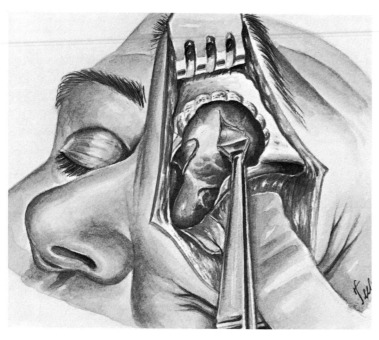

Fig. 8.13

The orbital periosteum is elevated medially and superomedially; part of the lamina papyracea is removed if it is fractured. The orbital periosteum is stitched if it has been torn. A double flap repair (Uffenorde 1952) is carried out after removing part of the nasal bone and the frontal process of the maxilla with Hajek's forceps, and smoothing of the junction of the nasal septum and the interfrontal septum (Fig. 8.12) (see also Vol.1, Chap. 7).

If there is a fracture of the posterior wall of the frontal sinus or the roof of the ethmoid, particular care should be exercised while removing the mucosa of the frontal sinus and clearing the ethmoid cells to avoid damaging the dura further. It is preferable to use the *operating microscope* for this removal and to open the ethmoid carefully from in front backward, cell by cell. In this way a prolapse of dura or brain in the region of the basal fracture is most easily differentiated from a cell. The bone of the base of the skull forming the roof of the ethmoids is whiter, and if it is not fractured, is also harder than the remaining ethmoidal labyrinth. The bone around the fracture or in the comminuted zone of the base of the skull is removed with fine forceps, chisel or diamond burr until the dura is exposed and it has been confirmed that there is no damage to the dura (Fig. 8.13) (if the dura is torn, additional procedures are used such as described on page 10).

Foreign bodies, often consisting of safety glass from a windshield, are removed from the sinus.

Large mobile parts of the base of the skull and crista galli are left alone in order to avoid tearing the dura further.

If a fracture or damage to the dura is suspected in the region of the anterior part of the cribriform plate (medial to the medial turbinate), the anterior attachment of the medial turbinate must be divided from the roof of the nose in order to be able to check the base of the skull lying under the mucosa of the roof of the nose (Fig. 8.14). This causes division of the filaments of the olfactory nerve, in this area.

Packing is unnecessary if repair of the dura has not been carried out, but a finger stall may be introduced from the nose into the frontal sinus and left in place for several days. The finger stall is filled with gauze strips and has a tape inferiorly; it is slit superiorly.

The skin wound is closed with subcutaneous catgut and skin sutures of 4×0 atraumatic Mersilene.

The incision is covered with a sterile dressing (Fig. 8.15), eye ointment is introduced and a head bandage is applied for 1 to 2 days.

Nasal packing is removed after 2 days; the dressing and stitches after 6 days.

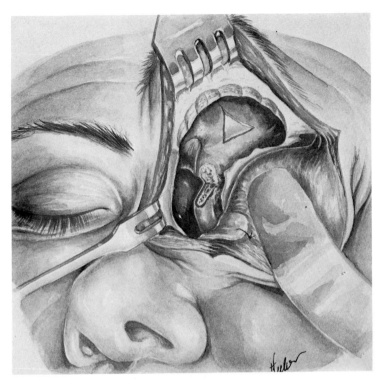

Fig. 8.14

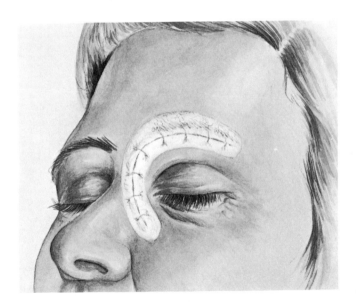

Fig. 8.15

Operation for Prolapse of the Dura or Brain

If the dura prolapses through a bony defect of the base of the skull, it must be reposed. A small dural tear often occurs at the apex of such a prolapse (occasionally after operative damage to the roof of the ethmoid cells).

If cerebral tissue is encountered on opening the frontal sinus or on clearing out the ethmoid cells, the dura has been torn. A small smooth prolapse of the brain less than 2 cm in size should be replaced if possible. This can be facilitated by suboccipital puncture and removal of cerebrospinal fluid; the brain then falls back into place.

Disorganized or necrotic brain tissue which has prolapsed into the sinus is carefully sucked out, foreign bodies and splinters of bone are removed and hemostasis is achieved with Gelfoam or diathermy.

After repositioning or removing the prolapsed dura or brain, the dura is repaired in order to close off the intracranial cavity. Open management is only considered for an early brain abscess (see p. 34).

Operation for a Dural Tear or Defect (Transbasal Extradural)

A transfrontal extradural (see p. 14) or transfrontal intradural (see p. 16) operation must be carried out for extensive trauma affecting the dura and extending into the sinuses and the orbital roof. The transfrontal intradural operation is usually carried out by a neurosurgeon.

In most Type II, III, and IV injuries (Escher 1969) the dural defect can be satisfactorily managed by the transbasal extradural procedure after fronto-orbital clearance of the sinuses. This is especially true of late complications such as a dural fistula with recurrent meningitis.

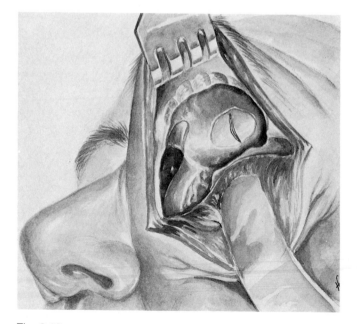

Fig. 8.16

Dural Suture for Dural Tears (Fig. 8.16)

It is only possible to introduce sutures in the region of the posterior wall of the frontal sinus; this is carried out with 5 × 0 atraumatic Mersilene. The dura is exposed first by removing bone with fine bone forceps or a diamond burr (Fig. 8.17). The suture line can also be covered with a free graft if necessary.

Dural Repair

This provides watertight closure of a dural defect (Fig. 8.18) in the region of the posterior wall of the frontal sinus, of the roof of the ethmoid cells or of the anterior part of the cribriform plate. Dural tears in the region of the posterior wall of the cribriform plate are extradural and are difficult to cover by an intradural operation. A cerebrospinal fluid fistula in the region of the sphenoid sinus is dealt with on page 14.

Repair of the dura can also be carried out in the usual way if a dural defect must be made during the course of a tumor operation on the sinuses.

After proceeding as described on page 6 and removing the damaged mucosa and the bony fragments which also occasionally stick into the dura from the base of the skull, the dura is exposed with a punch or a drill, using the microscope, until healthy tissue is reached.

The dura is now elevated carefully from the edges of the bone with a flat elevator (Fig. 8.18). In this way a ledge is prepared as a bed to receive the graft (preparation of the graft is described below).

The introduction of the graft can be facilitated by a sub-occipital puncture and removal of cerebrospinal fluid because this widens the space between the bone and the dura around the defect. The graft, which has been cut to size and compressed, is carefully introduced under the bone with a flat elevator. This produces a watertight closure of the dura (Fig. 8.19).

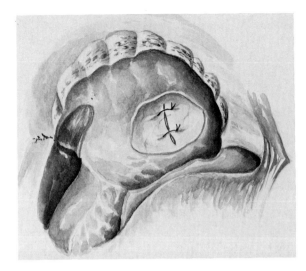

Fig. 8.17

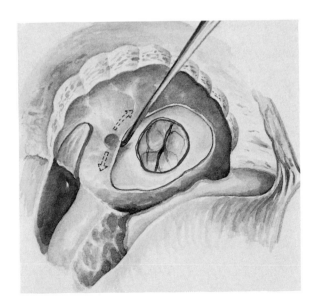

Fig. 8.18

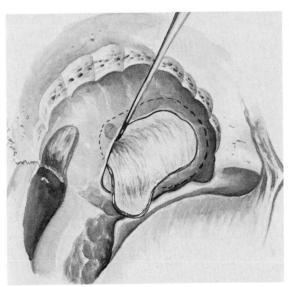

Fig. 8.19

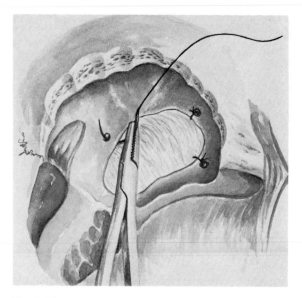

Fig. 8.20

The graft is held firmly in place between the dura and the bone by the intracranial pressure. Additional fixation can be provided by a fine suture introduced through bore holes (Fig. 8.20). Fixation with a tissue adhesive (Histoacryl) applied at multiple points between the dura and the graft has proved to be successful and, in contrast to suturing, can always be carried out. In this technique the previously flattened graft must be elevated briefly from that area to which the glue is to be applied. It is easy to fix the graft by introducing adhesive between the edges of the bone and the graft (Fig. 8.21). Tissue adhesive is especially useful for fixing grafts to the roof of the ethmoid because the bony edges can often not be satisfactorily undermined, particularly over the posterior part of the cribriform plate:

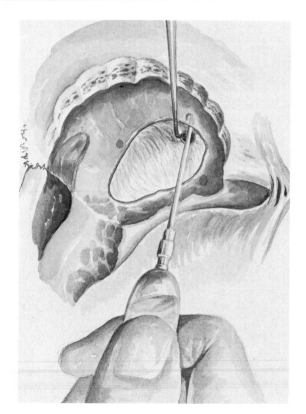

Fig. 8.21

Graft Material

A piece of galea is used as a free transplant. It is obtained from the forehead after incision and elevation of the skin of the forehead (Fig. 8.22).

If a larger graft is necessary, it can be obtained from the fascia lata. This, however, requires a separate operation on the thigh. The fascia is removed after making a long incision over the rectus femoris muscle followed by division of the subcutaneous fat. Refrigerated lyophilized cadaveric dura (available in different sizes) impregnated with saline has proved worthwhile. It is easy to introduce and adheres well (Pfalz 1969). Pieces of lyophilized dura must not be too thick or too stiff.

In the unusual case with a very large bony defect, the possibility of a postoperative dural prolapse must be kept in mind. To prevent this, a piece of septal cartilage is introduced into the bony defect after repair of the dura in the same way as a free graft. Large bony defects should not remain especially in children with a "growing" fracture (Kecht 1972).

The dural repair is covered with a layer of fibrin foam and is supported by packing which is led out through the nostril (Uffenorde's repair or median drainage, see p. 18 and Vol.1, Chap. 7) (Fig. 8.23). Gauze or foam rubber strips soaked in ointment are used for this; they are removed after 4 to 7 days.

After repair of the dura, the skin wound is closed as described on page 9.

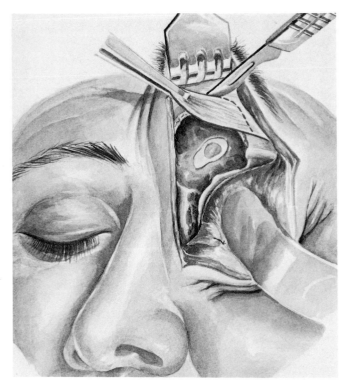

Fig. 8.22

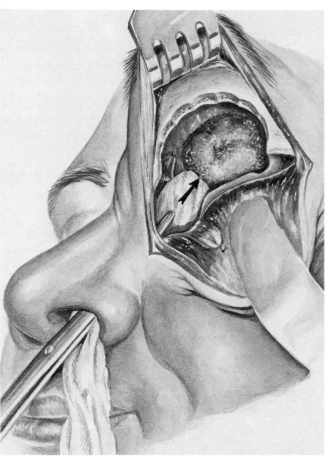

Fig. 8.23

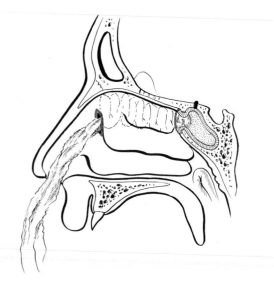

Fig. 8.24

Management of a Dural Fistula in the Region of the Sphenoid Sinus

If the fracture line extends into the sphenoid sinus, it is exposed by external ethmoidectomy, removal of the anterior wall of the sphenoid sinus and removal of the mucosa (a typical sphenoid operation is described in Vol. 1, Chap. 7). If cerebrospinal fluid is escaping from the fracture, the bone of the roof of the sphenoid sinus is *not* removed, but rather fascia is pressed into the fracture line. This can also be closed by using drops of tissue adhesive to line the entire sphenoid cavity which is then filled with a large fascial transplant held in place by moist Gelfoam (Fig. 8.24). The graft then adheres firmly to the wall of the sphenoid sinus (Kley 1968). A cerebrospinal fluid fistula into the sphenoid sinus following hypophysectomy is managed in the same way.

The packing is led out through the nose. If the sphenoid sinus is large, there is a danger that the large graft required can be extruded. In very large sinuses, one must be content with a piece of fascia or lyophilized dura fixed by tissue adhesive and supported by firm packing.

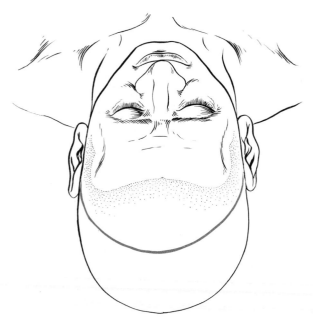

Fig. 8.25   Coronal incision.

Important Modifications and Surgical Alternatives

Unterberger's Transfrontal Extradural Procedure

In extensive frontobasal comminuted fractures with comminution of the frontal bone, the incision is made from ear to ear after having shaved the head (Fig. 8.25). The galea is elevated with the periosteum and an anterior scalp flap is turned down to the supraorbital ridge and the roof of the nose (Fig. 8.26). The elevation proceeds laterally as far as the insertion of the temporalis muscle. The scalp vessels are caught with hemostats. The fragments of the frontal bone are removed (Fig. 8.26) and are preserved so that they can be replaced after the operation. Alternatively, they may remain attached anteriorly to the periosteum.

Unterberger's procedure (1959) is to be used in the absence of extensive comminution when an osteoplastic bone flap is needed (Kecht 1965). Using irrigation and suction, holes are bored in the frontal bone with a Martell drill, Stryker cranial perforator or drill. The dura is elevated from the bone between the holes with a blunt elevator. The holes are then joined by a Stryker craniotome, narrow burr or Gigli saw and the flap is elevated, being freed simultaneously from the dura (bifrontal craniotomy, Fig. 8.26). The flap is replaced at the end of the operation.

The dura of the anterior cranial fossa is then elevated from the bone and pressed backward with the frontal lobe to expose the posterior wall of the frontal sinus, the roof of the orbit and the ethmoid sinuses on one or both sides and the fracture line (Fig. 8.27). The falx cerebri must be freed from the crista galli to expose the cribriform plate on both sides. This maneuver divides the fibers of the olfactory nerve.

Bone fragments of the base of the skull, the posterior wall of the frontal sinus, the roof of the orbit and the roof of the ethmoid sinuses are removed. Dural tears (Fig. 8.27) are now closed extradurally with sutures and are covered by a free graft which can also be fixed in place with adhesive.

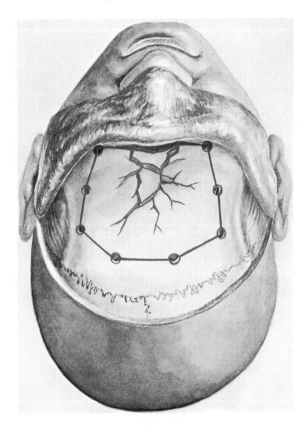

Fig. 8.26
Anterior scalp flap. Large bony fragments of the frontal bone are removed and replaced after the operation or form an osteoplastic flap.

More favorable access for ethmoidectomy and for creation of a wide drainage from the frontal sinus to the nose, with the usual mucosal repair, can be obtained with the fronto-orbital procedure (see p. 6), but the operation on the sinuses can also be carried out by this transfrontal extradural procedure. If the roof of the ethmoid sinuses is not comminuted, it should be preserved to support the dura. Clearance of the cells is then accomplished by the paranasal route (Kecht 1965).

Exposure of the orbital roof and the posterior wall of the frontal sinus is excellent with Unterberger's method. This method, however, does not permit such a good view of the roof of the ethmoid sinuses because the dura is easily torn when it is being elevated at this point. Exposure of the roof of the sphenoid sinus is also not possible with this method of access. The transfrontal intradural neurosurgical procedure (see p. 19) is recommended for extensive tears of the dura, which extend over the sinuses. In isolated injuries to the dura over the sphenoid sinus, the procedure is as described on page 14.

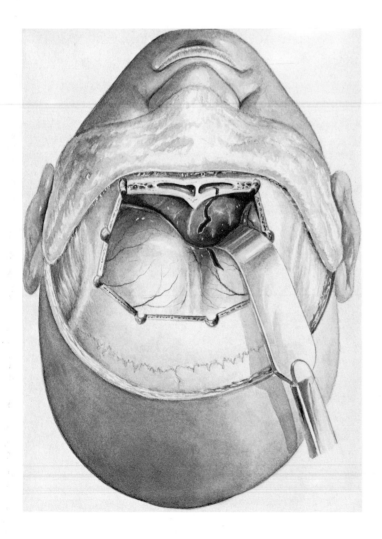

Fig. 8.27
The bony cover has been removed, the dura elevated from the bone and retracted posteriorly with the frontal lobe (extradural procedure). The fracture and the dural tear are exposed and dealt with extradurally.

Modifications of Dural Repair in the Transbasal Procedure

a) If there is a direct contact between the orbit and the dura after comminution of the orbital roof, this tear can be closed off by suturing the orbit and the dura.

b) After covering a dural tear with galea, fascia or lyophilized dura as described on page 10, mucoperiosteal flaps from the nose can be used as a second layer to ensure closure of the dural tear:

- By the superior Uffenorde flap (Berendes 1956).

- By a mucoperiosteal flap after removing the bone of the middle turbinate (Minnigerode 1967) (Fig. 8.28). After complete clearance of all the ethmoid cells, the bone of the middle and, if necessary, the superior turbinate is exposed with an elevator without tearing the mucosa and is removed with forceps (Fig. 8.28a). The mucoperiosteal flap can then be turned upward over the base of the skull within the nose and is held in place by packing (Fig. 8.28b).

- By a septal flap (Schreiner and Herrmann 1967) (Fig. 8.29). The mucoperiosteal flap based on the vomer is formed from the septum on the diseased side. The upper bony part of the septum is removed. A corresponding mucoperiosteal flap based on the roof of the nose is formed from the septum on the healthy side, drawn through the bony window, laid over the dural tear on the diseased side and is packed in place. The flap from the healthy side is turned over the bony bridge and covers the septum on both sides.

c) A large pedicled periosteal flap is developed from the vault of the skull after a coronal incision has been made. It is led in to the base of the skull through the superior recess of the frontal sinus, which is opened for this purpose.

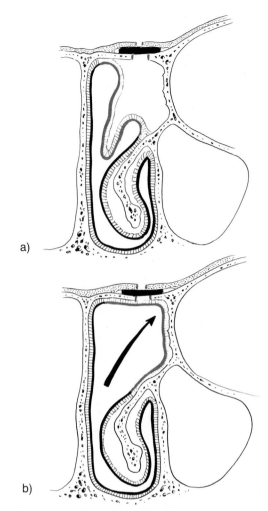

a)

b)

Fig. 8.28
Mucoperiosteal flap from the turbinate as a second layer for cover of a dural tear (Minnigerode).

a) Lyophilized dura (black) as the first layer. The turbinate (red) after removal of the bone.

b) Turbinate flap as a second layer packed on to the base of the skull.

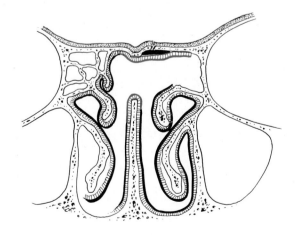

Fig. 8.29
Septal flaps from the healthy side packed in place as a second layer over the fracture and the dural tear (Schreiner and Herrmann).

d) In place of a graft (free or pedicled), Pfalz (1969) used tissue adhesive (Histoacryl) attached to a gel sponge to close a cerebrospinal fluid fistula, accepting the fact that foreign material is deposited in the sinus.

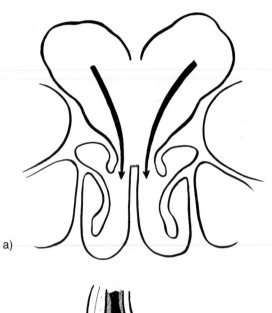

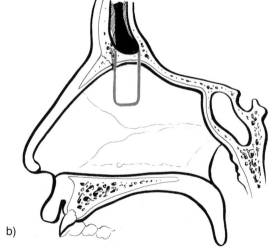

Fig. 8.30
Median drainage by O. Mayer's procedure (bilateral operation).

a) Permanent opening from the frontal sinus to the nose,

b) Thinning of the anterior wall of the frontal sinus and resection of the upper part of the septum.

Modification of the Access from the Nose to the Accessory Sinuses (Median Drainage) (Fig. 8.30)

Uffenorde's procedure can be combined with a bilateral fronto-orbital procedure, but it is easier to create a wide drainage into the nose after a bilateral frontal sinus operation using the median drainage procedure of O. Mayer (Fig. 8.30a). After removing the floor of the frontal sinus on both sides and the intersinus septum, the anterior wall of the frontal sinus is thinned from inside with a chisel or drill. The superior nasal spine is reached and the upper part of the perpendicular plate of the septum is removed (Fig. 8.30b). The removal should be kept as far forward as possible, to avoid damage to an anteriorly placed olfactory crest and crista galli (see also Vol. 1, Chap. 7). The wound in the septum is closed by rotation of parts of the previously elevated septal mucosa. The lateral surfaces of the entrance to the frontal sinus are covered on both sides with large inferior Uffenorde flaps from the lateral part of the nasal mucosa.

Obliteration of the Frontal Sinus

If the lumen of the frontal sinus cannot be reconstituted after a comminuted fracture of the anterior wall of the sinus, the lumen should be obliterated by Riedel's method (see Vol. 1, Chap. 7) in which the floor of the frontal sinus is also removed. The soft tissues of the orbit and the frontal skin then lie on the posterior wall of the frontal sinus, which is carefully cleared of as much mucosa as possible with the drill, or on the dura if the posterior wall must be also removed. Due to the unsatisfactory cosmetic results of this operation, the defect must be repaired about year later (see p. 25). The osteoplastic frontal operation in which the lumen of the frontal sinus is obliterated by fat (e.g., Goodale and Montgomery 1958) has not been generally accepted in Europe because of the increased danger of infection after comminution of the frontal sinus and tearing of the mucosa. Drainage of the infection is not possible since access to the nose and the ethmoid cells is closed off and the transplanted tissue then tends to shrink.

Transfrontal Intradural Operation (Neurosurgical Procedure)

The intradural procedure is preferred in more severe trauma to the base of the skull, especially over the frontal bone, in ramifying dural tears and in all deep injuries to the brain. Since this operation is not usually carried out by the rhinologist, only the principles will be illustrated here (Fig. 8.31).

After making a coronal incision and turning down the anterior part of the scalp in an osteoplastic flap, the dura is opened, the superior sagittal sinus is ligated and divided and the frontal lobe is retracted posteriorly. This procedure exposes the anterior cranial fossa and the dural floor which can now be dealt with from within the dura.

The *advantages* of this operation compared with the transfrontal extradural procedure are:

● Prevention of further tearing of the dura since it is not elevated;

● The possibility of inspection and treatment of a cerebral wound and of a pneumatocele;

● The possibility of plastic closure using fascia lata or a pedicled dural flap of a dural defect which ramifies and extends over the frontal sinus.

The *disadvantages* are that, in the intradural operation, operative trauma to the brain is certainly greater than via the extradural route. Furthermore, the sense of smell is lost and satisfactory treatment of the damaged or comminuted frontal sinus is not possible by this route. The aim of the operation must, therefore, be to carry out an operation on the frontal sinus and to remove bone splinters (as described on p. 6) when dealing with dural injury by an intradural procedure.

If the patient's condition permits, the operation on the sinus should be carried out simultaneously extradurally through the coronal incision by turning down an anterior scalp flap to expose the injured area. If there is a delay of days or weeks between the two operations, the rhinologist must be particularly careful to avoid further tearing of scars or adhesions when carrying out the fronto-orbital operation for repair of the dura over the roof of the frontal sinus.

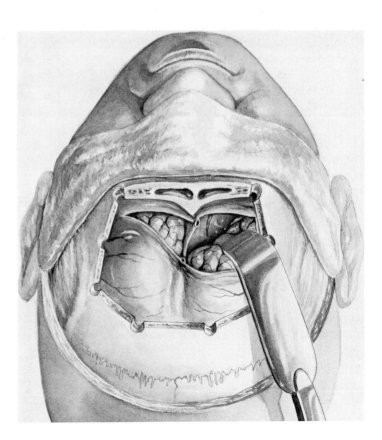

Fig. 8.31
Transfrontal intradural procedure as carried out by the neurosurgeon for dealing with damage to the dura and brain.

Orbital Fractures

In a typical fronto-orbital operation (see p. 6), it is possible to reach not only fractures of the medial wall of the orbit but also the roof of the orbit, which can be fully exposed after lateral extension of the incision in the eyebrow. Lehnhardt also recommends this access for decompression of the optic nerve in fractures of the base of the skull accompanied by deterioration of vision. Splinters of the bone are removed carefully from the orbital periosteum. In a retrobulbar hematoma, the lamina papyracea, the floor of the frontal sinus or the roof of the antrum may need to be removed in order to relieve the orbital contents. In a fresh hematoma, a medial orbitotomy (p. 39) may save the vision.

Tears in the orbital periosteum are sutured with fine atraumatic catgut. Prolapsed fat should be removed sparingly since excessive removal can lead to enophthalmos. Foreign bodies which have been driven into the orbit should be removed. During a search for a foreign body in the soft tissues of the orbit, great care should be exercised because of the danger of bleeding or of damage to the nerves and muscles. If a defect in the orbital periosteum cannot be sutured, an attempt should be made to cover it with a piece of fascia. It should be sewn if possible, but can also be fixed with tissue adhesive.

Fractures of the orbital roof (lateral to the frontal sinus) and tears of the dura can be overlooked at this point in an operation on the frontal sinuses. They can be the cause of infection extending through the ethmoids and the frontal sinuses via the orbit. If radiological examination (including tomograms) suggests that there may be a fracture or a tear of the dura at this site, an operation to explore this area is absolutely indicated. It can be easily carried out through a skin incision extended laterally in the eyebrow.

A fracture of the orbital roof can originate from isolated violence to the bulb, in the same way as the well known fracture of the floor of the orbit (blowout fracture, see Vol. 1, Chap. 7, 9) (Boenninghaus 1969).

An ophthalmologist should be consulted if damage to the orbital contents and the lacrimal drainage system is present (see Vol. 1, Chap. 4).

Wounds of the eyelids should be carefully closed with atraumatic sutures, if possible, without excising the skin in order to avoid later scar contraction and its results (epiphora, conjunctivitis and corneal ulcers).

Bullet Wounds

In *indirect* bony injuries (for example, from a ricochet) where the fracture line extends only into the upper part of the frontal sinus, the position is similar to that described above for frontobasal fractures mediated by blunt trauma.

In *direct* bony injuries, there is inevitably comminution and splintering of bone together with an impacted bullet as well as a great risk of infection and meningitis. Brain damage is often an important feature and the cooperation of a neurosurgeon is necessary.

The bullet is localized by radiographs in two planes and by tomograms; image intensification should be available during the operation for removal of the bullet. A bullet wound is an absolute indication for surgery.

In addition to removal of the bullet, debridement and a radical operation on the superior sinuses, this operation must provide a watertight closure of the dura.

Compared with the typical operation for blunt injury, the operation must often be extended or modified, depending on the extent of the damage. Obliteration of the frontal sinus by Riedel's method is more often necessary than after blunt trauma. Torn entry and exit wounds in the skin are carefully excised and should be included in the skin incision if possible. If there is loss of substance, the skin is closed with a mattress suture at the end of the operation. A brain abscess or a prolapse of the brain (if there has been unsatisfactory closure of the dura) is more common after this type of accident than after blunt trauma (see p. 10). Prophylaxis against tetanus is necessary after all bullet wounds.

Stabbing Injuries

Stab injuries caused by a knife, knitting needle, pencil or ski pole, for example, often have insignificant external wounds which conceal the seriousness, extent and danger of damage to the base of the skull and dura. Foreign bodies are often deflected by the nasal bones and then penetrate the medial part of the eyebrow. If there is the slightest suspicion that part of the foreign body still remains in the wound or that there has been comminution of the ethmoids, the wound must be explored by an external approach as described on page 6.

Postoperative Care

- Packing is removed after 2 days, or after 4 to 7 days following a repair of the dura.

- Antibiotics are given for 5 to 8 days.

- The patient is advised not to sneeze.

- In fresh injuries the patient is managed by the intensive care team. If this is not possible, the vital signs must be checked carefully (blood pressure, pulse and respiratory rate) and the usual laboratory investigations of renal function as well as fluid and electrolyte balance carried out.

- Neurological studies should be requested if there is trauma to the skull or brain.

- If a tracheotomy is necessary, the usual after-care is carried out.

- During the first few weeks, cotton swabs and later Ritter bougies (see Vol. 1, Fig. 7.5c) are used to check that the access to the operated sinus is open and that no blockage caused by secretions has formed.

Rules, Hints and Danger Points

- If obliteration of the frontal sinus is required, Riedel's procedure is used. Obliteration of the frontal sinus by filling it with Gelfoam, muscle or fat is dangerous because a hollow is left behind which can lead to the development of a mucocele or a pyocele.

- A mucocele can also be formed if clearance of the damaged mucosa in the frontal sinus is unsatisfactory or if the access to the nose is not sufficiently wide.

- Mucosa should only be used for the external second layer when closing the dura. If the dural tear is covered only with mucosa there is a danger of extension of mucosal inflammation to the meninges.

- Watertight closure of the dural defect with a graft is more secure than closure with Gelfoam or tissue adhesive alone.

Hemostasis after Damage to Blood Vessels

Anterior or posterior nasal packing (see Vol. 1, Chap. 6) is used for many cases of bleeding after trauma. If large vessels have been torn, they must be ligated. If the bleeding is from the posterior part of the nose, localization of the site of the bleeding is often difficult. The course of the fracture on radiographs may give an indication; angiograms may also be necessary.

Branches of the External Carotid Artery in the Nasal and Sinus Region (Maxillary Artery, Sphenopalatine Artery and Posterior Nasal Artery)

In bleeding of large vessels in the posterior part of the nose, the maxillary artery is ligated using Seiffert's method (1928) (Fig. 8.32).

The antrum is opened as in the Caldwell-Luc operation (see Vol. 1, Chap. 7). The posterior wall of the antrum is removed with the drill or chisel.

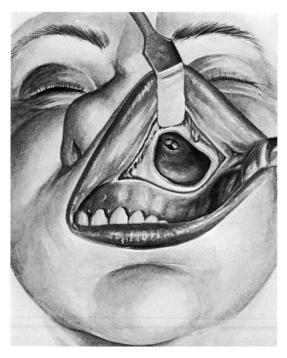

Fig. 8.32   Ligation of the maxillary artery (Seiffert).

The operation must be carried out medially in order to ligate the artery near its entrance into the nose. The periosteum is split and the fatty tissues are carefully divided with dissecting forceps and the maxillary artery is exposed. The artery can be drawn out slightly with a blunt hook and is then ligated with 4×0 Mersilene or is clamped with silver clips (see also Vol. 1, Chap. 7).

Ligature of the external carotid artery is less effective because of the collateral supply which is carried through the lingual artery. The incision lies along the anterior border of the sternocleidomastoid muscle (Fig. 8.33).

Medial Meningeal Artery

Hemorrhage from the middle meningeal artery, which passes through the foramen spinosum into the cranial cavity after leaving the maxillary artery, produces an extradural hematoma. Such a hematoma must, therefore, be considered in a skull fracture within the distribution area of the branches of the middle meningeal artery (Fig. 8.34).

The symptoms are increasing intracranial pressure, reappearance of unconsciousness after a symptom-free interval (this can be concealed by concussion), unilateral dilation of the pupil on the side of the hemorrhage, motor paralysis on the contralateral side and epileptiform attacks.

If this condition is suspected, an echoencephalogram or preferably a C.A.T. scan or a carotid angiogram should be carried out immediately.

The management consists of trephining the skull, draining the hematoma and hemostasis. If a neurosurgeon is not available, the ear, nose and throat surgeon may be forced to carry out this life-saving operation himself.

Operation: A longitudinal incision about 5 cm long is made over the origin of the zygoma through the skin and galea; a retractor is inserted. An exploratory burr hole is made with the electric drill in the vault of the skull; if necessary this can be extended by forceps (Fig. 8.35). The hematoma is sucked out or carefully removed. If bleeding does not stop, an attempt must be made to apply a suture ligature to the damaged vessel or to close the foramen spinosum with wax. Finally, the dura is sutured to the edges of the bone or to the outer periosteum.

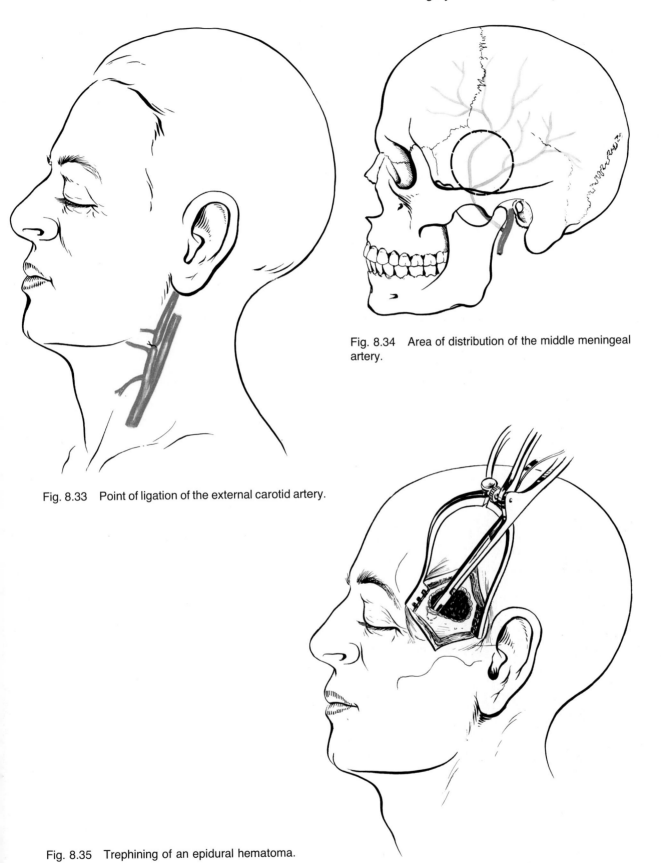

Fig. 8.33   Point of ligation of the external carotid artery.

Fig. 8.34   Area of distribution of the middle meningeal artery.

Fig. 8.35   Trephining of an epidural hematoma.

Internal Carotid Artery

If hemorrhage from the internal carotid artery is suspected, a carotid angiogram should be carried out to localize the source.

a) Damage within the bony canal or intracranially outside the cavernous sinus causes massive hemorrhage from the sphenoidal cavity or the roof of the pharynx. If only the intima has been torn, an aneurysm forms which then ruptures days or weeks after the accident and produces a torrential hemorrhage. Such a hemorrhage cannot be controlled for any length of time with packing.

b) Rupture within the cavernous sinus leads to an arteriovenous fistula. The principal symptom of this fistula is pulsating exophthalmos which begins several days after the accident and increases during the following days or weeks. Edema of the eyelids, chemosis with subjective disturbances of vision (even amaurosis) and a rushing or buzzing noise in the head synchronous with the pulse are also present. The buzzing noise can occasionally be reduced by careful pressure on the carotid artery in the neck.

Hemorrhage from the internal carotid artery is best controlled by ligature of the common carotid artery and possibly ligature of the internal carotid artery several days later. If circumstances permit, gradual compression of the vessels over minutes or preferably hours is recommended. Instead of supplementary ligature of the internal carotid artery, ligature of several branches of the external carotid artery as a second step has been recommended (Denecke 1968).

This treatment should be carried out in close cooperation with a neurosurgeon who should carry out an intracranial procedure to ligate the vessels if the hemorrhage is not controlled. A neurosurgeon is also the appropriate person to carry out Brooks' method, in which small pieces of muscle, or more recently barium-impregnated silicone spheres, are introduced into the carotid artery in the hope that these particles will be carried by the blood stream to the point of rupture of the vessel and will close the vessel by thrombosis.

Anterior and Posterior Ethmoidal Arteries

Hemorrhage from these vessels occurs in fractures of the ethmoids and the orbital roof. The origin of the hemorrhage is often difficult to diagnose.

The vessels can be reached in the apex of the orbit. A curved incision is made from the lateral part of

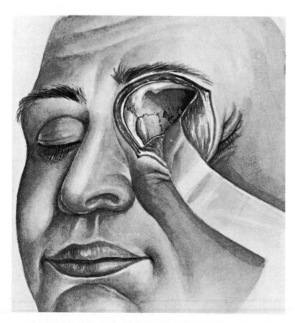

Fig. 8.36   Ligation of the anterior ethmoidal artery and the posterior ethmoidal artery 1 cm deeper.

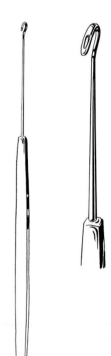

Fig. 8.37   Hessberg's ligation needle.

the nose into the eyebrow as in frontal sinus operations (see p. 6). The soft tissues are divided down to the bone and the orbital periosteum is elevated carefully from the lamina papyracea with a blunt elevator. The trochlea must often be detached also. The anterior ethmoidal artery passes across the field of vision about 1 cm behind the trochlea; the posterior ethmoidal artery lies a centimeter further behind this within the orbit (Fig. 8.36).

The arteries are ligated or sealed with clips shortly after their exit from the bone. The ligation is facilitated by Hessberg's retrograde ligature needle, as recommended by Mennig (1970) (Fig. 8.37).

Intranasal search for the artery, especially in the presence of established bleeding, is not indicated. During an external ethmoidectomy, the canals of the ethmoidal arteries can be occluded with wax.

Mucocele and Pyocele

Incomplete removal of damaged mucosa from the frontal sinus and cicatricial closure of the drainage of the frontal sinus or obliteration of the surgically created duct may be the cause of a mucocele (or a pyocele if the duct becomes infected) years after the accident.

Diagnostic Preoperative Procedures

In a mucocele, painless expansion of the floor of the frontal sinus leads to lateral and forward displacement of the eye. Radiographs in the occipitofrontal and occipitonasal projections show a balloon-shaped, distended frontal sinus with marked absence of loculi; it is opaque, due to thickened secretion. Eroded remnants of the bony septa within the frontal sinus or of the bony walls of the frontal sinus, especially of the floor, can sometimes be seen on tomograms. Old fractures or operative defects are also confirmed by such radiographs.

Operative Technique

The best operation to prevent recurrence is an obliteration of the frontal sinus such as Riedel's operation with careful removal of the mucosa of the

mucocele and creation of a wide drainage into the nose (details of an operation for mucocele are described in Vol. 1, Chap. 7).

Repair of Defects of the Frontal Bone

If obliteration of one of the frontal sinuses has been necessary, this can lead to unsightly prolapse of the forehead and eyebrows, particularly if the sinuses were large. Secondary repair is, therefore, advisable, at the earliest 6 months after treatment of the frontobasal fracture. Plastic materials, particularly polyethylene and Silastic, have proved to be the best for filling the defect, particularly with regard to tissue tolerance and malleability; pieces of bone or cartilage are less satisfactory in this regard.

Preparation of the Implant

A wax model of the necessary plastic implant is first made. This wax model may be formed on the patient, or, better on a plaster model of the patient's face. (Fig. 8.38). Using this model, the bar of plastic

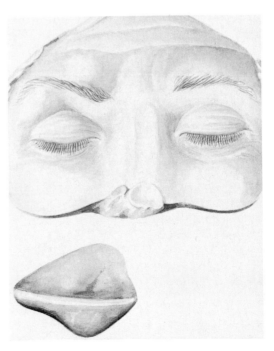

Fig. 8.38   Plaster cast of the frontal area and a wax model formed from this cast.

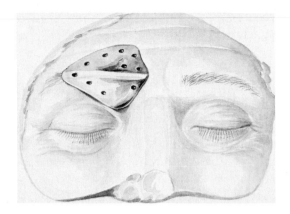

Fig. 8.39   Perforated plate prepared from the wax model.

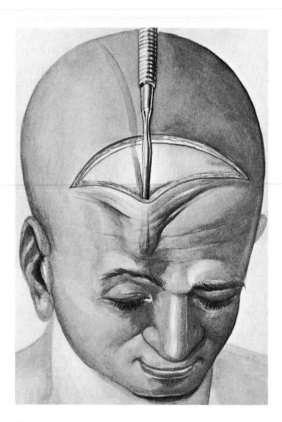

Fig. 8.40

is made from colorless artificial material by polymerization in a cuvette. The implant is polished and pierced at several points to allow penetration of the connective tissue and better fixation (Fig. 8.39). The prepared implant is then left in sterilizing solution for 12 hours.

Preparation for Surgery and Anesthesia

The operation can be carried out under local anesthesia or under general endotracheal anesthesia. If the incision lies above the hair margin, this area should be shaved.

Operative Technique

The incision is not made directly over the point where the artificial inlay will lie. If there are scars or a skin crease above this area on the forehead, the incision is made through them; otherwise, it is made above the hair margin (Fig. 8.40). The scalp is undermined by sharp dissection using a scalpel, scissors or elevator until the sunken area is reached (Fig. 8.40).

While forming the receptor area for the implant, the covering skin should not be thinned too much or the plate will lie too superficially. Any exposed dura or dura repaired at the first operation must not be damaged.

If the bony posterior wall of the frontal sinus is present, dissection proceeds close to the bone. If possible, the pocket should lie within the soft tissues so that the implant will be covered by soft tissue at all points after it has been introduced. The pocket should be small enough to prevent displacement of the plate (Fig. 8.41). The position of the plate can be checked by inspection and palpation. If the plate is properly positioned, an aluminum splint is placed over the nose and the defect. The incision is closed and a light bandage is applied for 1 week (Fig. 8.42).

The sutures are removed 1 week later. In many cases, a seroma forms which must be aspirated. Antibiotics are given for 5 days after the operation.

Rules, Hints and Typical Errors

Primary repair using artificial material to reconstruct the anterior wall of the frontal sinus at the same operation for treatment of a frontobasal fracture and for obliteration of the frontal sinus using Riedel's method is not recommended. Since the implant is not enclosed within the tissues on all sides, a foreign body reaction develops and, as a result, the implant does not settle.

In secondary repair, plastic implants are preferred to pieces of bone because they can be shaped better and a second operation to obtain the bone is not necessary. Furthermore, the bone changes in shape due to resorption. Plastic implants are inert and heal without incident since they are not under tension. Isografts should be used in children (Kecht 1972).

Filling the defect with self-hardening artificial material is not advised because the material only polymerizes in the tissues with considerable development of heat. This resulting heat damages the tissues and can injure the exposed dura.

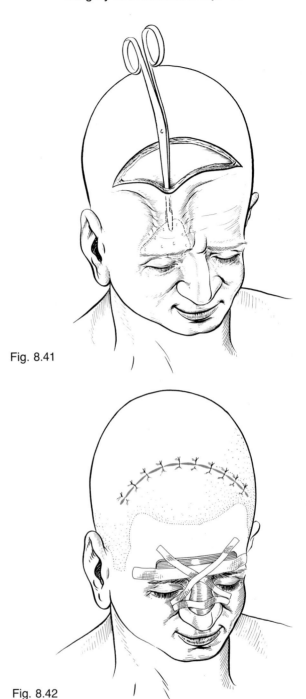

Fig. 8.41

Fig. 8.42

Surgery of Rhinogenic Intracranial Complications

Operation for Rhinogenic Meningitis (Suppurative Leptomeningitis)

Cause and Pathway of Spread

In trauma to the sinuses with tearing of the dura as just described, the pathway of spread of infection is determined by the injury. The early onset of meningitis (usually between the fifth and the seventh day after the accident) should be distinguished from meningitis of late onset occurring months or even years later. Rhinogenic meningitis can occur due to acute or chronic inflammation of the sinuses bordering on the base of the skull independent of trauma or operative damage to the dura. It usually arises from the ethmoid or the frontal sinuses and seldom from the sphenoid. Infection of the meninges occurs along perforating vessels from the roof of the sinuses or the posterior wall of the frontal sinus. It usually spreads via an intermediate stage of an extradural abscess. The same is true for meningitis following osteomyelitis of the frontal bone.

In a septal abscess, it must be remembered that the infection can spread via the cribriform plate, and inflammation of the orbit can extend via the venous route or along the optic nerve. Finally, meningitis can occur secondary to a subdural or cerebral abscess or in the course of a cavernous sinus thrombosis. In the latter case, the maxillary antrum may be the site of origin, and thrombosis of the pterygoid plexus may be the route of spread.

Diagnostic Preoperative Measures

The first symptoms of meningitis are elevation of temperature (possibly accompanied initially by chills), headache, vomiting, stiffness of the neck, sensitivity to light and sound, hyperesthesia and motor disturbances. Kernig's and Brudzinski's signs are positive.

At the earliest suspicion of a rhinogenic meningitis, the cerebrospinal fluid must be examined. The fluid may be obtained either by suboccipital or lumbar puncture. The suboccipital route, which is closer to the source of infection, is preferred both in rhinogenic and otogenic meningitis. Continuous check of pulse and respiration is necessary during the puncture.

Instruments for Obtaining Cerebrospinal Fluid

The following sterilized instruments should be available (Fig. 8.43):

a) A trochar and cannula. The cannula for suboccipital puncture is finer and shorter than for lumbar puncture.

b) A graduated and extensible glass tube with an attachment for the cannula to measure pressure.

c) A black receiver for carrying out Pandy's test. Universal containers should also be available to catch the fluid for cell counts, for protein and other chemical investigations as well as bacteriological examination.

Puncture can be carried out without anesthesia, under local anesthesia via a short general anesthetic or intubation anesthesia.

Suboccipital Puncture

The neck is shaved and the point of puncture cleaned.

Position of the patient. Two positions are possible:

a) Lateral with the head bent forward (Fig. 8.44);

b) Lying on the back with the head strongly flexed and held by an assistant (Fig. 8.45). A pillow is introduced under the shoulders for support.

The head must be positioned accurately in the midline and must not be turned to the side.

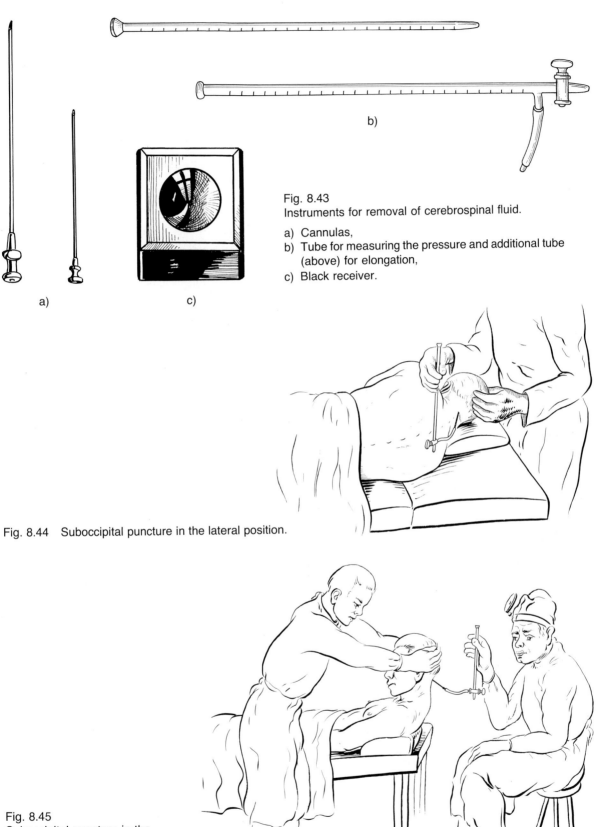

Fig. 8.43
Instruments for removal of cerebrospinal fluid.

a) Cannulas,
b) Tube for measuring the pressure and additional tube (above) for elongation,
c) Black receiver.

a)   c)

Fig. 8.44   Suboccipital puncture in the lateral position.

Fig. 8.45
Suboccipital puncture in the supine position.

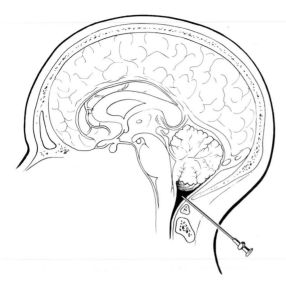

Fig. 8.46   Position of the needle in suboccipital puncture.

Puncture. The skin is pierced in the midline between the external occipital protruberance and the spinous process of the second cervical vertebra. The needle is then advanced obliquely upward. The operation proceeds by one of the following methods:

a) In Eskuchen's indirect method (1924), the needle is advanced until it meets the occipital bone

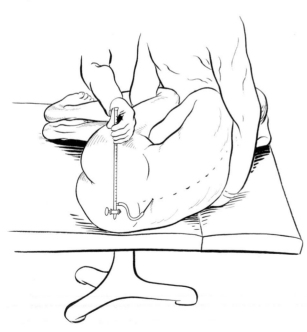

Fig. 8.47   Lumbar puncture.

above the foramen magnum. The needle is then withdrawn and the end elevated slightly. The point of the needle is thus depressed and is carefully advanced until the posterior atlanto-occipital membrane is reached.

b) Ayer's method (1926) is preferable for those who are skilled in this technique. In this method the needle is directly introduced in the direction of the posterior atlanto-occipital membrane. The area of elastic resistance is sought, the membrane is pierced and the cerebellomedullary cistern is reached immediately after the resistance has been overcome (Fig. 8.46). It is advisable to steady the little finger on the skull to prevent deeper penetration of the needle after the membrane has been pierced. The cistern is reached at a depth of 4−5 cm (as much as 8 cm in patients with a thick neck, but only 2−3 cm in children). The fluid drips out after the trochar is removed. After removal of the fluid, the trochar is introduced again and the needle is quickly removed. A pledget is pressed on the site of the puncture for a short time and a small bandage is then applied. If the fluid must be removed slowly, the trochar can be reintroduced several times to interrupt the flow of the cerebrospinal fluid.

Lumbar Puncture

Position of the patient. With the patient supported as firmly as possible in the lateral position, the back is strongly flexed. The assistant supports the patient in this position by holding the knees and the neck (Fig. 8.47).

Puncture. A horizontal line between the iliac crests crosses the spinal column between the third and fourth lumbar vertebrae. After cleaning the skin, the needle is introduced between the spinous processes of these two vertebrae (or through the intervertebral space one space higher or lower) and is carried obliquely upward. The point of the needle, which should not deviate laterally from the midline of the body, reaches the subdural space at a depth of 5−8 cm (in children at a depth of 2−4 cm). The needle can be advanced in steps. To test whether the subarachnoid space has been reached, the trochar is temporarily removed, holding the needle carefully in place until drops of fluid appear. A thin needle should be used to prevent headache, backache and possibly nausea and vomiting after the lumbar puncture. The patient should also lie flat on his back for 24 hours after the procedure.

Examination of Cerebrospinal Fluid

Pandy's test for protein. The first drops of fluid are received in a black receiver filled with Pandy's reagent (1 part carbolic acid crystals to 15 parts distilled water). If the protein content is increased, the fluid does not remain clear but, depending on the protein concentration, becomes opalescent, cloudy or milky.

Measurement of the pressure. After attaching the graduated tube to the cannula, the pressure is measured; the patient should not bear down during this maneuver. Variations with pulse and respiration are observed. In normal circumstances the pressure is between 100 and 200 mm water pressure; it is increased in pathological conditions.

Compression of the internal jugular vein on both sides (Queckenstedt's test) produces a rapid rise of pressure in the tube due to venous congestion if there is free communication within the subarachnoid space. Unilateral compression of the internal jugular vein (Kindler's test) causes the pressure to rise when compression is carried out on the healthy side in a patient with a sinus thrombosis.

Removal of the cerebrospinal fluid. The fluid is collected in a test tube. The color is normally clear, but in inflammatory conditions, it becomes opaque, and in traumatic conditions, it is bloodstained.

The amount of liquid drained off depends on the indication for the procedure. For diagnostic purposes, 20 ml suffices but if there is evidence of increased intracranial pressure (for example, in meningitis), a few drops must suffice. It is drained off with continuous check of the pulse and respiratory rate until the fluid drips slowly, and the pressure drops to 150 mm water pressure.

The fluid removed is used for the following tests:

Cell count. A Fuchs-Rosenthal counting chamber is used to count the leucocytes and lymphocytes after they have been stained with methylene blue. The normal values for fluid removed by the suboccipital route are up to 5 cells/mm^3 and, for fluid removed by the lumbar route, up to 10 cells mm^3. A marked increase in the number of cells, (especially granulocytes) is found in purulent meningitis; a moderate increase in cells (especially lymphocytes) is found in a brain abscess.

Bacteriological examination. The demonstration of bacteria is not always successful, even in purulent meningitis. The patient has often already been treated with antibiotics. If bacteria are present, appropriate treatment with antibiotics is possible depending on the degree of resistance.

Examination for admixture of blood. If *hemorrhage is due to trauma caused by inserting the needle,* the discoloration of the fluid is greater in the initial fluid specimen than in later specimens. The erythrocytes are well formed or crenated.

If there is *bleeding into the subarachnoid space,* the discoloration of all the fluid specimens is the same. The erythrocytes are leached. Bleeding into the subarachnoid space causes a meningeal reaction with a temporary resorption leucocytosis.

Examination for protein. Quantitative and qualitative examinations for protein, colloid reactions and a Wassermann reaction can be carried out; the glucose content is also measured.

Chemical investigation of the fluid is only of minor significance in the rhinogenic meningitis to be discussed here. Increase of protein, and thus of globulin, will already have been demonstrated by Pandy's test during removal of the fluid. The Wassermann and colloidal reactions allow a differential diagnosis to be made between nonspecific inflammation and syphilitic disease. The glucose content is reduced in tubercular meningitis and occasionally in nonspecific meningitis, but it is somewhat increased in cerebral tumors, encephalitis and intracranial bleeding.

Danger Points and Typical Errors

● The principal danger is impaction of the cerebellar tonsils during removal of the fluid if the intracranial pressure is increased. For this reason the optic fundi must always be examined to exclude papilledema before the puncture is carried out. With readings above 4 diopters, a few drops of liquid must be removed for examination and must be replaced by saline. If fluid does not drain off, this can indicate a cisternal block which constitutes a threat to the respiratory center. It should be taken as an indication for endotracheal intubation and controlled respiration.

● Puncture of a vessel in an atypical position, for example, the posterior cerebellar artery, can occasionally cause bleeding during suboccipital puncture.

● After the age of 60, suboccipital puncture should not be carried out because of the increased brittleness of the vessels.

● Intracerebral and medullary hemorrhage have been described on rare occasions after lumbar puncture.

● Postoperative discomfort is greater after lumbar puncture than after suboccipital puncture.

● Advancement of the needle in suboccipital puncture must stop immediately after the posterior atlantooccipital membrane has been pierced to avoid damaging the vital centers lying in the medulla oblongata.

● The main error leading to inability to find the subarachnoid space is lateral deviation of the needle from the midline of the body.

Indications

A rhinogenic meningitis demonstrated by clinical symptoms and confirmed by examination of the cerebrospinal fluid is an indication for operative treatment. The cerebrospinal fluid shows increased pressure, protein content and cell count, which can rise to more than $1,000/mm^3$ of granulocytes, and often positive bacterial cultures.

Principle of the Operation

The site of origin of the meningitis must be found and must be dealt with surgically. The routes of spread to the dura and the dura itself must be exposed, the damage to the dura must be treated and the epidural abscess must be exposed and drained.

Timing of the Operation

The necessary operation is carried out as soon as possible after the onset of meningitis. Postponing operation on the sinuses or repair of the dura in cases of traumatic meningitis under antibiotic cover until the meningitis has resolved cannot be recommended since the meningitis is maintained by the infected sinus.

If a late meningitis or a recurrent meningitis occurs in a long standing *cerebrospinal fluid fistula*, the meningitis can be controlled by high doses of antibiotics. The operation can then be carried out on the sinuses and the dura repaired a few days later. After resolution of the meningitis a check of the sinuses is necessary even if no cerebrospinal fluid leakage is present but the patient's case history indicates a frontobasal injury.

A delay of several days is permissible in *acute* inflammatory disease of the sinuses, if high doses of antibiotics are given, if the cerebrospinal fluid is checked daily and if the disease has not progressed beyond meningitic irritation with a slight elevation of cells (up to $100/mm^3$, primarily lymphocytes). If the meningitis is a result of a *chronic* inflammation of the sinuses, an operation must always be carried out immediately.

Operative Technique

The following operations are indicated in rhinogenic meningitis depending on the site of origin of the infection:

a) In *acute* or *chronic inflammation* of the superior sinuses (frontal, ethmoid and sphenoid sinuses, and occasionally of the latter sinus alone), a *radical operation* on the sinuses is indicated for meningitis. Pulsating discharge of pus from the sinus demonstrates that the dura is exposed. Otherwise a search must be made for collections of pus or fistulae in the bone of the posterior wall of the frontal sinus. Next, the *dura is exposed* even if the bone appears to be healthy. A drill or chisel is used to remove a part of the posterior wall of the frontal sinus or the anterior part of the roof of the ethmoid cells to allow inspection of the dura (Fig. 8.48).

Occasionally this exposes and drains an extradural abscess without which control of the meningitis is not possible. If the dura appears to be normal the operation is concluded. If alterations of the dura such as thickening, granulations or absence of pulsation are found, the dura is exposed by removing more of the neighboring bone, until healthy bone is obtained if possible. If a subdural abscess or brain abscess is suspected, further procedures are carried out as described on page 35.

b) In *traumatic meningitis* after frontobasal fractures or after surgical damage during a radical operation on the sinuses, the damaged area of the dura is exposed and dealt with as described on page 10.

c) In a *septal abscess* complicated by meningitis, the septum is incised. In an extradural abscess in this area, it is necessary to elevate the dura over the cribriform plate. This is best carried out from the area where the roof of the ethmoid cells has been removed.

d) In meningitis complicated by an *orbital abscess*, a radical operation is carried out on the frontal sinus and the ethmoids. The orbital periosteum is elevated and occasionally slit in the region of the lamina papyracea. The same operation is also carried out if a cavernous sinus thrombosis is present (see p. 38).

e) In meningitis complicated by *osteomyelitis of the bones of the skull*, removal of the outer table of the skull and the diploe (see Vol. 1, Chap. 7) along with the removal of the inner table around the diseased area to expose the dura is indicated. The procedure usually uncovers an extradural abscess. Removal of the inner table is accomplished with the drill; the defect in the bone is extended with Hajek's forceps or with sinus forceps. The dura is elevated from the bone with an elevator. If a brain abscess is suspected, an operation is carried out as described on page 34.

If a simultaneous thrombosis of the superior sagittal sinus is present, the sinus is exposed by removing the bone of the skull. It is then packed and slit. The thrombus is removed.

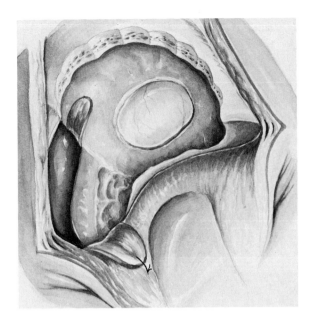

Fig. 8.48

Postoperative Care

Cerebrospinal fluid is removed by puncture every 2 days (see p. 29). If the findings on examination of the fluid are improving, the interval between punctures can be increased until the fluid becomes normal. Antibiotics are administered intravenously, preferably in high doses as a continuous infusion. The antibiotic is determined by the sensitivity of the organism. Penetration of the antibiotic solution into the subarachnoid space is made possible by the dural irritation. Recently, carbenicillin has become available for intrathecal use. The patient should also be managed by an internist.

Operation for Rhinogenic Brain Abscess

A frontal abscess usually arises from the frontal sinus and seldom from the ethmoid sinuses or from osteomyelitis of the vault of the skull. The cause is either a frontobasal injury with trauma to the dura which produces a preformed pathway or is inflammatory disease of the sinuses when there is direct spread of the disease. In a *traumatic abscess* an *early abscess* in the region of the cerebral injury with disorganized and infected brain tissue (often after a penetrating injury) must be differentiated from a *late abscess* which usually forms around foreign bodies or splinters of bone driven into the brain substance, or around an area of contusion. The late abscess possesses a capsule which forms over a period of from 4 to 6 weeks. It should be dealt with and removed by the neurosurgeon (see p. 37).

A brain abscess may result from an acute (occasionally necrotizing) infection or more often from an acute exacerbation of a chronic *inflammatory disease of the sinuses.* It can also arise by secondary spread from an extradural abscess, a subdural abscess or a circumscribed leptomeningitis.

Infection reaches the cerebrum either by continuity or along the vessel with or without thrombosis. Spread can also occur via the filaments of the olfactory nerve. The abscess usually occurs in the center of the cortex and arises from liquefaction of a circumscribed encephalitis.

A thorough neurological examination, especially of the optic fundi, should be carried out as the first step in the diagnosis. If there is the slightest suspicion of a brain abscess, a lumbar or suboccipital puncture should be carried out (see p. 29). The fluid is under increased pressure, has an increased protein content or shows only a moderate increase of cells (primarily lymphocytes but also granulocytes if there is an accompanying meningitis). Care should be exercised in the presence of papilledema because of the danger of impaction of the cerebellar tonsils (see p. 30).

If the suspicion is confirmed, the following series of neurological, neuroradiological and neurosurgical methods of investigation are available:

- An electroencephalogram demonstrates a perifocal inflammation.
- Echoencephalography provides evidence regarding the displacement of the brain (particularly in subdural hemorrhage, but also in a large subdural empyema).
- A C.A.T. scan is the most reliable method for confirming a brain abscess.
- Carotid angiography demonstrates the position of the cerebral vessels.
- Recently, brain scanning has been used.
- In an anaerobic infection, gas formation can be demonstrated radiologically by translucency in the abscess cavity.

Diagnostic Preoperative Measures

A brain abscess causes relatively few symptoms during its development. Headaches, sensitivity of the skull to palpation, nausea, attacks of vomiting, loss of interest and lack of drive are suspicious symptoms. A brain abscess should be suspected in a patient with meningitis who does not improve in spite of the treatment described above. Symptoms of increased intracranial pressure, papilledema, unilateral mydriasis and epileptiform attacks can be caused or exacerbated by accompanying cerebral edema. A large subdural abscess produces symptoms similar to a brain abscess.

Indications for Operation

If the suspicions are confirmed or if there is evidence of subdural abscess or a brain abscess, immediate surgery is indicated, first on the sinus (the primary site of the infection) and second on the abscess.

In inflammatory disease of the sinuses, a radical operation on the frontal sinus, ethmoid sinus or sphenoid sinus (see Vol. 1, Chap. 7) is carried out. In traumatic cases, the surgery described on pages 6 and 14 is necessary. If open management of the abscess is anticipated, Riedel's operation (see Vol. 1, Chap. 7) is carried out on the frontal sinus.

Operative Technique

After a thorough operation on the sinus, the dura is exposed. The further course of the operation is determined by the condition of the dura and the position of the abscess. Today the position of the abscess is usually confirmed before surgery. In the author's opinion, the previously used procedure of aspirating the brain via the sinus cavity to look for an abscess should not be used today (Bettag 1972).

Several possibilities are available for treating a brain abscess:

Open Management (Drainage via the Pathway of Spread)

If the dura posterior to the posterior wall of the frontal sinus or on the roof of the operated sinus is clearly discolored (usually whitish yellow), thickened, under tension, not pulsating or necrotic, if there are granulations, or a fistula at this site extruding pus, a brain abscess is present in the immediate neighborhood of the dura. It should be managed by superficial aspiration (no deeper than 1 cm), splitting of the dura and drainage or packing. This procedure should also be used for a subdural abscess.

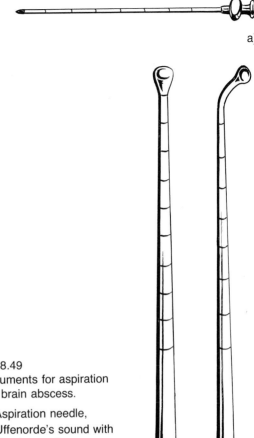

Fig. 8.49
Instruments for aspiration of a brain abscess.

a) Aspiration needle,
b) Uffenorde's sound with centimeter marks.

Technique. The dura is cleaned with iodine and is then punctured with a short, thick, beveled brain needle marked off in centimeter bands (Fig. 8.49 a). The pus is removed with a 10 ml syringe, thus providing material for bacteriological examination. The aspiration must be carried out slowly to prevent tearing the thin wall of the ventricle. If tearing should occur, it can be recognized by the aspiration of a mixture of cerebrospinal fluid and pus.

Next, the dura is incised (Fig. 8.50). The incision is made with a pointed, double-sided scalpel which is carried along the cannula if it is still in position. The point of the incision is extended in a cross-shape. Before doing this, the dura must be exposed by removing sufficient bone, with Hajek's forceps or a drill. A hammer and chisel are not used because they can further damage the already diseased brain tissue.

The cruciate incision in the dura is now carefully opened with a medium-sized Killian's nasal speculum and the pus is sucked out. To prevent further injury to the brain, suction inside the abscess should be omitted.

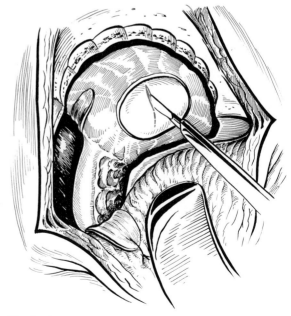

Fig. 8.50

Alternatively, a curved or straight sound may be carefully introduced into the abscess cavity (Fig. 8.51) (Uffenorde 1952). The sound (see Fig. 8.49 b) has centimeter marks along its length and sinks under its own weight into the abscess cavity. The extent and the form of the abscess cavity can be assessed by gentle palpation; foreign bodies and bone fragments in a traumatic abscess can be confirmed. Probing with the sound generally produces a further flow of pus. The older the abscess, the more clearly its capsule can be felt.

While the pus is being sucked out of the abscess cavity, the pulse and respiratory rate of the patient, who is under general endotracheal anesthesia, should be continuously checked.

Open aftercare of the abscess cavity is carried out either by a polyethylene tube or by gauze strips which are soaked with antibiotic solution. Tubes, particularly of polyethylene, secured with a safety pin are particularly recommended for a subdural abscess but not for an acute brain abscess.

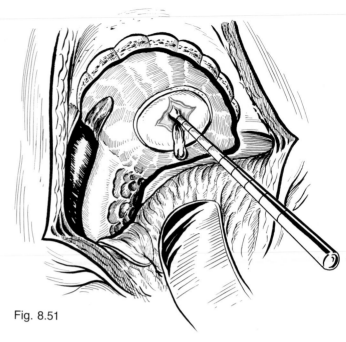

Fig. 8.51

Packing with Gelfoam (Fig. 8.52), gauze, or a gauze packed finger stall should hold the abscess open (the abscess cavity should not be completely filled with the packing) and should ensure drainage. The external skin wound remains open since further treatment is carried out via the incision (in the eyebrow or in the lateral part of the nose).

The packing is first changed after 3 or 4 days. Further change of packing, which must be carried out carefully in order not to damage the brain, is advisable every 2 or 3 days depending on the amount of drainage. The abscess cavity gradually contracts over a period of several weeks and granulates from within outward, as can be shown by palpation with the sound during the dressing change. As long as the abscess cavity still has a lumen, the opening in the dura must not be closed; it must be kept open by packing. The abscess will heal within 4 to 6 weeks. At this time the skin is closed secondarily over the frontal sinus, which is obliterated by Riedel's operation. During the postoperative phase, cerebrospinal fluid should be removed by puncture to relieve the pressure and to check the progress of the meningitis which develops in most of these cases. Cerebrospinal fluid removal should be carried out every few days; the interval should be determined by the pressure and cell count of the fluid. To prevent cisternal blockage, puncture should only be carried out after the abscess has been drained. A sudden increase in the cell count indicates that the abscess has penetrated into the subarachnoid space. If this occurs, cerebrospinal fluid drains from the abscess cavity. Penetration of the ventricle can be recognized on X-rays as a pneumatocele.

Operative treatment is supplemented by high dosage of parenteral antibiotics, if possible determined by the sensitivity. Increased intracranial pressure is managed by hyperosmolar solutions such as sorbitol or mannitol.

If an inflammatory prolapse of the brain occurs during treatment caused by progressive encephalitis, the prolapsed brain tissue should not be removed. Intensive antibiotic treatment, hyperosmolar therapy and release of the pressure by removing cerebrospinal fluid should bring about resolution of the inflammation and the cere-

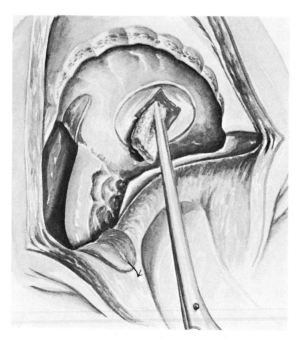

Fig. 8.52

bral prolapse. Mechanical removal is only advisable for necrosis of brain tissue. The disorganized tissue should be carefully removed or sucked out. A cerebral prolapse should also lead to suspicion that a further abscess has formed. Close cooperation with a neurosurgeon is obviously required for every patient with a brain abscess, in particular those with cerebral prolapse, or with meningoencephaloceles which extend into the accessory sinuses. Here a joint operation performed by the rhinologist and the neurosurgeon may be required.

Closed Management

If the abscess does not have an obvious pathway of spread with clear alterations of the dura, but rather is an abscess which was previously diagnosed and localized neuroradiologically as a deep cerebral abscess (metastatic abscess, traumatic late abscess or an abscess around a foreign body), and a thick layer of brain tissue is located between the accessory sinus and the brain abscess, treatment should be by "closed" management. There are two methods of closed management:

a) *Aspiration and instillation*: The neurosurgeon makes a small opening in the cranial vault (if possible close to the abscess) and exposes normal dura. The previously localized abscess is aspirated and an antibiotic is instilled into the abscess cavity (penicillin should not be used since this produces irritation, Gerlach 1968). This treatment is repeated several times during the next few days until the abscess heals. Puncture of the dura is not carried out via the diseased sinus, although this is possible (Mündnich 1964) (Fig. 8.53). Aspiration of an abscess arising by direct extension from the sinus is performed by the rhinologist after he has carried out the operation on the sinus. Deep aspiration may spread infected material through healthy brain tissue when the aspiration needle is withdrawn from the abscess. If the suspicion of a subdural abscess arising, for example, from secondary infection of a subdural hematoma is confirmed, the dura is exposed via a frontoparietal burr hole. The abscess is then aspirated and irrigated with an antibiotic solution; a fine drain is left in place if necessary. One complication of an acute abscess is progressive encephalitis which ruptures into the ventricle during the third week. For this reason aspiration treatment is particularly advisable for acute abscesses which do not

have a definite capsule. This allows time for the capsule to form. If a capsule has formed or an abscess heals by aspiration alone, the capsule or the scar of the abscess can be excised if the patient develops epilepsy. If the abscess heals by aspiration and instillation, this is unquestionably the best method of treatment for such an abscess.

b) *Extirpation of the abscess* (radical operation): The abscess is sought by the neurosurgeon via a transfrontal osteoplastic craniotomy and is removed with the abscess capsule. After this operation, cerebral scars can occur which may lead to epilepsy. The advantage of extirpation compared with open treatment is that the abscess is removed in toto; after care is not necessary. It is also particularly recommended for loculated or multiple abscesses with a capsule. If the neurosurgeon utilizes either of these methods of treatment, an operation on the sinuses must be carried out if the brain abscess arose from disease of the sinuses.

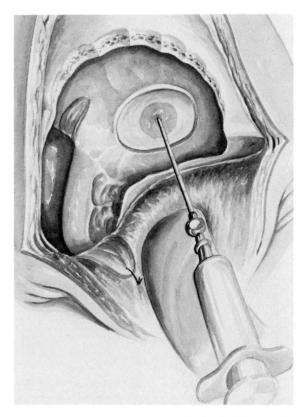

Fig. 8.53 Aspiration treatment of a brain abscess via the frontal sinus.

Typical Errors and Danger Points

● Attempts at deep aspiration in the search for a suspected abscess by introducing the needle at multiple points from the diseased sinus into the brain is contraindicated today because of the danger of infecting healthy brain tissue by spreading infected material, of bleeding and of damage to the ventricle. The neurological and neuroradiological methods of examination described on page 34 have now replaced this method.

● Slow removal of pus from the abscess is important to prevent rapid changes of pressure within the skull and to prevent tearing the wall of the lateral ventricle, which is often thin. Breaching of the ventricle can be recognized by the sudden appearance of a mixture of pus and cerebrospinal fluid. The tear can heal spontaneously (Kecht 1965) if the pus can drain externally and has not ruptured into the ventricle. If the ventricle has been ruptured, the patient should be positioned on his healthy side in order to facilitate escape of the air (Herrmann 1968).

Operation for Thrombosis of the Cavernous Sinus

A thrombosis of the cavernous sinus can arise:

a) By an ascending thrombosis (thrombophlebitis) via the angular vein and the superior ophthalmic vein from an infection arising, for example, from a furuncle of the upper lip.

b) From nasal disease, for example, inflammation of the frontal, ethmoid or sphenoid sinuses and, on rare occasions, from the maxillary sinuses via the pterygoid plexus.

c) From otogenic causes by ear disease spreading from the sigmoid sinus via the superior and inferior petrosal sinus.

Ascending thrombophlebitis via the angular vein presents with redness, thickening and tenderness of the inner canthus. The following signs of cavernous sinus thrombosis occur successively and rapidly:

Edema of the eyelids, chemosis, proptosis, ocular paralyses, alterations of the optic fundi (neuritis of the optic nerve, retinal hemorrhages and papilledema) or generalized signs of sepsis, as well as meningitis. After a short time, similar local symptoms can appear in the other orbit.

In thrombosis of the superior sagittal sinus, subgaleal or subperiosteal abscesses over the cranial vault occur due to spread via the parietal emissary veins.

Diagnostic Preoperative Measures

Radiology of the sinuses provides evidence of the site of origin of the disease. The patient should be examined by an ophthalmologist, neurologist and radioneurologist. Examination of the cerebrospinal fluid reveals an increased protein content and cell count depending on the degree of the accompanying meningitis. Alterations in the cerebrospinal fluid do not occur in solitary orbital inflammation not involving the cavernous sinus.

Purpose of the Operation

The purpose of the operation is to find the source of the infection and to drain or eliminate it. Surgical intervention on the cavernous sinus itself should be omitted.

Operative Technique

- In ascending thrombophlebitis of the angular vein, an operation is carried out as early as possible before the onset of cavernous sinus thrombosis. The vein is divided in the inner canthus through a skin incision and divided or coagulated (Fig. 8.54).

- If the infection arises from one of the sinuses, a radical operation on the appropriate sinus is necessary (see Vol. 1, Chap. 7). The orbital periosteum is exposed and elevated by removing the lamina papyracea. This uncovers the route of access from the ethmoid sinus to the orbit.

- In an orbital abscess or orbital cellulitis, the orbital periosteum is slit in a T-shape with a septal knife (medial orbitotomy). Next, the soft tissues are carefully opened (Fig. 8.55).

- Decompression of the orbit can be achieved by removing the roof of the maxillary sinus and the floor of the frontal sinus as well as the lamina papyracea. It is questionable whether exenteration of the orbit – a method advocated in earlier times in desperate cases – can prevent the fatal outcome in inflammatory processes in the orbit accompanied by cavernous sinus thrombosis and sepsis.

Supplementary Procedures

A very high dose of antibiotic (for example, 30 million units of penicillin) is given daily by continuous infusion.

Treatment by anticoagulant and fibrinolytic therapy for a sterile thrombus can be carried out in cooperation with the internist. The patient must often be managed in the intensive care unit.

Hints

A medial orbitotomy (Fig. 8.55) may also be necessary for an orbital hematoma. This operation is urgently indicated and should not be delayed if there is damage to the orbital soft tissues, bleeding into

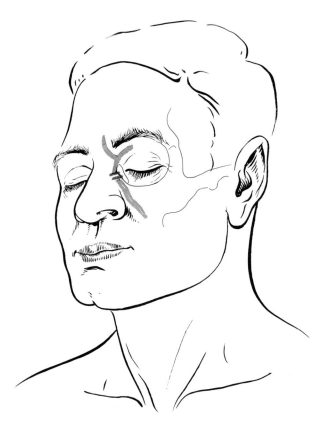

Fig. 8.54   Division of the angular vein in impending cavernous sinus thrombosis.

the orbit or decrease in vision after an ethmoidal operation either by the intranasal or transmaxillary route. The orbit should be decompressed within 30 minutes at the latest.

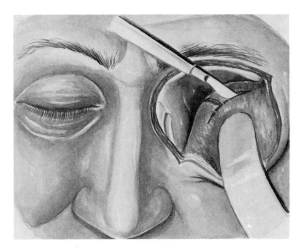

Fig. 8.55   T-shaped incision of the orbital periosteum (medial orbitotomy) for orbital abscess or hematoma.

Bibliography

Albrecht, H. R.: Cavernosusthrombose und Orbitalphlegmone, Änderung der chirurgischen Indikationen durch die neuzeitliche Chemotherapie. Z. Laryng. Rhinol. 29: 12, 1950

Aubry, R. M., J. Calvet, E. J. Piquet, E. J. Terracol: Les traumatismes des cavités annexes des fosses nasales. Librairie Arnette, Paris 1963.

Ayer, J. B.: The analysis of spinal fluid test. J. Am. Med. Assoc. 87: 377, 1926

Beickert, P.: Die oto-rhinologische Indikation zur Operation bei endocraniellen Erkrankungen. Arch. Ohren-, Nasen, Kehlkopfheilk. 183: 164, 1946

Berendes, J.: Doppelter autoplastischer Verschluß größerer Duradefekte in Nähe der Mittellinie bei Liquorrhoea nasalis. H.N.O. 6: 220, 1956

Bettag, W.: Der derzeitige Stand von Klinik und Behandlung der otogenen und rhinogenen Hirnkomplikationen. Neurochirurgische Betrachtungen. H.N.O. 20: 47, 1972

Boenninghaus, H.-G.: Die Behandlung der Schädelbasisbrüche. Thieme, Stuttgart 1960

Boenninghaus, H.-G.: Recidivierende Meningitiden als Folge früherer Schädelbasisbrüche. H.N.O. 16: 1. 1968

Boenninghaus, H.-G.: Blow-out Fraktur des Orbitadaches. Z. Laryng. Rhinol. 48: 396, 1969

Boenninghaus, H.-G.: Die operative Behandlung der frontobasalen Frakturen, insbesondere der Duraverletzungen durch den HNO-Arzt (Dokumentation über 66 Patienten). Z. Laryng. Rhinol. 50: 640, 1971

Boenninghaus, H.-G.: Rhinochirurgische Aufgaben bei der Chirurgie des an die Schädelbasis angrenzenden Gesichtsschädels. Arch. Oto-Rhino-Laryng. 207: 1–228, 1974

Brawley, B. W., W. A. Kelly: Treatment of basal skull fractures with and without cerebrospinal fluid fistulae. J. Neurosurg. 26: 57, 1957

Colas, J., M. Collet, R. Sartre, H. Dano, J. Fave, L. Toscler: Les rhinorrhées posttraumatiques. Réflexions à propos de 52 cas. Rev. Oto-neuro-ophtal. 36: 51, 1964

Denecke, H.-J.:Die oto-rhino-laryngologischen Operationen. In: Allgemeine und spezielle Operationslehre, Vol. V, ed. by M. Kirschner. Springer, Berlin 1953

Denecke, H.-J.: Unfallchirurgie des Gesichtes und Halses. Arch. Klin. Exp. Ohren-, Nasen-, Kehlkopfheilk. 191: 217, 1968

Dietz, H.: Die frontobasale Schädelhirnverletzung. Springer, Berlin 1970

Escher, F.: Clinic, classification and treatment of the fronto-basal fractures. Almqvist u. Wiksell, Stockholm 1969

Escher, F.: Les fractures fronto-basales ouvertes. Cah. Oto-Rhino-Laryng. 6: 515, 1971

Eskuchen, K.: Die bisherigen Erfahrungen mit der Cisternenpunktion. Zbl. Nervenheilk. 38: 323, 1924

Fischer, W.: Instrumentelle neurochirurgische Untersuchungsmethoden. In: Hals-Nasen-Ohren-Heilkunde, Vol. III/2, ed. by J. Berendes, R. Link, F. Zöllner. Thieme, Stuttgart 1966 (p. 1509)

Fremel, F.: Der otogene Hirnabszeß. Mschr. Ohrenheilk. 105: 521, 1971

Ganz, H.: Der derzeitige Stand von Klinik und Behandlung der otogenen und rhinogenen Hirnkomplikationen. H.N.O. 20: 33, 1972

Ganz, H.: Komplikationen der unspezifischen Nasen- und Nebenhöhlenentzündungen. In: Hals-, Nasen-, Ohrenheilkunde, Vol. 1, ed. by J. Berendes, R. Link, F. Zöllner, Thieme, Stuttgart 1977 (p. 14.1)

Gerlach, J.: Die neurochirurgische Beurteilung und Behandlung basaler Schädelhirnverletzungen. Arch. Klin. Exp. Ohren-, Nasen-, Kehlkopfheilk. 191: 419, 1968

Goodale, R., W. Montgomery: Experiences with the osteoplastic anterior wall approach to the frontal sinus. Arch. Otolaryng. 68: 271, 1958

Gotham, J. E., S. Meyer, I, Gilroy, R. Bauer: Observations on cerebrospinal fluid rhinorrhea and pneumencephalus. Ann. Otol. (St. Louis) 74: 215, 1965

Gross, Ch. W.: The diagnosis and treatment of cerebrospinal fluid rhinorrhea. Plast. Reconstr. Surgery 2.: 11, 1972

Herrmann, A.: Gefahren bei Operationen an Hals, Ohr und Gesicht und die Korrektur fehlerhafter Eingriffe. Springer, Berlin 1968

Kahrweg, A., W. Dorndorf: Das subdurale Empyem als Komplikation von Nasennebenhöhlenentzündungen und operativen Eingriffen an der Nase. Nervenarzt 40: 488, 1969

Kecht, B.: Die Oto-Rhino-Laryngologie bei Schädelverletzungen. Maudrich, Wien 1965

Kecht, B.: Operativer Zugangsweg und Defektplastik bei Frontobasalverletzungen im Kindesalter. Z. Laryng. Rhinol. 51: 309, 1972

Kindler, W.: Liquordiagnostik bei Komplikationen im Schädel nach Entzündungen, Verletzungen, Geschwülsten im Nasen-, Augen- und Ohrgebiet. In: Ophthalmologische Operationslehre, ed. by R. Thiel. VEB Thieme, Leipzig 1950 (p. 1343)

Kley, W.: Die Unfallchirurgie der Schädelbasis und der pneumatischen Räume. Arch. Klin. Exp. Ohren-, Nasen-, Kehlkopfheilk. 191: 1, 1968

Krahl, P.: Liquordiagnostik von Ohren-, Nasen- und Halserkrankungen. In: Hals-Nasen-Ohren-Heilkunde, Vol. III/2, ed. by J. Berendes, R. Link, F. Zöllner, Thieme, Stuttgart 1966 (S. 1495)

Lange, G. Operative Behandlung der entzündlichen Nasennebenhöhlenkrankheiten. In: Hals-Nasen-Ohrenheilkunde Vol. 1 ed. by J. Berendes, R. Link, F. Zöllner, Thieme, Stuttgart 1977 (p. 13.1)

Lehnhardt, E.: Die Dekompression des Nervus opticus bei Fraktur der Rhinobasis. H.N.O. 21: 158, 1973

Lewin, W.: Cerebrospinal fluid rhinorrhea in closed head injuries. Br. J. Surgery 42: 1, 1954

Lewin, W., H. Cairns: Fractures of the sphenoidal sinus with cerebrospinal rhinorrhea. Br. J. Ser. 4696: 1, 1951

Matzker, J.: Beitrag zur kosmetisch befriedigenden operativen Versorgung von schweren Zertrümmerungsfrakturen der Stirnhöhlenvorderwand. Monatsschr. Ohrenheilk. 95: 242, 1961

Mennig, H. Geschwülste der Augenhöhle und ihre operative Behandlung. VEB Thieme, Leipzig 1970

Messerklinger, W.: Über die mikroskopische intraoperative Funktionsprüfung der Nasen- und Nebenhöhlenschleimhaut als ein Hilfsmittel zur Lokalisation kleinster Liquorfisteln. Monatsschr. Ohrenheilk. 101: 355, 1967

Messerklinger, W.: Nasenendoskopie: Nachweis, Lokalisation und Differentialdiagnose der nasalen Liquorrhoe. H.N.O. 20: 268, 1972

Minnigerode, B.: Zur Technik der extraduralen rhinochirurgischen Deckung von Liquorfisteln nach frontobasalen Schädelverletzungen. Monatsschr. Ohrenheilk. 101: 441, 1967

Montgomery, W.: Surgery for cerebrospinal fluid rhinorrhea and otorrhea. Arch. Otolaryng. 84: 538, 1966

Mündnich, K.: Ist der Otologe heute noch zur Behandlung der Hirnabszesse berechtigt? Arch. Ohren-, Nasen-, Kehlkopfheilk. 183: 205, 1964

Oeken, F. W.: Spätfolgen nach frontobasaler Schädelverletzung. H.N.O. 14: 30, 1960

Pfalz, R.: Zur operativen Behandlung der Rhinoliquorrhoe. H.N.O. 17: 178, 1969

Pirsig, W., H. H. Treeck: Rhinochirurgische Behandlung von rhinobasalen Liquorfisteln. In: Hals-Nasen-Ohrenheilkunde Vol. 1 ed. by J. Berendes, R. Link, F. Zöllner, Thieme, Stuttgart 1977 (p. 9.1)

Riechert, T.: Klinik und operative Therapie der intracraniellen infektiösen Erkrankungen. Arch. Klin. Ohrenheilk. 183: 147, 1964

Rollin, H.: Glucose- und Eiweißstreifen in der Diagnostik der nasalen Liquorfisteln. H.N.O. 18: 18, 1970

Schreiner, L., A. Herrmann: Die operative Behandlung der nasalen Liquorrhoe mit der Septum- und Muschelschleimhautplastik. Arch. Klin. Exp. Ohren-, Nasen-, Kehlkopfheilk. 188: 418, 1967

Schürmann, K.: Operative Hämatombehandlung bei Schädelhirnverletzungen. Langenbecks Arch. Klin. Chir. 319: 576, 1967

Seiferth, L. B.: Die Unfallverletzungen der Nase, der Nasennebenhöhlen und der Basis der vorderen Schädelgrube. Arch. Klin. Ohrenheilk. 165: 1, 1954

Seiferth, L. B., F. Wustrow: Verletzungen im Bereich der Nase, des Mittelgesichts und seiner Nebenhöhlen sowie frontobasale Verletzungen. In: Hals-Nasen-Ohrenheilkunde Vol. 1. ed. by J. Berendes, R. Link, F. Zöllner, Thieme, Stuttgart 1977 (p. 8.1)

Seiffert, A.: Unterbindung der A. maxillaris int. Z. Hals-, Nasen-, Ohrenheilk. 22: 323, 1928

Simon, H.: Die Fluorescinprobe zur Diagnostik der oto- und rhinogenen Liquorfisteln. Z. Laryng. Rhinol. 49: 54, 1970

Uffenorde, W.: Anzeige und Ausführung der Eingriffe an Ohr, Nase, Hals. Thieme, Stuttgart 1952

Unterberger, S.: Neuzeitliche Behandlung von Schädelverletzungen mit Beteiligung der fronto- und laterobasalen Räume. Z. Laryngol. Rhinol. 38: 441, 1959

Wullstein, H. L., S. R. Wullstein: Die Verletzungen der Rhino- und Otobasis unter dem Gesichtspunkt des pneumatischen Systems im Schädel. Chirurg 41: 490, 1970

Zülch, K. J.: Neurologische Diagnostik bei endocraniellen Komplikationen von otorhinologischen Erkrankungen. Arch. Ohren-, Nasen-, Kehlkopfheilk. 183: 1, 1964

9 Surgery of Injuries of the Skeleton and the Soft Tissues of the Face

By G. Mårtensson

General Principles of Management of Injury of the Face and Jaws

In the management of serious injury of the soft tissues and the skeleton of the face, a differentiation must be made between:

● *Primary*, immediate, often life-saving procedures;

● *Secondary*, definitive procedures carried out in a special department.

Primary Management of the Injured Patient

A first-aid slogan, the "ABC of traffic accidents" has been introduced in Sweden by Aldman (1965). A refers to "airway", B to "bleeding" and C to "circulation". About 20% of deaths can be prevented if attention is paid to these vital factors at the site of the accident.

The most serious complication is **obstruction of the airway**. This must be prevented by immediately removing blood clots, fragments of bone and teeth, dentures, etc., from the mouth. **Bleeding** must be controlled with pressure or by compression bandages at the site of the accident. In order to prevent **shock**, the injured patient should be protected from loss of body temperature by blankets, warm clothes, etc., in addition to the usual antishock treatment.

Transporting the patient from the site of the accident to the hospital can also cause certain problems. It is important that the patient is placed in the prone position or on his side with the head downward to prevent blood and secretions from blocking the airway and to prevent the tongue from falling back into the throat (Fig. 9.1).

Management in the Hospital

The definitive management of a patient with serious injuries to the face or jaws usually requires the close cooperation of one or more of the specialists involved in head and neck surgery (oral surgeon, rhinologist, neurosurgeon, ophthalmologist, plastic surgeon). Bronchoscopy (an emergency bronchoscope should always be available!), intubation, tracheostomy or laryngotomy may often be necessary to guarantee a *clear airway*.

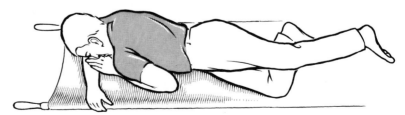

Fig. 9.1 Transportation position of a patient with injuries of the jaw.

The next most serious complication is *severe hemorrhage*. It can be caused by damage to the soft tissues of the mouth, tongue, palate, or pharynx. Hemorrhage may also occur from the base of the skull of from the intracranial vessels. A fracture of the neck of the mandible can cause bleeding into the external auditory canal if the canal has been ruptured by the bony fragments. Epistaxis can occur in fractures of the upper jaw due to rupture of the branches of the ethmoid arteries. Such an epistaxis is managed initially by the usual anterior nasal packing, but in many cases it is necessary to introduce a postnasal pack. If there has been excessive damage to the soft tissues and the skeleton of the face with profuse hemorrhage it may be necessary to ligate the external carotid artery (see Vol. 1, Chap. 6). For the *management of shock,* the reader is referred to an appropriate textbook.

Diagnostic Preoperative Procedures

After the above, often life-saving, procedures have been carried out, a careful examination is made including inspection and palpation of the face and jaws (Fig. 9.2) and a radiological examination. If there are other injuries (for example to the skull, chest or abdomen), the priority of the individual steps of management must be determined.

If there is simultaneous damage to the soft tissues and the skeleton of the face, the question of priority also arises. Here the degree and extent of the soft tissue injury must be considered as well as whether the soft tissue injury communicates with the mouth, pharynx or sinuses (see also Chapter 8). As a general principle, all complicated injuries of the facial skeleton should be managed "from within outward," a principle formulated by Ganzer in 1943.

Principles of Management

There are three objectives in the management of fractures of the jaw:

1. Restoration of normal appearance,
2. Restoration of normal occlusion,
3. Restoration of normal functions.

The principle of treatment is usually clear in fractures of the mandible. The fracture should be fixed with intermaxillary wiring to the intact upper jaw in correct occlusion. A fracture of the upper jaw cannot generally be managed with intermaxillary fixation alone, thus a fracture of the central middle third of the face usually requires extraoral fixation.

In a fracture of the jaw, there is usually considerable displacement of the fragments. Management consists of the following:

● *Reduction*, that is, manipulation of the displaced parts to their normal position;

● *Fixation*, that is, immobilization of the fragments firmly to each other and to the other jaw;

● *Retention*, that is, fixation of the fragments in the desired position during the healing process.

Usually the same apparatus can be used for the reduction as is used for the fixation and retention. There are, however, exceptions, as shown in the following section.

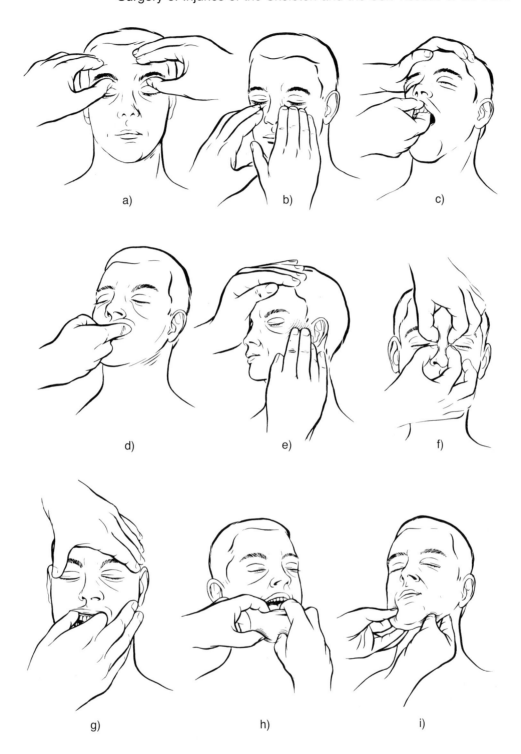

Fig. 9.2   Position of the hands for palpation of
a) Superior orbital ridge,
b) Inferior orbital margin,
c) Front teeth and the neighboring part of the upper jaw,
d) Lateral teeth, lateral part of the upper jaw and its connections to the zygoma,
e) External palpation of the zygoma,
f) Bony and cartilaginous infrastructure of the nose,
g) Maxilla and its connections to the remaining part of
   the middle third of the face,
h) Mobility and contour of the mandible palpated from
   the vestibule,
i) Contour of the mandible palpated externally.

Special Instruments

Figure 9.3 shows several instruments which are suitable for treating fractures of the jaw. They are:

- Bristow's elevator (Fig. 9.3 a),
- Howarth's raspatory (Fig. 9.3 b),
- Kilner's zygomatic elevator (Fig. 9.3 c),
- Rowe's disimpaction forceps (Fig. 9.3 d),
- Kelsey Fry's straight and curved bone awls (Fig. 9.3 e),
- Cannula (Fig. 9.3 f),
- Mathieu-Stille's needle holder (Fig. 9.3 g),
- Crown scissors (Fig. 9.3 h),
- Hillerström and Öquist's modification of Belzer-Langflach's splint removing forceps (Fig. 9.3 i),
- Hillerström and Öquist's modification of Mathieu-Stille's needle holder (Fig. 9.3 k).

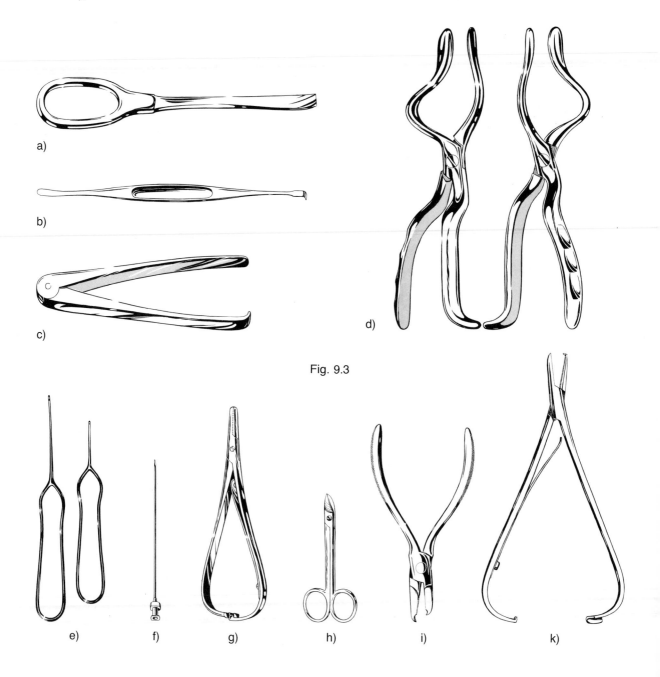

a)

b)

c)

d)

Fig. 9.3

e)   f)   g)   h)   i)   k)

Fractures of the Mandible

Classification of Fractures

During the last eight years, 1,210 patients with fractures of the jaws have been managed in the Department of Oral and Jaw Diseases and the Ear, Nose and Throat Department of the Karolinska Sjukhuset, Stockholm. Of these, 788 were fractures of the mandible and 422 fractures of the upper jaw. This distribution corresponds to the figures presented in the literature.

Although a fracture may occur in any part of the mandible, there are certain *sites of predilection*. In most statistics concerned with the localization of fractures, *fractures of the condylar process* are the most common. They comprise about one-quarter of the entire number (Schuchardt et al. 1966, quote 25% and Müller 1969, 26%). Next in frequency are fractures *in the area of the angle of the jaw*, and then *in the area of the canine tooth*.

Most fractures of the mandible demonstrate dislocation of the fragments which can be caused by the type and direction of the trauma but is essentially determined by the pull of the muscles inserted into the mandible.

In a fracture of the body of the mandible, the anterior fragment is usually drawn inferiorly and posteriorly by contraction of the suprahyoid and infrahyoid muscles, and the posterior fragment is retracted superiorly and medially by the masseter, medial pterygoid and temporal muscles (Fig. 9.4).

The central fragment of a double fracture in the mental region is displaced inferiorly by the contraction of the suprahyoid and infrahyoid muscles (Fig. 9.5).

There is usually relatively little displacement in a fracture of the ascending ramus of the mandible because of the powerful muscles which surround and fix the fragments.

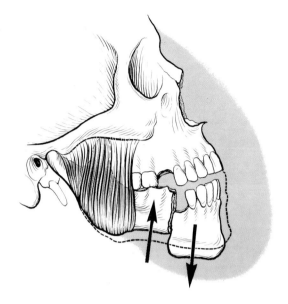

Fig. 9.4   Displacement of the fragments in a fracture of the body of the mandible.

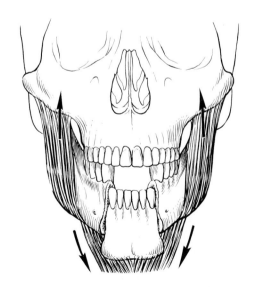

Fig. 9.5   Displacement of the fragments in a bilateral fracture of the mandible in the mental region.

Technical Methods

There are many different methods for fixation of the bony fragments. The best one depends on several factors, such as the extent of the fracture, number of remaining teeth, soft tissue damage, personal preferences and experience of the surgeon, etc.

In certain hospitals, direct interdental wiring is used for patients with sound teeth; in other hospitals, arch bars of metal or acrylic material or cap splints are preferred. Acrylic splints (Gunning splints) are generally used for the edentulous patient.

A detailed description of the different methods will not be given in this book. One of the special textbooks listed in the references should be consulted for further information. Only those principles of management used at the Karolinska Sjukhuset, Stockholm, will be presented here.

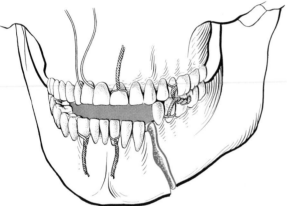

Fig. 9.6   Simple wire fixation.

Fractures of the Tooth-Bearing Mandible

Intraoral Fixation

If the dentition of the jaw is relatively good and the fragments are in good position, simple wiring can be used. A stainless steel wire (0.4 mm thick) is introduced around the appropriate tooth and is tightened around its neck. It is preferable to fasten separate wires around 2 or 3 teeth of the upper and lower jaw on both sides. Intermaxillary fixation is then produced by twisting the wires together (Fig. 9.6).

More secure fixation is produced by interdental eyelet wiring. A small loop is formed from steel wire (Fig. 9.7 a). The doubled wire is inserted from the buccal side between two teeth. One end of the wire is then turned forward and carried out again in the buccal direction in the immediately anterior interdental space. The other end is brought out through the immediately posterior interdental space. The wire is then passed anteriorly through the loop on the buccal side of the tooth. Both ends of the wire are then twisted together. The loop provides for intermaxillary fixation (Fig. 9.7b) with wires. Both of these fixation methods using wire are easy to carry out, but they provide unstable fixation and, therefore, are used only for emergency fixation or in cases as mentioned above.

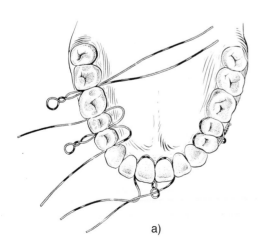

a)

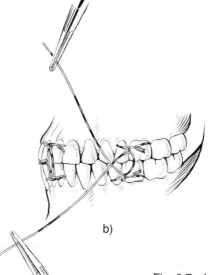

b)

Fig. 9.7   Interdental eyelet wire.

Obwegeser's fixation method (1952) is more reliable and more stable. It has also the advantage that the fixation can be applied directly to the teeth. Stainless steel wire is also used for this method.

The technique is illustrated in Figures 9.8–9.12. Kjellman's acrylic plate (1962) (Fig. 9.8c) is particularly helpful for forming the wire. The pillars on the plate correspond to the teeth in one-half of the jaw.

The stainless steel wire is passed around the pillars and then around the pins between the pillars (Fig. 9.9a).

If a tooth is missing, the corresponding pillar on the acrylic plate is not used. A wire splint, which is easy to release from the plate, can be made quickly and easily with this method.

The small arcs are bent vertically with a needle holder (Fig. 9.10) to form small loops. Lengths of cotton thread are drawn through these loops, facilitating the introduction of the wire between the teeth

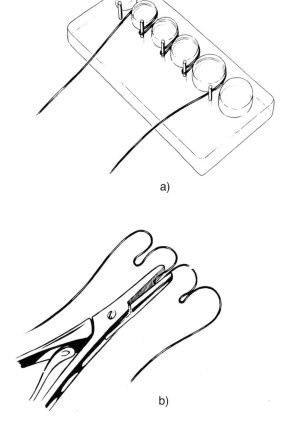

a)

b)

Fig. 9.9
Formation of the wire loops.
a) On the acrylic plate,
b) With a needle holder.

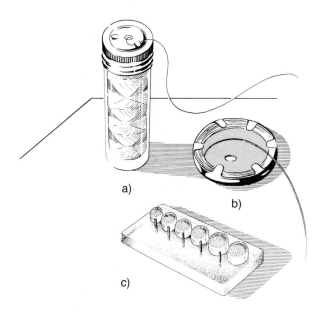

a)

b)

c)

Fig. 9.8   Material for making Obwegeser's wire ligatures.

a) Cotton thread,
b) Wire thread,
c) Acrylic plate.

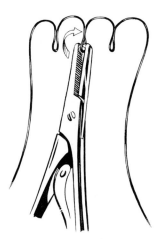

Fig. 9.10   Vertical bending of the loops.

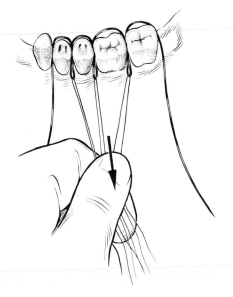

Fig. 9.11 Introduction of the wire loops between the teeth.

(Fig. 9.11). The wire should be applied closely to the lingual side of the teeth. The distal end of the wire is carried through the loops on the buccal side (Fig. 9.12a). The loops are then twisted 3 or 4 times (Fig. 9.12b) with forceps (Fig. 9.3k) so that the wire is fixed securely to each tooth. Finally, both ends of the wire are twisted together. The loops are then used for intermaxillary fixation (Fig. 9.12c).

Obwegeser's method is simple and reliable, requires no technical assistance, and can be used for most fractures of the mandible when dentition is good.

If several teeth are missing, other methods must be used to fix the mandibular fragments, for example metal arch bars fastened to the teeth. Arch bars of several different types and materials can be bought ready made. Figure 9.13 shows one type made of stainless steel (Wall's fracture splint, Rocky Mountain). While these manufactured metal arch bars do not provide secure fixation, they do provide a good method of emergency fixation.

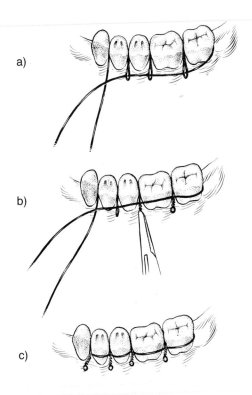

a)

b)

c)

Fig. 9.12 The individual steps for fixation of the wire ligatures.

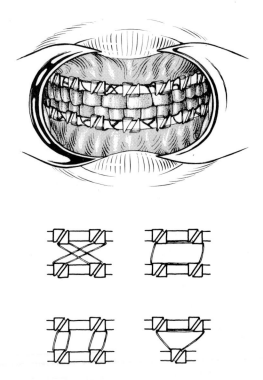

Fig. 9.13 Metal arch bars and their method of fixation.

Individually made arch bars provide secure fixation. Impressions are made in alginate of the upper and lower jaw, and a model is made from these in plaster of Paris. One material recommended for the arch bar is semicircular nickel-silver wire (2 mm thick). This is bent around the buccal surface of the teeth and shaped in such a way that it follows the gingival margins. Hooks made from silver material are soldered at appropriate points on the arch bar. This is fastened to the teeth with 0.4 mm stainless steel wires (Fig. 9.14). The ligation is easy to make (Fig. 9.15a). The wire is introduced between the teeth above the arch bar, bent over the palatal or lingual surface of the teeth and brought out in the immediately anterior interdental space beneath the arch bar. The ends of the wire are then twisted together.

An even more secure ligature can be achieved with the following method: A wire is introduced between the teeth, bent forward as described above and then brought out on the buccal side *above* (that is, *gingival*) to the arch bar. It is then bent backward over the buccal surface of the tooth, reintroduced *occlusal* to the arch bar, bent anteriorly on the palatal side and is brought out between the teeth. The wire thus forms a cross over the bar (Fig. 9.15b). It is particularly important that the wire be always turned in a *clockwise* direction to facilitate later corrections and removal of the wires at the end of the treatment.

If there is more severe displacement of the fragments or the dental condition is bad, the best fixation is achieved by *metal* (Fig. 9.16) or *acrylic cap splints* (Fig. 9.17). This method has many advantages but requires the assistance of a well trained technical staff.

If there is little or no displacement of the fragments of the jaw, an impression of the entire jaw is made in alginate. A model is then made in plaster of Paris by the technical staff. A wax splint is modeled, invested and cast in splint metal. A high quality silver alloy (silver 90%, copper, zinc and tin) is used. The splint is fastened to the teeth with copper cement. After this has hardened, traction can be applied by intermaxillary rubber bands to place the teeth in the correct occlusal position. When the correct occlusal position has been achieved, the rubber bands are replaced by fine stainless steel wires.

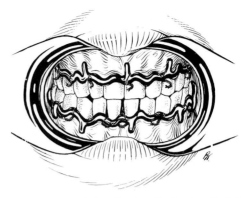

Fig. 9.14   Metal arch bar fixed to the teeth with 0.4 mm steel wire.

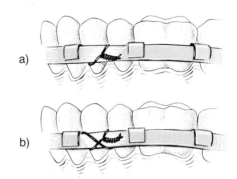

a)

b)

Fig. 9.15   Arch bar wiring

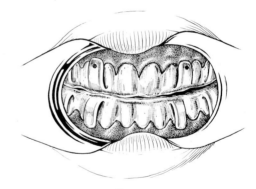

Fig. 9.16   Metal cap splint.

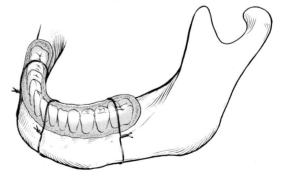

Fig. 9.17   Acrylic cap splint.

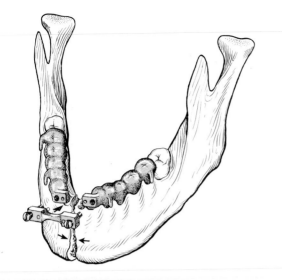

Fig. 9.18   Partial splint and locking device.

If there is a severe displacement of the fragments, it is advisable to take impressions from each fragment and prepare separate splints for each of them. After fixing the *partial splints* to the corresponding fragments of the jaw, the fragments are repositioned and fixed to the upper jaw in normal occlusion. A satisfactory permanent splint in one piece is made by locking the two individual parts of the splint together with a special locking device (Fig. 9.18).

It is helpful to provide an extension to each of the individual parts of the metal splint (Fig. 9.19a). After repositioning of the fragments (Fig. 9.19b), these extensions provide good retention for the acrylic (Fig. 9.19c). This is a simple and satisfactory method of retaining the splint in one piece.

In many hospitals, acrylic splints are used rather than metal ones (Fig. 9.20).

Acrylic splints can be made individually according to the principles described above for cast-metal cap splints. After making a model, the wax splint is invested, boiled out, and then acrylic is pressed and polymerized in the flask. The splint is fastened to the teeth with self-polymerizing acrylic.

A suitable method has been described by Schrudde (1956) using Palavit; it has the advantage of being simple and quick. The technique is as follows: The plaster of Paris model is made from alginate impression. Metal wires are fixed with wax interdentally on the buccal and lingual sides. A thin layer of wax is laid on the gingival side, and wires to fasten the intermaxillary fixation are secured in this. A thin plate serving as a cuff is made of wax around the model. The space between the model and the wax-cuff is then filled with fluid Palavit. When polymerization is complete, the splint is cleaned, polished and fastened to the teeth with fluid

a)

b)

c)

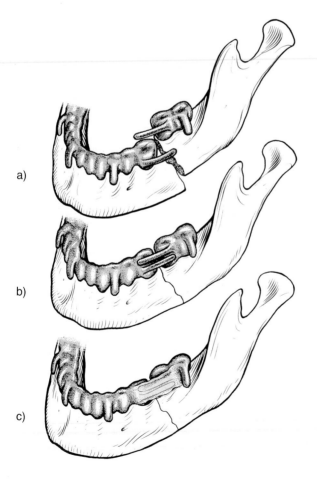

Fig. 9.19   Combination of metal splint and acrylic.

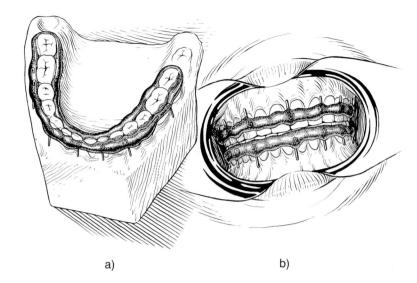

Fig. 9.20   Palavit splints.
a) On the plaster of Paris model,
b) Fastened to teeth of the upper and lower jaws.

Palavit. "In our opinion the greatest advantage is the fact that the artificial splints can be fixed to the fragments as separate splints and, after successful reduction of the fragments, they can be converted into a permanent splint in one piece by the use of fluid Palavit in the fissure between the parts" (Schrudde 1956).

Schuchardt (1956) has described a method of making arch bars which has several advantages: It can be carried out directly within the mouth and thus requires no technical assistance. The bar is very stable and can be used for fractures of the upper and lower jaw. The material used for the bar is Randolf metal (aluminium alloy, 2 mm thick) or stainless steel. This is provided with six wire pegs (1.4 mm thick) fixed at right angles to the bar. The arch bar is contoured exactly to the dental arch. The upper part of the wire pegs is bent over the occlusal surfaces (Fig. 9.21a) to prevent the splint slipping on the gingiva. It is then fixed with stainless steel wire (0.4 mm) to the teeth as described above. The bars and the wires are covered with self-polymerizing acrylic. The pillars over the occlusal surface are cut with metal scissors. The vestibular part is left in place to serve as hooks for the intermaxillary fixation (Fig. 9.21b).

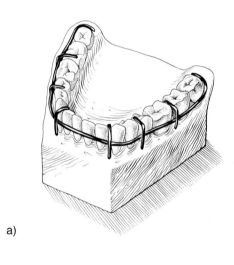

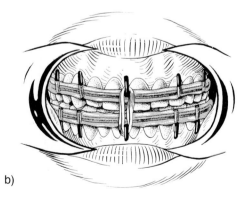

Fig. 9.21   Schuchardt's arch bar (a) covered with self-polymerizing acrylic (b)

Extraoral Fixation

Nowadays extraoral fixation is seldom indicated for treating fractures of the mandible since it has many disadvantages. The indications are restricted to fractures where a defect of the mandible is present and to patients with severe infection in the fracture line.

Roger-Anderson's method of skeletal pin fixation (Fig. 9.22) is one of the best known methods of extraoral fixation. The apparatus consists of steel pins, a locking device and connecting bars made from steel. Two pins are introduced through the skin into each bone fragment. They are then connected by the locking device and the connecting bars. Another variation on extraoral fixation is that of Becker (1958). This method has been described as a percutaneous intraosseous fixation for fractures of the mandible; it requires the use of a special Becker's apparatus. Screws are used instead of steel pins and a bridge of acrylic is made to connect the screws (Fig. 9.23).

The advantages of these methods of extraoral fixation are that the apparatus is available ready made and that it is relatively easy to apply – be it under general or nerve block anesthesia. Another advantage is that no intermaxillary fixation is required. Many authors, however, have described the disadvantages of extraoral methods: The pins or screws can damage vessels or nerves in the mandibular canal as well as the roots of the teeth; drilling the already damaged jaw can cause splintering of the bone; the fixation is inadequate and very susceptible to pressure or blows. A particularly important disadvantage is the psychological disturbance of the patient by the apparatus.

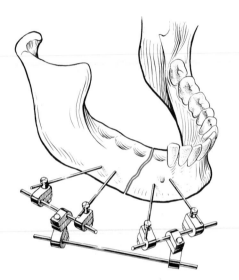

Fig. 9.22   Roger-Anderson's pin fixation.

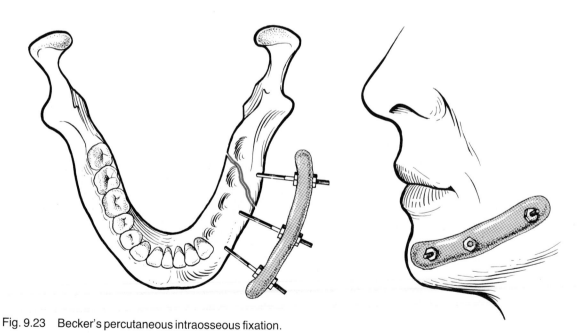

Fig. 9.23   Becker's percutaneous intraosseous fixation.

Fractures of the Edentulous Posterior Fragment

As described above, the posterior fragment is often displaced superiorly due to contraction of the masseter, the medial pterygoid and the temporal muscles (see Fig. 9.4). This displacement is the most severe in fractures of the body of the mandible, particularly of the angle of the jaw if the posterior fragment is edentulous. The severity of the displacement depends on the course of the fracture line and is most pronounced if the fracture line proceeds inferiorly and posteriorly (a socalled unfavorable fracture). In such a case, *intermaxillary fixation should be combined with transosseous wiring*.

Technique of transosseous wiring. The operation is carried out under nasotracheal anesthesia; an oral tube must not be used because the occlusion cannot be checked.

The incision is made 2 cm inferior to the lower border of the mandible (Fig. 9.24) in order to preserve the mandibular branch of the facial nerve (Fig. 9.25).

The incision divides the skin, platysma and superficial fascia. Depending on the position of the fracture, it may be necessary to dissect out, ligate and divide the facial artery and vein (Fig. 9.26).

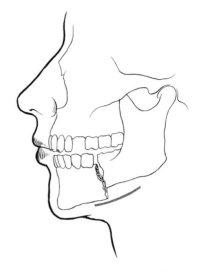

Fig. 9.24   Incision for transosseous fixation.

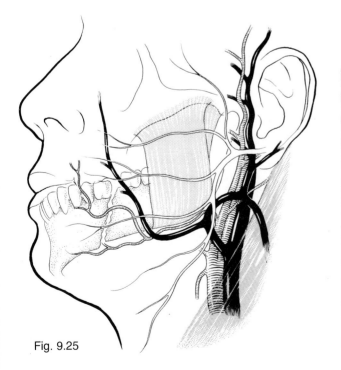

Fig. 9.25

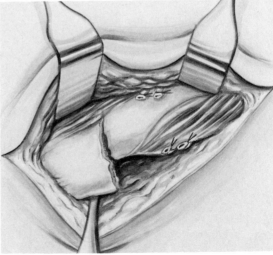

Fig. 9.26

The fracture is exposed and the periosteum is slightly elevated. Holes are drilled in the bony fragments as shown in Figure 9.27. Irrigation with saline solution is used to reduce the heat produced by the drill.

After exact reduction, the fragments are fixed with transosseous stainless steel wire (0.4 mm thick) (Figs. 9.28, 9.29). The ends of the wire are twisted on the buccal side of the mandible for exact control. It may be difficult to introduce the wire from the medial side through the drill holes. To overcome this difficulty, the following technique can be used: A wire is introduced through the distal hole (Fig. 9.28 a). A second wire is bent so that it forms a loop and is introduced through the anterior hole. This anterior wire is then used to grasp the first wire and bring it out (Fig. 9.28 b). Another technique is the so-called figure-of-eight "pannier" method (Fig. 9.29). This method provides greater stability since the wires also surround the lower border of the mandible.

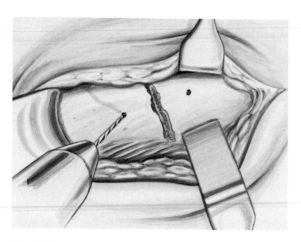

Fig. 9.27

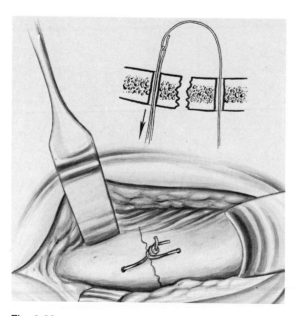

Fig. 9.28

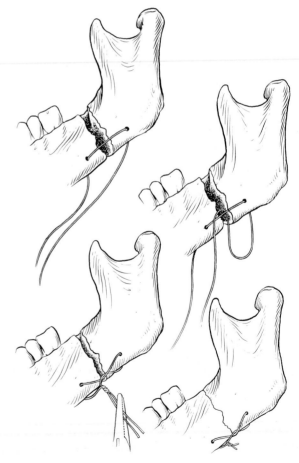

Fig. 9.29

The wound is now closed in layers. The great advantage of this extraoral method is that it is carried out under absolutely sterile conditions and allows reduction to be checked under direct vision.

During the last few years, intraosseous fixation has been carried out in several hospitals using *metal plates* (Fig. 9.30). This method has been used with good results for fractures of the body and the angle of the mandible by Spiessl et al. (1971). The advantage is that no intermaxillary fixation is required. Other authors indicate that there are certain disadvantages to this method, for example, damage to large parts of the periosteum caused by the metal plate which delays healing.

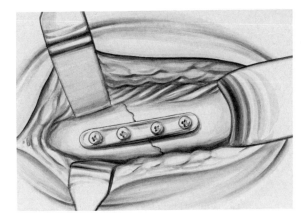

Fig. 9.30

Fractures of the Edentulous Mandible

Several different methods of treatment are available for fractures of the edentulous jaw. In general they can be divided into *orthodontic, surgical* and *combined methods of fixation of the jaw.*

In the orthodontic method of repair, the patient's own dentures (after they have been repaired if they were broken) or acrylic splints are used (Gunning splints) (Fig. 9.31).

The denture or the splint is fixed to the *lower jaw* by circumferential wiring with a special awl (see Fig. 9.3e). A good technique for circumferential fixation utilizing a cannula has been described by Björn (1952).

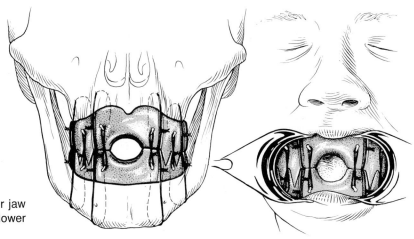

Fig. 9.31
Gunning splints fixed to the upper jaw by peralveolar wiring and to the lower jaw by circumferential wiring.

Technique. The operation is carried out under general or nerve block anesthesia. The cannula is introduced through the skin toward the inferior margin of the mandible and is then brought out into the mouth close against the lingual side of the bone (Figs. 9.32, 9.33). A stainless steel wire (0.4 mm) is then introduced through the cannula.

The cannula, with the wire within it, is withdrawn around the lower border of the mandible and is then inserted into the mouth on the vestibular side of the mandible (Figs. 9.34, 9.35). The end of the wire is now secured by a hemostat and the cannula is brought out inferiorly through the skin.

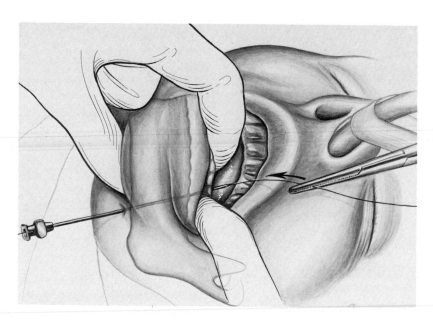

Fig. 9.32

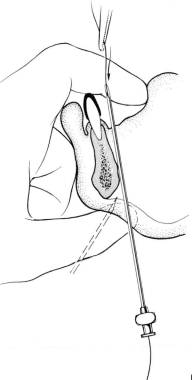

Fig. 9.33

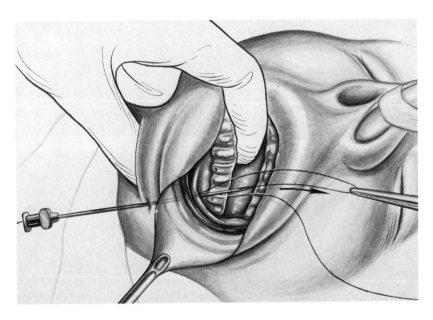

Fig. 9.34

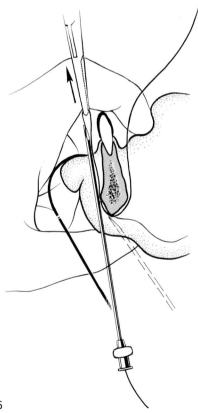

Fig. 9.35

The two ends of the wires are twisted together within the oral cavity over the cap splint (see Fig. 9.17), the denture or the Gunning splint (Figs. 9.36–9.39). The circumferential wiring is carried out twice on both sides. This method is simple and causes little bleeding or scarring.

If the patient has a well-fitting denture, treatment is simple; intermaxillary fixation with rubber bands or steel wire is usually not indicated but a simple chin bandage is applied. A mild degree of displacement of the fragments is not significant; it can be compensated by treatment with a new denture later.

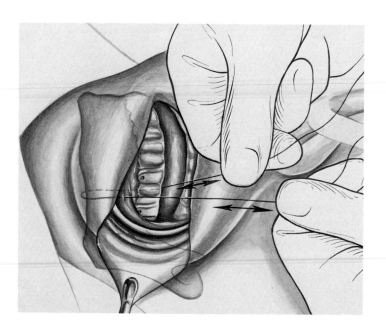

Fig. 9.36

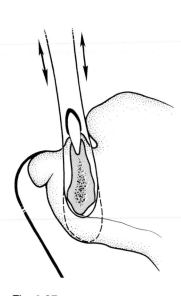

Fig. 9.37

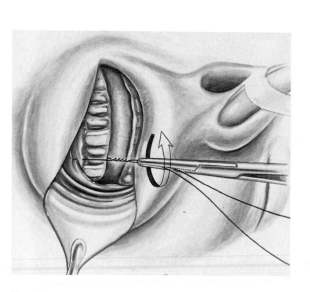

Fig. 9.38

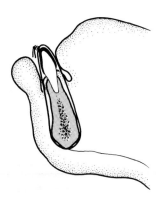

Fig. 9.39

Fractures of the Condyle

As already mentioned, this is the most common type of fracture of the mandible. This is particularly true for children in whom such a fracture can be easily overlooked.

Opinions regarding the correct management of this fracture vary. Several authors recommend active treatment while others favor a more conservative approach. The conservative treatment is generally used in Sweden and with good results to judge from the many reports and follow-up studies.

The principle of management is to obtain good occlusion and articulation. If there is little or no displacement of the mandible, an elastic chin bandage is the only support necessary.

If there is more severe deviation of the mandible, it must be replaced in the correct occlusion with arch bars or splints and intermaxillary rubber bands.

The length of time which the intermaxillary fixation must be maintained depends on the extent of the deviation of the mandible. Usually 2 to 3 weeks is sufficient and rubber bands are usually adequate. Regular checks must be carried out.

Active surgical management carries a considerable risk of damage to the facial nerve, and fixation of the head of the mandible with a wire suture or a metal plate often causes great technical difficulties. For this reason most authors warn against surgical procedures for fractures of the condyle.

See also surgery of the temporomandibular joint, Chapter 12.

Fractures in Children

The principles of management of mandible fractures in children are the same as for adults, but considerable difficulty arises when it is necessary to fix splints to the teeth. The period of eruption of the permanent teeth is a particularly difficult one. Many of the milk teeth frequently have caries; the permanent teeth are still not properly erupted or their roots are not completely developed. Circumferential wiring (Figs. 9.32–9.39) and suspension from the zygomatic arch (see Figs. 9.50–9.58) provide stronger fixation for the splint; these methods do not damage the permanent teeth.

Rules, Postoperative Care and Complications

Rules, Hints and Typical Errors

The majority of fractures of the mandible heal within 4 to 6 weeks and even earlier in children. The intermaxillary fixation is removed after 3 or 4 weeks to check whether the fracture has healed, and the stability of the fracture line is tested by palpation. If the jaw appears to be unstable, it is left in fixation for a further 1 to 2 weeks. Even if the mandible is stable, the fixation apparatus should not be immediately removed. The patient may chew soft food and is instructed how to perform intermaxillary fixation with rubber bands during the night. If no instability of the jaw fragments is found after an additional week, the splints can be removed. Healing of the fracture cannot be radiologically determined at this time because the callus can only be recognized a few months later on an x-ray. Special forceps (see Fig. 9.3 k) can be used to remove the cap splints. The short limb is placed on the gingival side of the splint and the longer limb on the occlusal side as shown in Figure 9.40. The splint can be easily bent outward with this technique and is then removed from the teeth.

Postoperative Care and Complications

Delayed healing (*a pseudoarthrosis*) can have several different *causes*; they may be *general* or *local*. General causes include poor general condition, diabetes, tuberculosis and advanced age.

Local causes can be a local disease such as infection, tumors or cysts of the jaw, previous radiotherapy or a wide defect between the fragments. The most common causes of pseudoarthrosis are infection, unsatisfactory fixation and interposition of the surrounding soft tissues. To prevent infection, an antibiotic should be given for all compound fractures and also if an extensive hematoma is present.

Management of Pseudoarthrosis

First, rigid and secure fixation must be provided. The apparatus used for fixation of the mandibular fragments depends on many factors:

- Number of remaining teeth,
- Localization of the pseudoarthrosis,
- Size of the bony defect.

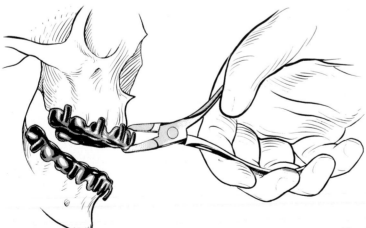

Fig. 9.40   Removal of cap splints.

The extraoral percutaneous method of splinting (see p. 54) can be used, but it has many disadvantages which have already been described. These disadvantages can be avoided and adequate stability can be achieved with the use of intraoral splints.

If there is a small bony defect in a tooth-bearing mandible, the fixation used is the same as that already described for severe displacement of the mandibular fragments (see p. 52, Figs. 9.18, 9.19). In the presence of a bony defect behind the teeth (for example, of the angle of the mandible), cap splints are cemented over all of the teeth remaining in the upper and lower jaw. If the mandible is edentulous, a Gunning splint (see Fig. 9.31), is fixed around the mandible with circumferential wiring as described on page 57. To secure stability, intermaxillary fixation with stainless steel wires should always be applied after the operation. The operation is carried out under general anesthesia.

The bony fragments are exposed by a submandibular incision (see p. 55). Soft tissue impacted between the bony fragments is removed. The ends of the bony fragments are freshened to provide bleeding surfaces. A segment of the iliac crest or the tibia is used as a bone graft to fill the defect in the mandible. The graft is fixed to the neighboring mandibular fragments with intraosseous wires (Fig. 9.41).

Teeth in the Fracture Line

The management of teeth in the fracture line is very controversial. If there are signs of pulp necrosis or of apical infection, the tooth should be extracted because of the danger of infection of the fracture line. In other cases the question of extraction must be decided individually. In principle, healthy teeth in the fracture line should be preserved, particularly in the posterior fragment, since even a wisdom tooth can prevent a more severe displacement (see p. 55).

Functional Sequelae

Several teeth may feel loose after the fixation has been removed. Usually they become fixed again after several weeks.

In spite of exact intermaxillary fixation, the teeth must often be ground off to achieve good occlusion. If teeth were knocked out at an accident, they must be replaced by a permanent bridge or a denture.

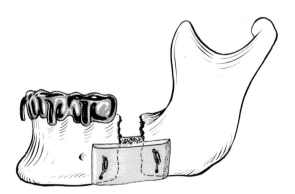

Fig. 9.41   Bone graft.

Fractures of the Upper Jaw

Classification

As already mentioned on page 47, our statistics show that out of 1,210 fractures of the jaw, the upper jaw was affected in 422 cases. Of the latter, 63 were fractures of the middle third of the face, 246 were fractures of the zygoma and 113 were fractures of the alveolus of such an extent that they required some form of fixation. Fractures of the middle third of the face are classified in different ways by different authors. The best known is that of the French surgeon Le Fort (Figs. 9.42, 9.43).

● The *Le Fort Type I* (Guerin's fracture or low-level fracture) is characterized by separation of the hard palate and the alveolar process. The fracture line passes through the piriform aperture and the floor of the antrum posteriorly into the lower third of the pterygoid process of the sphenoid bone.

● In the *Le Fort Type II* (pyramidal fracture), the fracture line proceeds through the nasal bone, the lacrimal bone and the frontal process of the maxilla and then through the inferior orbital fissure and the zygomatic process of the maxilla so that the zygoma is divided from the upper jaw. It finally passes posteriorly through the pterygoid process.

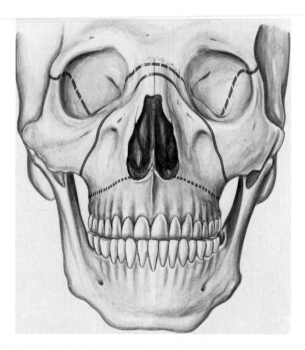

Fig. 9.42   Le Fort's classification of fractures of the upper jaw (front view).

..... = Le Fort Type I
———— = Le Fort Type II
------ = Le Fort Type III

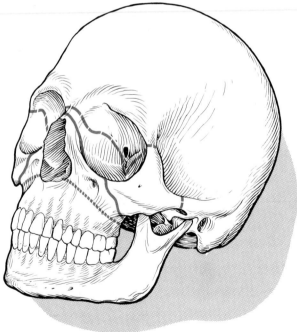

Fig. 9.43   Fractures of the upper jaw as shown in Figure 9.42, (lateral view).

- In the *Le Fort Type III* (suprazygomatic fracture) the fracture line passes through the nasal bone, the orbit and the ethmoid and just below the base of the skull through the frontal process of the zygomatic bone and the temporozygomatic suture and the posteriorly through the pterygoid process. This fracture completely separates the entire midfacial bones from their cranial attachments. It is often combined with a frontobasal fracture (see Chapter 8).

Pape (1969) differentiates between two large groups in his classification:

- "Central midfacial fractures" and
- "Lateral midfacial fractures".

Rowe and Killey (1968) follow similar principles in their classification. They divide fractures of the upper jaws into two groups:

- Fractures not involving the teeth and the alveolus,
- Fractures involving the teeth and alveolus.

Within these two groups, fractures are further divided into central and lateral groups. Even if most fractures of the upper jaw can be included in one of these principal types, other forms do occur (e.g., sagittal fractures and comminuted fractures).

The purpose of these anatomical classifications is to provide guidelines for treatment.

Central upper midfacial fractures are comprised of fractures of the nose and the nasoethmoidal complex. These are dealt with in Chapters 6 and 8. Lateral midfacial fractures involve the zygomatic region particularly (see p. 78).

Fractures Involving the Alveolar Process and the Teeth

Symptoms

Fractures of the middle third of the facial skeleton are usually combined with some degree of damage to the soft tissues and hematoma. Since the upper jaw is usually displaced posteroinferiorly, the result is an open bite. Epistaxis usually occurs also. Fractures of the Le Fort Type II and Type III often have ophthalmological and intracranial complications (see Vol. 1, Chap. 4 and 7 and Chap. 8).

Palpation is particularly important for the clinical diagnosis in order to determine abnormal movement of the upper jaw (see Fig. 9.2). The diagnosis is confirmed by radiology, including tomography.

General Principles of Management

First, all life-threatening complications should be prevented or treated (see p. 43). This requires close cooperation with all specialists concerned with the head and neck. The purpose of treatment is to restore normal anatomy, physiology and function.

It has already been stated that the principle of management of a *fracture of the mandible* consists of fixing the mandible to the intact upper jaw. This principle usually *cannot* be applied in *fractures of the upper jaw* because the fractured upper jaw follows the movement of the mandible when the patient speaks or eats if the upper jaw is only fixed to the mandible. If the upper jaw is mobile, it must be fixed by a combination of intraoral and extraoral methods.

Technical Adjuncts

Intraoral Fixation

The intraoral fixation for immobilization of a fracture of the upper jaw requires greater stability than for a fracture of the mandible. For this reason, wire ligatures and arch bars are usually not adequate. Generally metal or acrylic splints are used in patients with good dentition and acrylic splints for edentulous patients.

The methods for extraoral fixation are very different. In some hospitals the "antler" (Kingsley) splint (Fig. 9.44) is used. This consists of intraoral and extraoral splints with a metal bar running around the angle of the mouth. This bar can be either soldered to the splint or fixed by small tubes. Effective and constant traction is provided by rubber bands between the metal bars and the plaster of Paris head cap (Fig. 9.45). Another method uses

steel wires passed transcutaneously through the cheeks to fix the splints to a head cap (Fig. 9.46).

Extraoral Splints

There are several different sets of apparatus available for extraoral fixation of a fracture of the upper jaw.

Plaster of Paris Head Cap and Metal Head Band

A plaster of Paris head cap is often used for anchoring the splint. There are many different ways in which the head cap can be connected to the splint fixed on the teeth. Metal rods of different material are used, usually aluminum, because it is light. These rods are connected by stainless steel universal joints to nickel-silver rod soldered to the cap splint (Fig. 9.47).

A plaster of Paris head cap has many disadvantages. It is unstable, heavy, uncomfortable and occasionally causes pressure sores; furthermore it cannot be used if there is extensive damage to the skull.

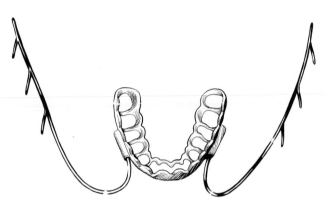

Fig. 9.44   "Antler" (Kingsley) splint.

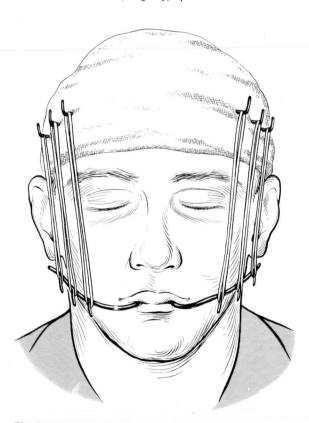

Fig. 9.45   "Antler" (Kingsley) splint with a plaster of Paris head cap.

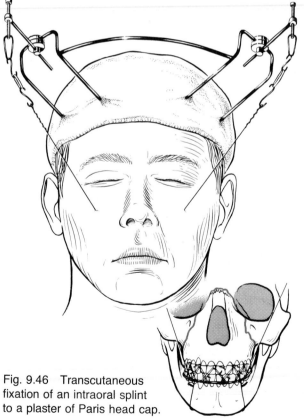

Fig. 9.46   Transcutaneous fixation of an intraoral splint to a plaster of Paris head cap.

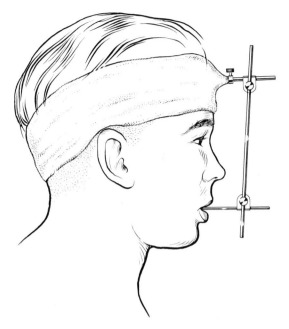

Fig. 9.47   Plaster of Paris head cap with metal rods.

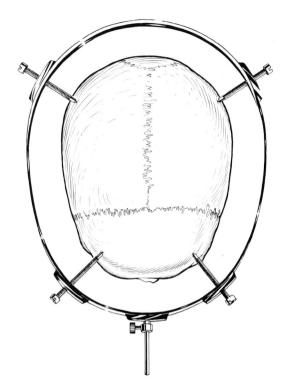

Fig. 9.48   Crewe's metal head band.

Crawford (1943, 1948) and Crewe (1963) among others have constructed a *metal head band* in an attempt to overcome these disadvantages (Figs. 9.48, 9.49). Crawford's head frame consists of a band cast in aluminum which is fixed to the bones of the skull with vitallium screws. One advantage of this metal band is the greater stability, which guarantees sound anchoring of the splints. Furthermore, it weighs only one-half as much as a head cap.

A metal head band of this sort is easy to apply, even in ambulant treatment. Its screws are fixed only superficially to the bones of the skull and do not penetrate deep into the cortical bone. This fixation can be carried out under local anesthesia. Small incisions are made in the skin where the screws are to be introduced. In order to ensure stability, it is important that no soft tissue is interposed; the screws should come into direct contact with the bone.

All external methods of fixation, such as the plaster of Paris head caps and metal bands, have some disadvantages in treatment of fractures of the upper jaw. (The same is also true of extraoral pinning of the bone in fractures of the mandible.) The patient finds it embarrassing to appear in public with his fixation apparatus, and he is unable to work for a long time. Naturally, the method to be used for treatment of all injuries to the jaws should be that

which yields the best functional and esthetic results. But there are methods of fixation of maxillary fractures which have certain advantages compared with the methods of extraoral fixation just described.

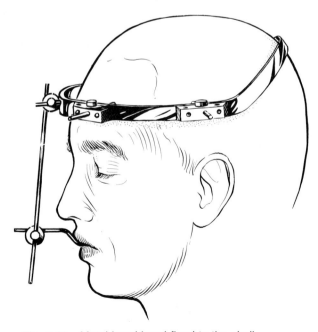

Fig. 9.49   Metal head band fixed to the skull.

Treatment by Intraosseous Fixation

Treatment of a fracture of the upper jaw by means of intraosseous fixation or the socalled subcutaneous suspension has many advantages over extraoral fixation. Adams described the principle of subcutaneous suspension in 1942; the principle has been further developed by Thoma: "Internal wiring fixation" (1948), Lesney: "Circumzygomatic wiring" (1953), Schwenzer: "Drahtaufhängung bei Mittelgesichtsfrakturen" (1967), Rowe and Killey: "Internal skeletal fixation" (1968) and others.

Zygomaticomaxillary suspension can be used for a Le Fort I or II fracture when the zygoma is intact.

Technique of zygomaticomaxillary suspension. The operation is best carried out under general anesthesia with nasal endotracheal intubation. Steel wire (0.4 mm) is used for the suspension, and an awl is used to introduce the wire. The other instruments are the same as those used for circumferential wiring around the mandible (see Fig. 9.3 e).

The zygoma is palpated with the left hand. The awl is introduced from the mouth medial to the zygoma and emerges through the skin (Fig. 9.50). The wire is passed through the opening in the awl and is then drawn into the oral cavity (Fig. 9.51). The end of the wire is held with a

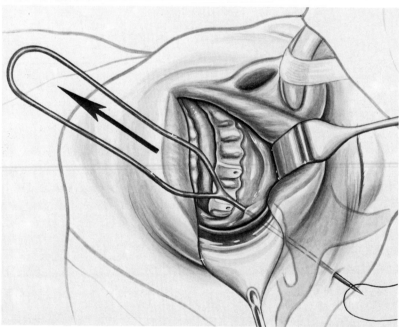

Fig. 9.50

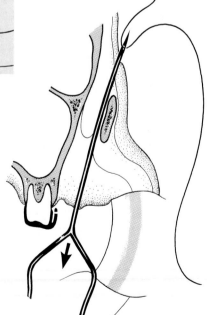

Fig. 9.51

hemostat. The awl is then pierced on the lateral side of the zygoma through the same perforation in the skin (Fig. 9.52), the upper end of the wire is passed into it and is then drawn back again into the oral cavity (Fig. 9.53).

In this way the wire sling is passed closely around the zygoma (Fig. 9.54). Both ends of the wire are now twisted together in the mouth and fastened to the splint (Fig. 9.55).

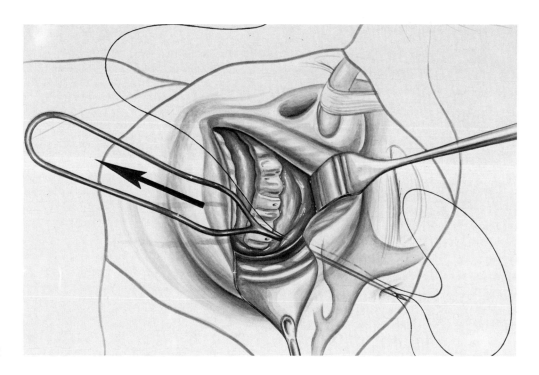

Fig. 9.52

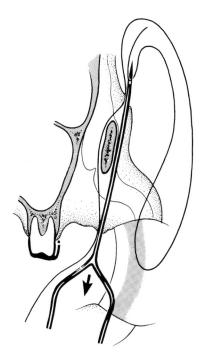

Fig. 9.53

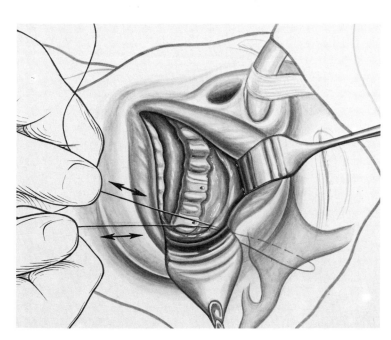

Fig. 9.54

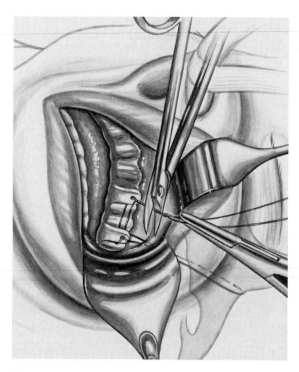

Fig. 9.55

A satisfactory alternative method of zygomaticomaxillary suspension is the following: A cannula is introduced through the skin of the cheek medial to the zygomatic arch and is passed into the oral cavity. A 0.4 mm thick stainless steel wire is then passed through the cannula (Fig. 9.56a).

The end of the wire is fixed with a hemostat. The needle is now drawn upward subcutaneously, passed around the zygoma (Fig. 9.56b) and down its lateral side to emerge in the oral cavity (Fig. 9.56c). The wire is held with a hemostat and the needle is withdrawn. Both ends of the wire are then fixed to the splint. This method is simple and causes only an insignificant cheek wound. The principle is similar to that of the method described by Björn (1952) where wire slings are passed around the mandible.

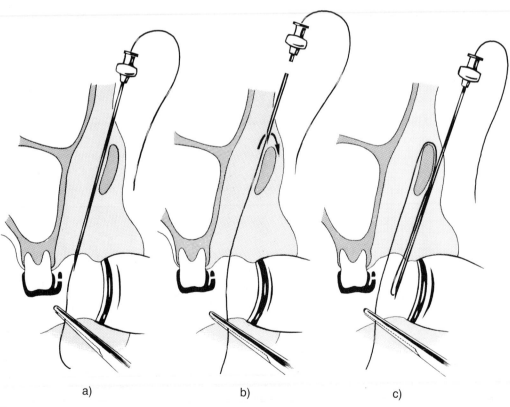

a)   b)   c)

Fig. 9.56

It is important that the steel wire be suspended as far forward as possible on the zygoma and that it be fixed as far posteriorly as possible on the splint, (Figs. 9.57, 9.58) to prevent dorsal dislocation of the jaw. It is also helpful to provide the hooks intended for intermaxillary fixation with holes for the fixation of the suspension wires (Figs. 9.55, 9.58).

A simple procedure is as follows: When the ends of the wire have been drawn into the mouth, they are twisted into a loop. A further piece of wire is then introduced between this loop and the hole in the hook (Fig. 9.58 a). The advantage of this procedure is that fixation can be carried out more easily and, if the intermediate piece of wire breaks, it can be removed and replaced by another similar small piece of wire.

Suspension is carried out on both sides (Fig. 9.57) to ensure optimal stability. Intermaxillary fixation is then achieved to provide correct occlusion, preferably by rubber bands.

In a *Le Fort Type III fracture of the middle third of the face* in which the zygoma and the zygomatic arch have been fractured, another method of wire suspension, the socalled *frontomaxillary fixation*, must be used.

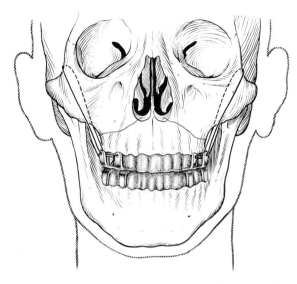

Fig. 9.57 Schematic representation of zygomatico-maxillary suspension, from the front.

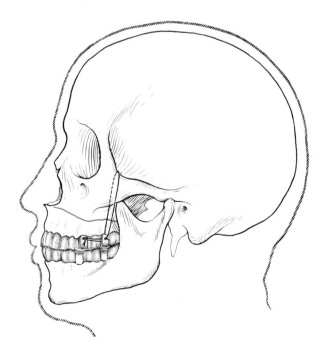

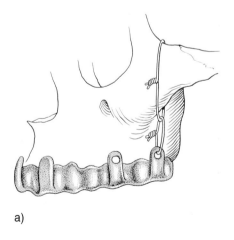

a)

Fig. 9.58 Lateral view of suspension shown in Figure 9.57. Diagram a) shows a modification of this method of wiring by means of an additional piece of wire.

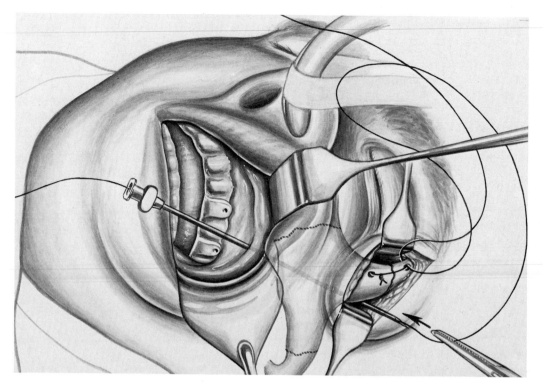

Fig. 9.59

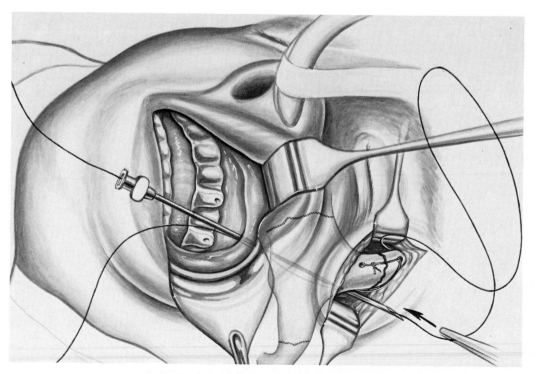

Fig. 9.60

Technique of frontomaxillary suspension. The operation is carried out under general anesthesia. The wire and instruments used are the same as those used for zygomaticomaxillary suspension. The incision is made through the skin at the lateral end of the supraorbital margin. The periosteum at this point is then incised. A hole is drilled through the orbital ridge about 1 cm superior to the frontozygomatic suture, the wire is passed through the hole and is then passed into the oral cavity with an awl or a cannula on the medial side of the zygomatic arch (Figs. 9.59, 9.60).

Finally the wire is fastened to the splint as described above (Fig. 9.61). Suspension is carried out on both sides. The wound is closed with subcutaneous catgut and the skin with silk. The periosteum need not be sutured.

In many cases there is a simultaneous fracture of the region of the frontozygomatic suture which should be managed by a simultaneous burr hole through the frontal process to allow adequate stabilization of the zygoma by intraosseous fixation (Figs. 9.59–9.61).

This method of surgical exposure and intraosseous fixation has many advantages, and avoids the use of an extraoral apparatus, with all its disadvantages.

Wire suspension should not be used uncritically. Rowe and Killey (1968) state that: "Internal skeletal fixation is not universally applicable, however, for the maxillae are not rigidly supported but only *suspended* from the intact portion of the facial skeleton and it is impossible to exert adequate lateral or anterior traction by these means."

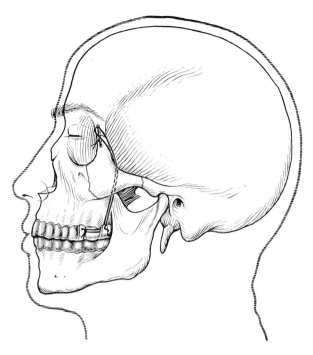

Fig. 9.61   Schematic representation of frontomaxillary suspension.

If it is not possible to restore exact occlusion with this gradual orthodontic traction method, an operation must be carried out to allow active mobilization of the displaced maxilla and reduction and fixation in the correct occlusion.

Reduction

The upper jaw is usually displaced posteroinferiorly in a fracture of the central middle third of the face. This produces an open bite and a flat face ("dish face").

The upper jaw must be replaced in the correct position before it is immobilized, if possible by conservative measures using rubber bands between the splints on the upper and lower jaws. For this reason the rubber bands proceed obliquely downward and forward from the splint on the maxilla to the mandibular splint (Fig. 9.62). The force and direction of traction can be altered with the rubber bands. When normal occlusion has been restored, the rubber bands are replaced with 0.4 mm thick stainless steel wire.

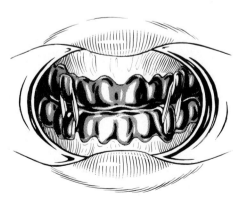

Fig. 9.62   Reduction with rubber bands.

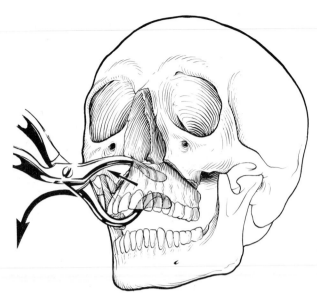

Fig. 9.63   Reduction of the upper jaw by "rocking".

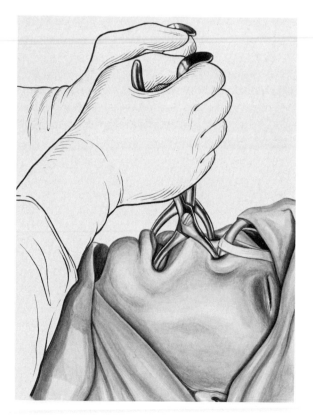

Fig. 9.64   Bimanual operative reduction of the posteriorly displaced jaw.

If there is also a simultaneous frontobasal fracture, or such a fracture is suspected, an operative repositioning must always be carried out. The upper jaw is replaced *first* and the upper part of the face and the base of the skull are reconstructed on this "basis". If the order of the operation is reversed (reconstruction of the base of the skull first followed by reduction of the central middle third of the face), there is a danger that those structures of the base of the skull which have already been replaced will be damaged again by reducing the maxilla.

Operative Reduction

This is carried out with special forceps (see Fig. 9.3 d).

Technique. The operation is carried out under general anesthesia with nasoendotracheal (not oral endotracheal) *intubation* in order to facilitate checking of the occlusion. One shank of the forceps is introduced along the floor of the nose and the other grasps the palate through the mouth (Fig. 9.63). Forceps may be placed on each side to exert maximum traction. The operator grasps the forceps with each hand and replaces the maxilla by means of powerful forward traction combined with rotatory movements (Fig. 9.64). Obwegeser (1956) calls this the "rocking" method and states: "The socalled rocking of the upper jaw, i.e., forced mobilization and simultaneous reduction of all displaced pieces of the midfacial bones, is indicated in the vast majority of cases of midfacial fractures accompanied by displacement to restore not only occlusion but also the contour of the middle third of the face."

Fractures of the Alveolus

Fractures of the alveolar process vary greatly in degree and extent, but are most common in the area of the incisor teeth of the upper jaw (Fig. 9.65a). The patient's history often reveals relatively minor trauma such as a blow or a push.

Typically, the teeth and the affected part of the alveolar process are displaced toward the oral cavity. Irrespective of the clinical picture, the diagnosis is confirmed by radiology.

Treatment consists primarily of repositioning the dislocated fragments and of suturing the wounds of the gingiva.

The fragments can be fixed in the acute phase using self-polymerizing acrylate between the teeth.

If the fracture is more extensive, stable fixation with retention should be carried out using a cast splint of metal or acrylic (Fig. 9.65b) which should be fastened to at least two teeth on each side of the fracture if possible. Intermaxillary fixation is not carried out in fractures of the alveolar process.

The fracture usually heals within 4 weeks and the splint can then be removed. It is important to test the sensitivity of the damaged or loosened teeth. Reduced sensitivity is not equivalent to deficient vitality and does not require endodontic treatment. Such treatment should only be instituted if there are clinical and radiological signs of nonvitality of the pulp.

Sensitivity is an index of innervation; vitality is an index of the blood supply. Thus, a tooth can be vital in the presence of reduced sensitivity as is often found during the first few months following a Caldwell-Luc antrostomy.

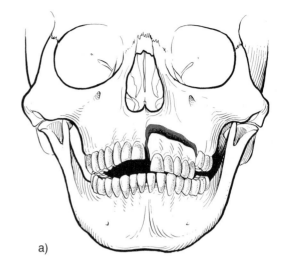

a)

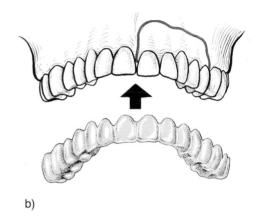

b)

Fig. 9.65   Fracture of the alveolus.
a) Typical situation,
b) Fixation with metal splint.

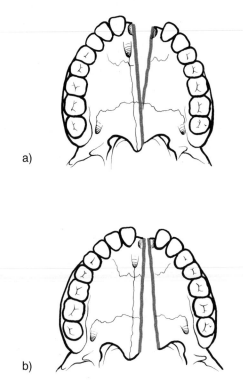

Fig. 9.66   Sagittal fracture.
a) Anterior cleft,
b) Posterior cleft.

Sagittal Fractures

Sagittal fractures in the midline of the palate can occur either alone or in combination with other fractures of the central middle third of the face. The first is often caused by a powerful blow to the chin. The pressure is transmitted to the alveolar process and the teeth so that both halves of the hard palate are forced apart (Fig. 9.66). The technique of reduction and fixation of a sagittal fracture is the same as that already described for a fracture of the mandible with severe displacement of the fragments (p. 50).

An alginate impression is taken of each segment of the upper jaw and of the mandible. A plaster of Paris model is then made from this impression. Separate splints are fashioned from this model in metal or plastic material and are attached to the teeth. The maxillary fragments are replaced in accurate occlusion by the use of intermaxillary rubber bands. The parts of the splint are then united with locking bars or self-polymerizing acrylate (Fig. 9.67). It is important that the *medial* side of the central incisors is not included in the splint; this can make exact reduction impossible.

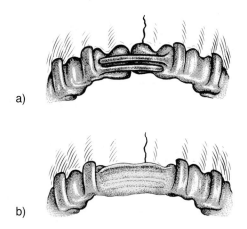

Fig. 9.67   A divided metal splint used for a sagittal fracture.

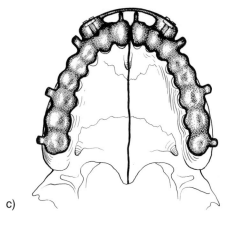

a) Divided splint in position,
b) Connecting the divided splint with acrylic,
c) Connecting the two halves of the splint by means of a locking device.

Rules, Postoperative Care and Complications

Rules, Hints and Typical Errors

It is impossible to draw up simple, universally applicable rules for the management of maxillary fractures. In many cases different methods must be combined in order to obtain the best functional and cosmetic results.

Pseudoarthroses are uncommon in maxillary fractures. Most of the fractures stabilize after 6 to 8 weeks, but the intermaxillary fixation can be removed after about 3 to 4 weeks. The stability can be determined at that time by palpation.

It is extremely important that intermaxillary fixation for all fractures of the upper jaw is always carried out in correct occlusion. The only exception to this rule is the edentulous patient. Here a slight displacement persisting after the fracture has healed can be compensated by a new denture. In patients with good dentition, incorrect occlusion must be corrected by detailed, time consuming and expensive prosthetic procedures.

Postoperative Care and Complications

When healing is complete it is relatively easy to remove the interoral and extraoral fixation as well as the suspension wires; cap splints are removed with special forceps (see p. 62). Before removing the suspension wires, the oral cavity is carefully irrigated and cleaned. If the upper jaw has been fixed by *zygomaticomaxillary suspension,* local anesthesia is used; 3 to 4 ml of anesthetic is injected from the oral cavity into the zygomatic region. The wires are loosened from the splint. One end of the wire is grasped with a needle holder and the entire wire is drawn out through the oral cavity.

In *frontomaxillary suspension,* local anesthesia of the operative scar and of the oral cavity must be in-

duced as described above. The wire is exposed through an incision in the scar and divided; the wound is then sutured again. It is important to finish this part of the procedure first since it must be carried out under sterile conditions. It is then easy to pull both halves of the wire out through the oral cavity. This minor operation seldom causes complications, but antibiotics should be given before and after operation to prevent infection.

Functional Sequelae

If the patient has brain damage, he should be checked in the postoperative period by a neurologist. Severe midfacial fractures can also cause ophthalmological lesions. These should be assessed and treated by an ophthalmologist if necessary (see Vol. 1, Chap. 4).

Reduction and fixation of the fractured jaw may need to be delayed because of severe cerebral complications or poor general condition. Diagnosis of the fracture must not be overlooked because, after 2 to 3 weeks, the upper jaw becomes fixed in a posteroinferior position by fibrous union of the fragments. The result is a deformed flat face (dish face) which causes severe psychological problems. Incorrect relationships between the upper and lower jaw also produce serious functional disorders. It is, therefore, very important that *reduction* and *fixation* of a fracture of the upper jaw are carried out *as soon as possible.*

After 2 to 3 months, the fragments are completely fixed and exact reduction requires refracturing with osteotomy. Pseudoprognathism can result from incorrect healing of the upper jaw in the displaced posteroinferior position; pseudoprognathism indicates that the mandible is normal but that the upper jaw has sunk inward. Normal configuration of the face and functional occlusal relationships can often be restored by an operation on the mandible (osteotomy on the ascending ramus or the body of the mandible).

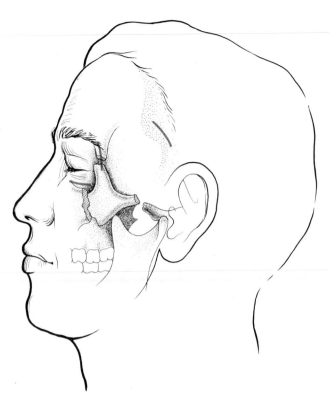

Fig. 9.68   Incisions for access to fractures of the zygoma.

Fracture of the Zygoma

Classification of fractures of the upper jaw varies depending on the author. As already mentioned, one of these classifications differentiates between central and lateral midfacial fractures. Fractures of the zygoma belong to the latter group, but most authors regard them as a separate type.

Etiology

Most fractures of the zygoma are caused by direct violence. Therefore the neighboring soft tissues are usually bruised extensively. The most common causes of fractures of the zygoma are traffic accidents and fighting; about 10% of fractures of the zygoma arise from sport injuries (football and ice hockey).

Preoperative Diagnosis

Symptoms

The symptoms of a fracture of the zygoma depend on the extent and the displacement. Two types can usually be differentiated:

● Those affecting only the *zygomatic arch.*

● Those of greater extent which affect all three *processes,* that is the maxillary process, the temporal process and the frontosphenoid process (Fig. 9.68). The frontal process is a constituent part of the infraorbital margin and the floor of the orbit.

In severe cases in which the floor of the orbit has also been damaged, orbital fat can prolapse into the antral cavity; the eye is displaced inferiorly and double vision occurs. A hematoma within the orbital cavity can also cause displacement of the globe and double vision. The frequency of double vision, according to most authors, is about 10%. A fracture of the infraorbital margin often leads to loss of sensation around the bridge of the nose, the cheek and the upper lip on the same side due to damage to the infraorbital nerve. This symptom occurs in about one-third of all cases.

If the zygomatic arch is depressed against the coronoid process, limitation of movement of the mandible results.

Experience shows that a fracture of the zygoma is easily overlooked. Due to simultaneous hematoma or edema of the soft tissues, the depression of the zygoma may not be recognized. The diagnosis is made by careful palpation which often reveals a step in the infraorbital margin. The diagnosis is confirmed by radiology (including tomography) of the floor of the orbit.

Treatment

Treatment of a fracture of the zygoma is determined by the severity of the symptoms. Insignificant depression of about 1 mm without marked displacement and loss of sensitivity does not require surgical correction. If a fracture of the zygoma occurs in association with a middle third fracture, reduction and fixation of the fracture of the zygoma is carried out simultaneously. This can be combined with intraosseous wiring as described above (see p. 73). Treatment should be carried out as soon as possible since the fracture consolidates within 10 to 12 days.

Several methods of reduction of a separate zygomatic fracture have been described. Basically, there are *internal* and *external* methods.

1. A hook is introduced around the zygomatic arch through a small skin incision in the cheek; the displacement is corrected by traction. The disadvantages of this method are that it can be difficult to localize the fracture line accurately and that a scar remains on the cheek.

2. Very good results can be achieved with Gillies' *external temporal method* (1927).

Technique. The operation is best carried out under general endotracheal anesthetic. A 2 to 3 cm long incision is made in the temporal region above the hair line; it is carried through skin and temporal fascia (Fig. 9.69).

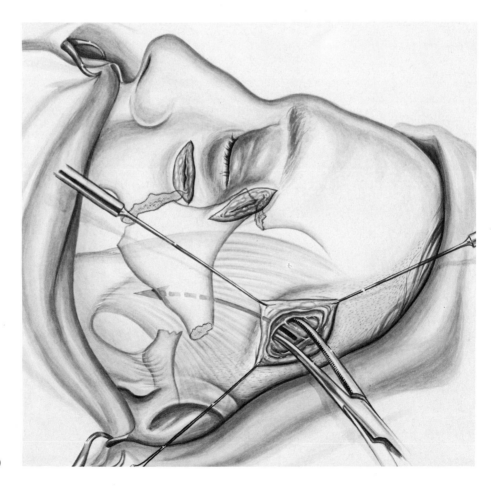

Fig. 9.69

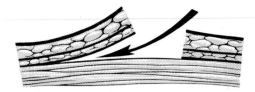

Fig. 9.70

The depressed bony fragments are elevated with the zygomatic elevator introduced via this external approach between the temporalis muscle and the temporal fascia medial to the zygoma (Figs. 9.70, 9.71).

Since a considerable force is developed with the elevator, this operation is particularly valuable in consolidated defects. Reduction must be done carefully to prevent injury to the surrounding soft tissue.

3. Thoma (1963) has described a method of access through the mouth. An incision is made in the vestibule behind the zygomatic process of the maxilla and a powerful elevator is introduced. Fixation is seldom necessary with this method since it is generally used if only the zygomatic arch has been depressed.

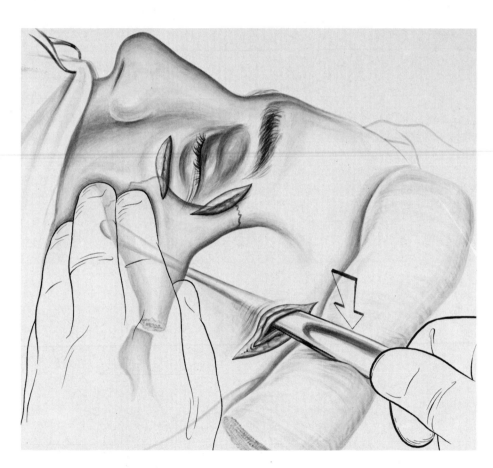

Fig. 9.71

Fig. 9.72 Search for the infraorbital margin to allow reduction and transosseous fixation of the bony fragments.

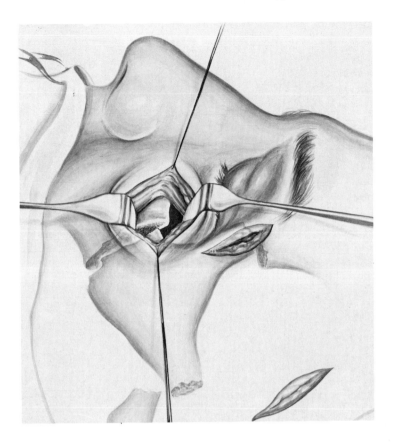

4. In severe fractures of the zygoma affecting the lateral wall of the antrum as well as the floor of the orbit, the maxillary sinus must be opened to allow removal of bony fragments and blood clots and to allow repositioning of the prolapsed orbital fat. The most common method for such cases is either a Caldwell-Luc or a Denker's antrostomy (see Vol. 1, Chap. 7). After the displaced bony fragments have been repositioned, they must still be fixed in the desired position. Several materials are available, for example, metal or plastic props. Tight packing may also be used; it is retained within the cavity under antibiotic cover for about 1 week (see Vol. 1, Chap. 7). The plastic prop can remain in the maxillary sinus for several weeks.

5. If it is difficult to fix the fragments exactly, intraosseous fixation with wire must be carried out, particularly for fractures of the infraorbital margin and the frontozygomatic suture (Figs. 9.72–9.75). The technique of intraosseous fixation is described on page 73.

The blow-out fracture with a marked defect of the walls of the orbit is a special problem. A bone transplant must often be used for support. The graft can be taken from the iliac crest, the tibia or a rib. Montgomery (1971) and other authors have recommended pieces of bone from the walls of the antral cavity to provide a graft of adequate thickness (see also Vol. 1, Chap. 4, 7).

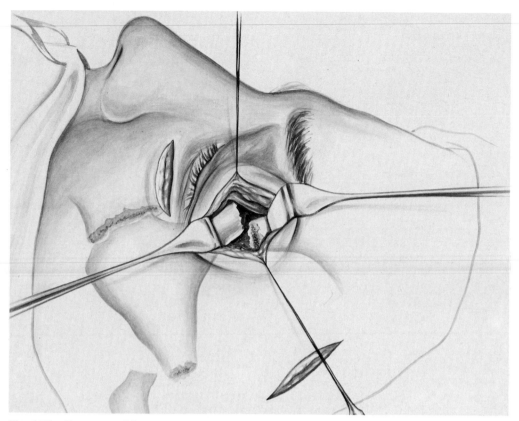

Fig. 9.73   Exposure of frontozygomatic suture and the bony fragments.

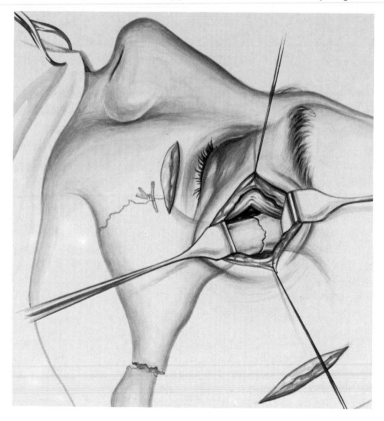

Fig. 9.74   Reduction of the zygomatic fractures.

Fig. 9.75   Final position after reduction of the zygomatic fractures.

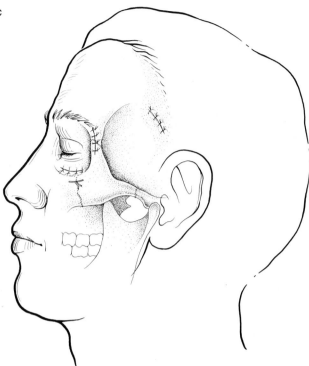

Combined Injuries of Soft Tissues and Facial Skeleton

Many problems are caused by simultaneous fractures of the jaw and extensive damage to the soft tissues of the face.

If facial injury is combined with a fracture of the jaws, the repair should proceed from within outward (Ganzer 1943).

In fresh injuries small fragments of the jaw can be replaced easily and can be stabilized by intraosseous wiring. The situation is more difficult if fragments of the jaw need to be fixed at the same time as treatment of the soft tissue injuries. Time consuming methods should not be used in such a case.

Such fractures of the mandible can be treated by arch bars or prefabricated metal bars (see Fig. 9.13). The fixation can be carried out quickly and does not require technical assistance.

If necessary, an impression of the teeth and the jaws can be made before the soft tissues are treated. A cap splint is then made by a technician and can be fixed in place several hours later.

Schuchardt (1956) has developed a method of fixation of the jaw for such acute cases. This method consists of a combination of arch bars and self-polymerizing acrylic (see p. 51). Other procedures used for fixation of the jaw in the presence of extensive soft tissue injury are those described above: Percutaneous transosseous fixation in mandibular fractures (see p. 52) and a metal head band in fractures of the upper jaw (see p. 67).

Soft Tissue Injuries

The surrounding parts of the head must be carefully cleaned before the wound is closed. Grease is removed with benzine or ether. Pieces of gravel or asphalt must also be thoroughly removed to prevent a disfiguring tattoo. Dirt of this nature may need to be removed with a brush and mild soap. Particles of dirt driven into the surrounding skin can be removed by dermabrasion. The open wound surfaces are irrigated with normal saline and then with 1% hydrogen peroxide solution. Strong antiseptic solutions should not be used for wounds of the face since all injured facial tissue should be treated with extreme care.

The extent of the injuries and the general condition of the patient determine whether the operation should be carried out under local or general anesthesia.

Wounds of the face heal better if the treatment is carried out as soon as possible. The *time limit* for *primary closure of the wound* is 10 to 12 hours, but experience has shown that good results can be achieved after a delay of as long as 24 hours. Schultz (1970) writes: "Most soft-tissue wounds of the face, properly cleansed and dressed, can await primary repair up to 24 hours, without serious risk of infection and without jeopardizing the final esthetic results." Thoma (1963) confirms: "Contaminated, lacerated wounds of less than 24 hours standing may be closed by primary suture."

Necrotic and torn wound edges are excised carefully. The deeper layers of the soft tissues are closed carefully with 3×0 or 4×0 catgut. The skin is closed by 4×0 or 5×0 nylon on a fine atraumatic needle.

Facial sutures should be removed at the latest on the fifth day.

Plastic procedures for soft tissue defects of the face are described in Vol. 1, Chap. 2.

As stated above, all bony fragments of the jaws must be covered with soft tissue to prevent the development of a sequestrum. It may be necessary to suture the oral mucosa over the edges of the bone to the skin.

In many cases, a delayed plastic reconstruction may be easier to carry out and may provide a better cosmetic result than primary suture which can produce extensive and disfiguring scar contractures.

Finally, it must be emphasized that the management of the patient with severe injuries of the facial skeleton and the soft tissues of the face requires the close cooperation of many specialists in order to obtain the best possible functional and esthetic result.

Bibliography

Adams, W. M.: Internal wiring fixation of facial fractures. Surgery 12: 523, 1942

Aldman, B.: ABC vid trafikolycka. Läkartidningen 62: 1005, 1965

Becker, E.: Ein Instrumentarium zur extrakutanen Osteosynthese bei Unterkieferfrakturen unter Verwendung plastischer Kunststoffe. Chirurg 29: 63, 1958

Björn, H.: Circumferential wiring. Dtsch. Zahnaerztl. Z. 7: 302, 1952

Crawford, M. J.: Appliances and attachments for treatment of upper jaw fractures. Nav. Med. Bull. 41: 1151, 1943

Crawford, M. J.: Selection of appliances for typical fractures. Oral Surg. 1: 442, 1948

Crewe, T. C.: Facial transfixion in maxillo-facial injuries. N. Z. Dent. J. 59: 201, 1963

Dingman, R., P. Natvig: Surgery of Facial Fractures. Saunders, Philadelphia 1964

Ganzer, H.: Die Kriegsverletzungen des Gesichts und Gesichtsschädels. Barth, Leipzig 1943

Gillies, H., T. P. Kilner, D. Stone: Fractures of the malar zygomatic compound with a description of a new x-ray picture. Br. J. Surg. 14: 650, 1927

Kazanjian, V. H., J. M. Converse: The Surgical Treatment of Facial Injuries. Williams & Wilkins, Baltimore 1959

Kjellman, O.: Mall för Stout's fortlöpande ögleligatur i Obwegesers version. Svensk Tandläk.-T. 9: 487, 1962

Lesney, T. A.: Method of immobilizing a common type of maxillary fracture. J. Oral Surg. 11: 49, 1953

Lesney, T. A.: Skeletal head frame. In: Oral Surgery, ed. by H. Arche. Saunders, Philadelphia 1969

Montgomery, W. W.: Surgery of the Upper Respiratory System, Vol. I. Lea & Febiger, Philadelphia 1971

Müller, W.: Häufigkeit, Sitz und Ursachen der Gesichtsschädelfrakturen. In: Traumatologie im Kiefer-Gesichts-Bereich, ed. by E. Reichenbach. Barth, Munich 1969

Obwegeser, H.: Über eine einfache Methode der freihändigen Drahtverschienung von Kieferbrüchen. Z: Stomat. 49: 652, 1952

Pape, K.: Die Frakturen des zentralen Mittelgesichts und ihre Behandlung. In: Traumatologie im Kiefer-Gesichts-Bereich ed. by E. Reichenbach. Barth, Munich 1969

Rowe, N. L., H. C. Killey: Fractures of the Facial Skeleton. Livingstone, Edinburgh 1968

Schrudde, J.: Die Behandlung der Kieferfrakturen mit Hilfe von Kunststoffschienen. In: Fortschritte der Kiefer- und Gesichts-Chirurgie, Vol. II, ed. by K. Schuchardt. Thieme, Stuttgart 1956

Schuchardt, K.: Ein Vorschlag zur Verbesserung der Drahtschienenverbände. Dtsch. Zahn-, Mund- u. Kieferheilk. 24: 39, 1956

Schuchardt, K., N. Schwenzer, B. Rottke, J. Lentrodt: Ursachen, Häufigkeit und Lokalisation der Frakturen des Gesichtsschädels. In: Fortschritte der Kiefer- und Gesichts-Chirurgie, Vol. XI, ed. by K. Schuchardt. Thieme, Stuttgart 1966

Schultz, R. C.: Facial Injuries. Year Book, Chicago 1970

Schwenzer, N.: Zur Osteosynthese bei Frakturen des Gesichtsskeletts. Thieme, Stuttgart 1967

Spiessl, B., K. Schroll: Spezielle Frakturen- und Luxationslehre. vol. I/1, Schädel – Gesicht – Kiefer, ed. by H. Nigst. Thieme, Stuttgart 1972

Spiessl, B., G. Schargus, K. Schroll: Die stabile Osteosynthese bei Frakturen des unbezahnten Unterkieferastes. Schweiz. Monatsschr. Zahnheilk. 81: 39, 1971

Thoma, K.: Oral Surgery. Mosby, St. Louis 1948, 1963

10 Transsphenoidal Surgery of the Pituitary Gland

By C.-A. Hamberger and J. Kinnman

All rhinological methods of hypophysectomy are based on the transsphenoidal access first described by Schloffer (1906). Three different methods of approach to the sphenoid bone and the sella turcica are now used:

1. Transseptal route (Hirsch 1910) often combined with a sublabial incision;

2. Paranasal route (Chiari 1912).

3. Transantrosphenoidal (transmaxillary) route (Denker 1921, Lautenschläger 1928, Hamberger et al. 1959–1964).

The transantrosphenoidal route is not only suitable for the removal of a normal pituitary gland but also for the removal of tumors, even in the presence of moderate suprasellar extension. The access is very good, there is no visible scar and this method allows the operation to be repeated if necessary. We have used this operation on 425 patients.

Diagnostic Preoperative Procedures

The case history is recorded. A routine otolaryngological and a general examination is performed to ensure that the patient is fit for surgery.

The endocrinological examination includes:

a) Measurement of tropic functions, particularly ACTH, the thyrotropic hormone (TSH), the gonadotropins and growth hormone.

b) Antidiuretic hormone (ADH).

c) Measurement of the secretory hormones of the target organs (thyroid gland, adrenal gland and gonads).

An ophthalmoneurological examination is extremely important and must always include evaluation of the visual fields, in which small objects (0.25 mm) at low relative intensity (0.10 – 0.315) should be used.

Infected foci of the teeth, nose and throat must always be managed before the operation. The thrombocyte count, bleeding and clotting time and prothrombin time are assessed. A considerable degree of thrombocytopenia is often found in patients with widespread skeletal metastases; diabetics usually have an increased tendency to bleed.

The **radiological examination** includes the skull, skeleton, heart and lungs; tomographs are taken of the sella and the sphenoidal sinuses with special reference to the degree of pneumatization, irregularities and asymmetry.

Pneumoencephalograms and possibly carotid angiograms are done to demonstrate suprasellar extension.

With regard to the transsphenoidal approach the sphenoidal sinuses may be divided into three main types (Fig. 10.1): (a) conchal, (b) presellar and (c) sellar type according to the degree of pneumatization of the sphenoid bone.

The *conchal type* should be regarded as a contraindication for a transsphenoidal operation on a normal sized pituitary gland. In tumors which expand the sella anteriorly and inferiorly, this type of sphenoidal cavity does not appear, however, to constitute a contraindication. Radiographs must be taken during the operation in such cases.

The *presellar type* of sinus does not extend posteriorly beyond a vertical plane passing through the tuberculum sellae. A transsphenoidal hypophysectomy can be carried out through this type of sphenoidal sinus.

The *sellar type* occurs bilaterally in 59% of the patients and unilaterally in 86%. Only one sellar

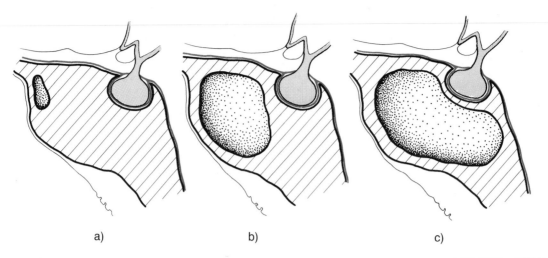

a)   b)   c)

Fig. 10.1   Pneumatization of the sphenoidal sinus.
a) Conchal type, b) Presellar type, c) Sellar type.

sphenoidal cavity is necessary to obtain good access for transsphenoidal hypophysectomy.

The thickness of the anterior wall of the sella turcica is usually determined by **serial tomograms** in the lateral projection. The position of the intersinus septum and any other bony septa is most easily recognized on an axial projection.

Indications

● Removal of the pituitary gland in patients with *breast carcinoma with metastases*. In young women it is done after a previous oophorectomy; in menopausal patients, it can be recommended as the first endocrinological measure.

● The indications have not yet been clarified in *other* hormone-dependent *malignant tumors* (chorionepithelioma, ovarian carcinoma, adrenal tumors, malignant melanomas, prostatic carcinoma).

● *Severe diabetic retinopathy*: Hypophysectomy causes increased sensitivity to exogenous insulin so that the progress of a diabetic retinopathy is partially or completely halted. Satisfactory vision must be present in at least one eye; progressive renal disease with a glomerular filtration rate less than 60 ml/min is regarded as a *contraindication* (Luft 1969).

● *Removal of pituitary tumors*: In acromegaly there is seldom pure suprasellar extension of the tumor; more often, the sella is expanded inferiorly and anteriorly. Hypophysectomy has also been tried in *Cushing's syndrome*; 10% of all patients with this syndrome have an ACTH producing pituitary tumor. Pituitary tumors with suprasellar extension (*chromophobe adenomas* and *craniopharyngiomas*) can also be removed by the transsphenoidal route. Naturally transsphenoidal exposure of these pituitary tumors cannot replace that by the cranial route but should be used under certain circumstances (e.g., if there is a prefixed chiasma, and in operations for recurrence).

Principle of the Operation

After opening the maxillary sinus, its bony medial wall is removed (Fig. 10.2). This is achieved by removing the lateral nasal wall, dislocating the inferior and middle turbinates medially, carrying out an ethmoidectomy (Fig. 10.3), opening the sphenoid cavity, and removing its anterior wall and the sphenoidal septum (Fig. 10.4). Next, the bony inferior wall of the sella turcica is removed and the capsule of the pituitary gland is divided by a cruciate incision (Fig. 10.4). The pituitary gland or the tumor is then removed.

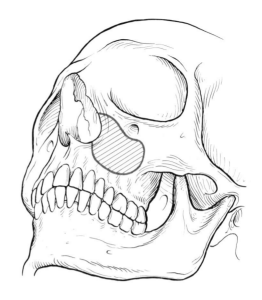

Fig. 10.2 Bony medial wall which is removed in the operation.

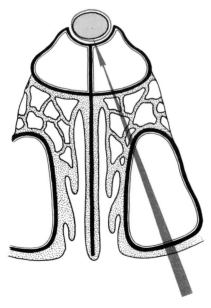

Fig. 10.3 Excision of the ethmoid cells.

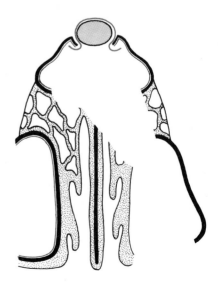

Fig. 10.4 Removal of the anterior wall of the sphenoid sinus and the sphenoid septum.

Preparation for Surgery

Premedication is given on the evening before the operation and immediately before the operation.

Shortly **before the operation**, 100 mg of cortisone acetate is given intramuscularly and, at the beginning of the operation, an intravenous infusion of 5.5% glucose is administered with 100 mg hydrocortisone acetate added to it.

To **cleanse the nasal cavities**, gauze strips infiltrated with protargol are inserted. They are removed after the medial wall of the maxillary sinus has been taken away.

The **position of the patient**, the placement of the surgical team and the larger pieces of apparatus are shown in Figure 10.5.

A **self-retaining urethral catheter** and a **feeding tube** are introduced at the beginning of the operation.

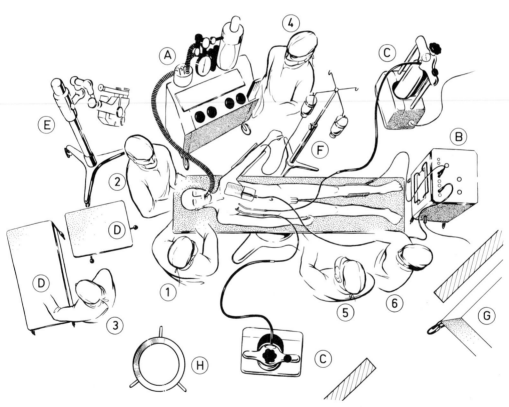

Fig. 10.5

1. Surgeon
2. First assistant
3. Scrub nurse
4. Anesthetist
5. Second assistant
6. Scrub nurse

A) Anesthetic machine
B) Diathermy
C) Suction apparatus
D) Mobile instrument table

E) Operating microscope
F) Infusion stand
G) Mobile x-ray unit
H) Washbowl

Special Instruments

The instruments illustrated in Vol. 1, Fig. 7.17, can be used for opening the maxillary, ethmoid and sphenoid sinuses.

Figure 10.6 shows the special instruments necessary to expose the pituitary gland, make the cruciate incision and dissect the capsule as well as for the hypophysectomy itself.

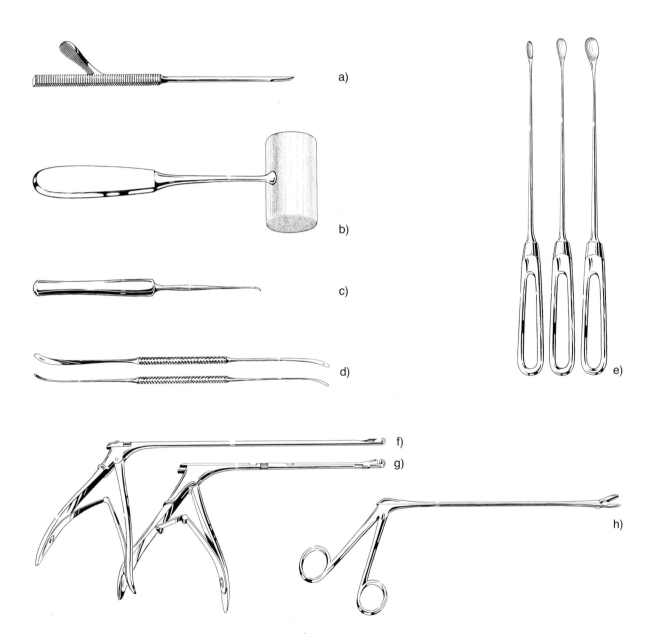

a)

b)

c)

d)

e)

f)

g)

h)

Fig. 10.6 Special instruments for operation on the pituitary gland:

a) Frenckner's chisel for the anterior wall of the sella;
b) Hammer;
c) Trigeminal knife;
d) Two dissectors 24 cm long (large and small);

e) Three malleable gall stone scoops 27 cm long in widths of 5 mm, 8 mm and 10 mm;
f) Frenckner's pituitary rongeurs;
g) Kofler's sphenoidal rongeurs;
h) Olivecrona's pituitary forceps;

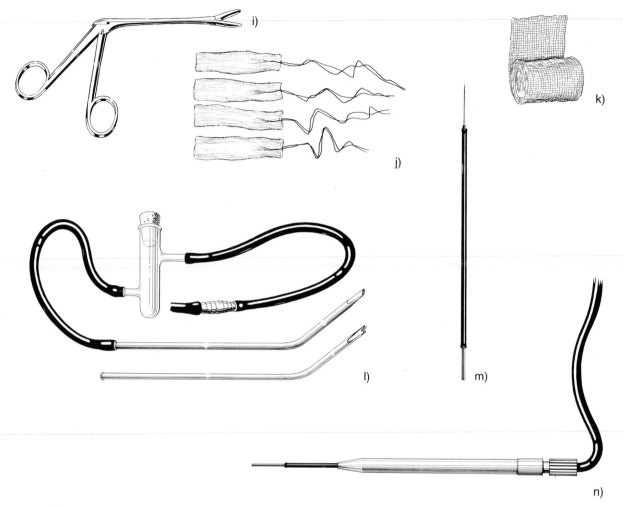

Fig.10.6

i) Watson-Williams' nasal forceps;
j) Gauze strips for hemostasis within the sella;
k) Gauze packing 4 cm wide;

l) Glass suction tubes and aspirator for removing pieces of the tumor;
m) Needle electrode for incision of the pituitary capsule;
n) Handpiece and electrode for hemostasis.

Anesthesia

Transsphenoidal hypophysectomy is nowadays always carried out under endotracheal general anesthesia using a respirator.

A blood transfusion should be given throughout the entire operation since in many patients a sudden, but usually moderate hemorrhage, can occur from the wide veins of the pituitary capsule.

About 40 g mannitol is given via intravenous infu-sion immediately before opening the capsule of the pituitary gland. This is done to reduce intracranial pressure.

In a patient with normal adrenal function, cortisone is not given before the operation but a dose of 200 mg must be administered by infusion after removal of the pituitary gland.

The canine fossa and surrounding tissue should be infiltrated with local anesthetic to reduce the bleeding and reflex swelling (see Vol. 1, Fig. 7.18).

Operative Technique

An incision is made in the superior buccal sulcus from the last molar to the frenulum; this incision passes through the mucosa and the periosteum (Fig. 10.7). The mucosa and the periosteum are elevated, preserving the vessels and the infraorbital nerve emerging from the infraorbital foramen (Fig. 10.8).

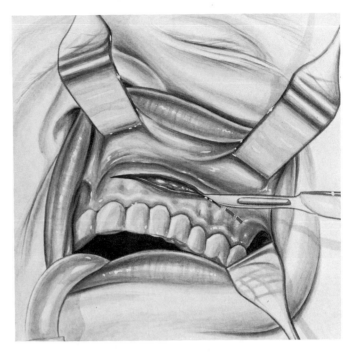

Fig. 10.7

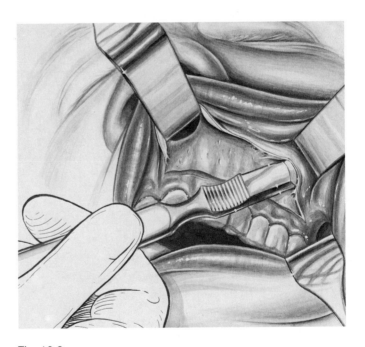

Fig. 10.8

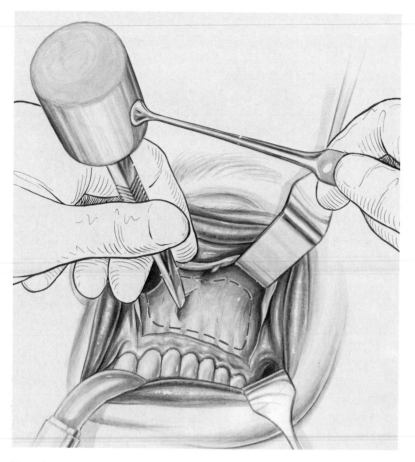

Fig. 10.9

Fig. 10.10

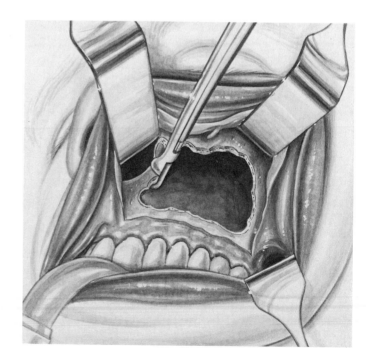

The part of the bone of the anterior wall of the antrum to be removed is marked out with a hammer and chisel, laterally as far as the zygomatico-alveolar crest and superiorly as far as the lacrimal bone avoiding the infraorbital foramen. The area of bone thus defined is then removed. The edges of the bony defect are smoothed with bone forceps and sharp curettes (Fig. 10.9).

The soft tissues are elevated anteriorly as far as the piriform aperture and the anterior nasal spine as well as along the floor of the nasal vestibule. The whole of the bony wall between the nasal cavity and the floor of the antral cavity is cleared of soft tissue and is removed as far as the posterior wall of the antrum (Fig. 10.10).

The lateral wall of the nose is now mobile and can be displaced medially. It is held in this medial position with a long retractor (Fig. 10.11), thereby improving the surgical access; the nasal cavity should be kept intact as much as possible.

The ethmoid cells are now removed, preserving the lamina papyracea (Fig. 10.11). The bony crest separating the antral cavity from the ethmoids is removed without damaging the retromaxillary vessels.

The sphenoidal cavity abuts immediately onto the posterior ethmoid cells at the level of the middle turbinate. Usually both ostia of the sphenoid sinuses can be identified, and the mucosa emerging from the ostium can be clearly recognized. The entire anterior wall of the sphenoid, including the rostrum, is removed working from the ostium outward with forward biting rongeurs (Fig. 10.12).

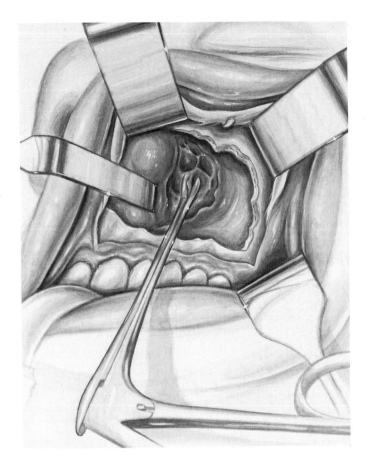

Fig. 10.11

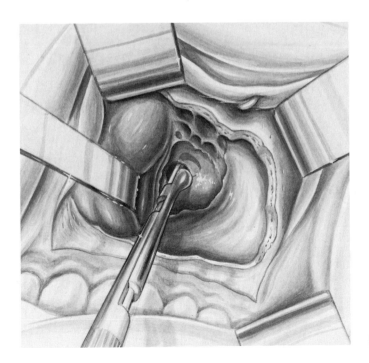

Fig. 10.12

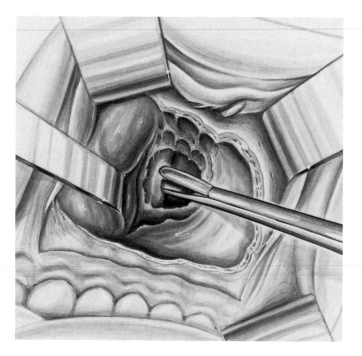

Fig. 10.13

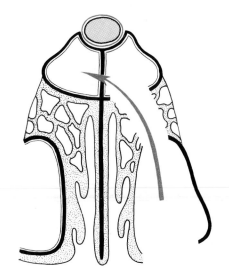

Fig. 10.14

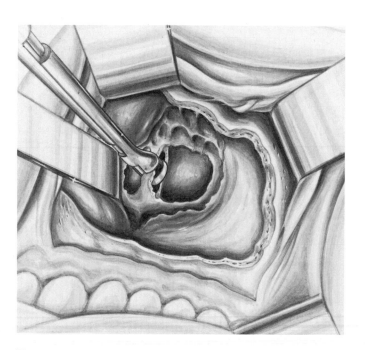

Fig. 10.15

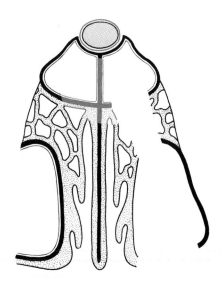

Fig. 10.16

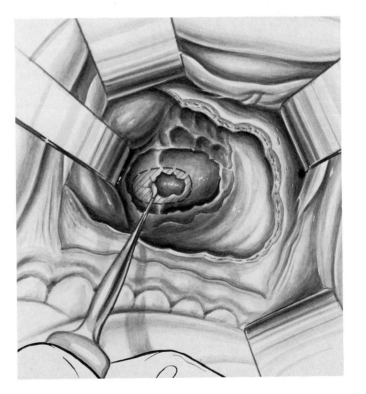

Fig. 10.17

The sphenoidal septum and any other septa are now removed (Figs. 10.13–10.15).

The posterior part of the nasal septum and the vomer must often be removed (Fig. 10.16). It is very important that the soft tissues of the nasal cavity are now retracted maximally to the opposite side.

After both sphenoidal cavities have been opened widely, a good view is obtained of the sella turcica. The anterior wall of the sella is usually about 11 mm wide (7–16 mm). The ridge produced by the internal carotid artery arches forward along the side of the sphenoidal cavity. Once an accurate picture has been obtained of the extent of the anterior wall of the sella, removal of the bone is started. In most cases the bone is very thin. It is removed with a chisel, beginning at the thinnest point. A small hole is made with the hammer and chisel (Fig. 10.17). The remaining part of the bony wall is elevated with a small hook and is then removed piecemeal (Fig. 10.18). At this stage it is helpful to introduce a packing soaked in hydrogen peroxide in order to maintain a dry operative field.

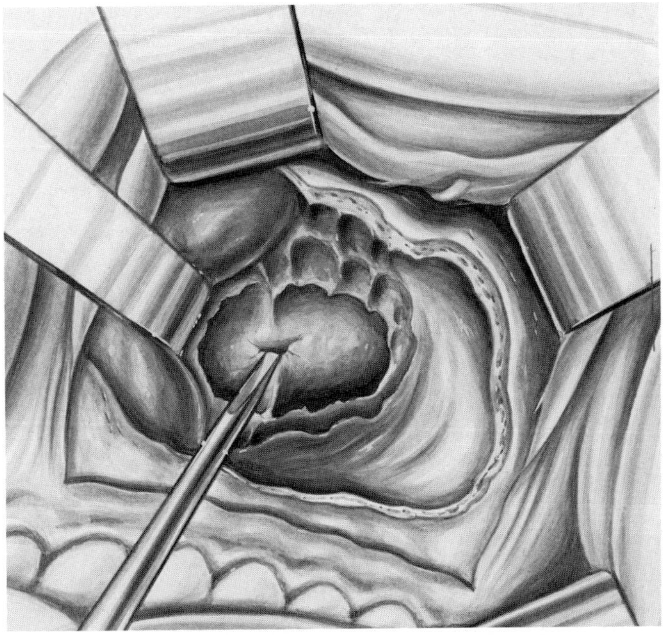

Fig. 10.18

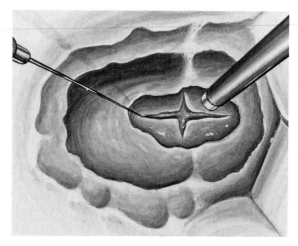

Fig. 10.19

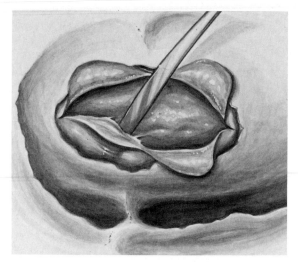

Fig. 10.20

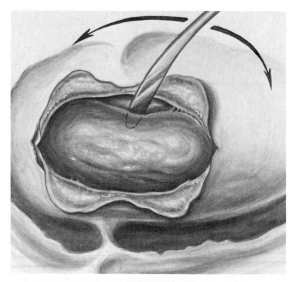

Fig. 10.21

The capsule of the pituitary gland is now opened through a cruciate incision. A large annular branch of the cavernous sinus usually lies at the base of the bulging part of the capsule and large vessels can be seen along its superior part.

If possible, the capsule of the pituitary gland should be opened at the point which is free from veins. The incision is then extended toward the transverse veins and the branches of the cavernous sinus with a vertical and a horizontal incision (using a trigeminal knife, see Fig. 10.6 c). The opening in the capsule of the pituitary gland is preferably made by means of a fine diathermy needle with an insulated shaft to reduce the bleeding (Fig. 10.19). Bleeding from smaller vessels is controlled by packing.

The pituitary gland or the tumor is now exposed by elevation of the edges of the capsule with a fine dissector (Fig. 10.20). The diaphragma sellae and the branches of the cavernous sinus can occasionally be seen. Often there are adhesions between the pituitary gland and the capsule, particularly laterally at the junction between the anterior and the posterior lobes. As a result a certain amount of damage to the gland cannot be avoided. At this stage there can be a certain amount of bleeding from the internal surface of the capsule, but this can usually be controlled by light pressure.

If a *normal pituitary gland* is being removed, it is now displaced inferiorly with a dissector so that its stalk becomes visible and can be stretched (Fig. 10.21).

A cerebrospinal fluid leak can easily occur at this stage of the operation.

If the pressure from above is now increased with the elevator (Fig. 10.22), the stalk tends to tear so that a few millimeters of the stalk can remain adherent to the gland.

When the stalk has been torn, the cerebrospinal fluid leak will usually cease.

The stalk now projects through the diaphragma into the sella and pulsates in a superoinferior direction (Fig. 10.23). The sella is explored with an elevator and a glass suction tube to ensure that the entire gland has been removed. The operating microscope can be used advantageously for this inspection.

If the operation has been carried out for removal of an *adenoma*, the tumor mass may present when the capsule is first incised. It should be removed with a gallstone scoop (Fig. 10.24) and a glass suction tube (Fig. 10.25). This stage of the operation should be carried out under magnification with the operating microscope.

The sella is now probed as described above. It is often possible to define and preserve the normal pituitary gland.

If the operation has been carried out for a tumor, a fairly large sellar cavity remains (Fig. 10.26). The diaphragma prolapses into this cavity if there has been suprasellar extension.

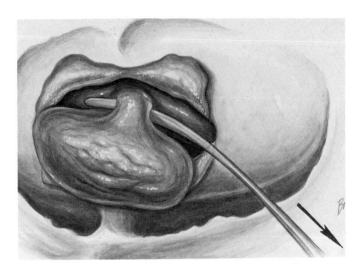

Fig. 10.22

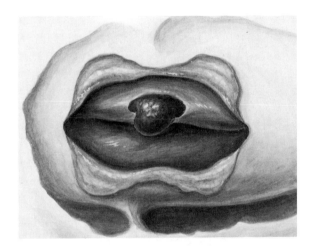

Fig. 10.23

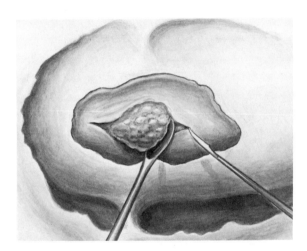

Fig. 10.24

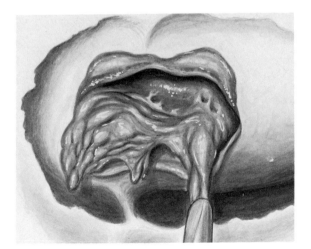

Fig. 10.25

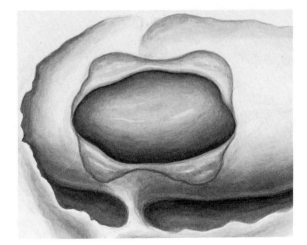

Fig. 10.26

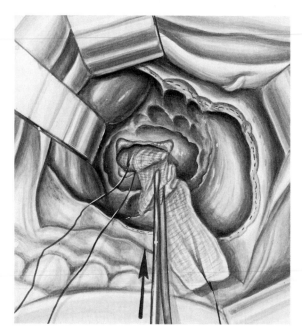

Fig. 10.27

After hemostasis has been achieved with small gauze strips (Fig. 10.27), the sellar cavity is filled with a piece of muscle removed from the antrolateral side of the thigh (Fig. 10.28). This piece of muscle should be about $3 \times 1.5 \times 1.5$ cm large (larger in patients with a tumor and especially in acromegaly).

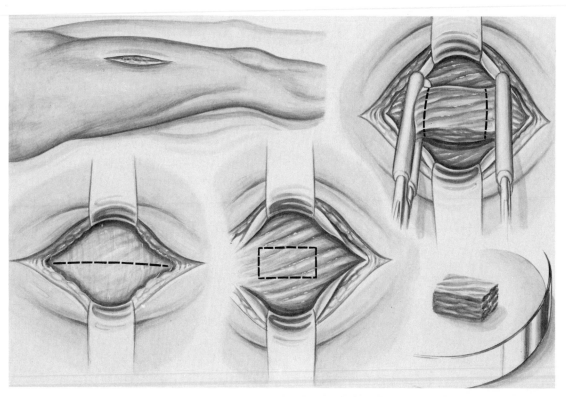

Fig. 10.28

The piece of muscle is introduced with the left hand. Packing with gauze (4 cm wide) soaked in benzyl penicillin is immediately introduced on top of this (Figs. 10.29, 10.30).

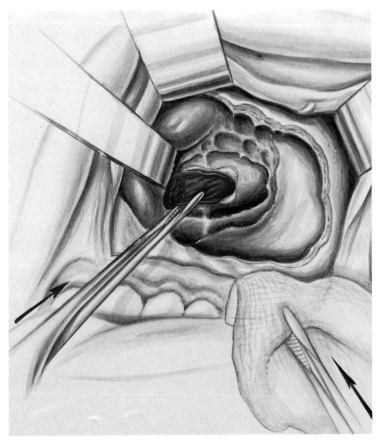

Fig. 10.29

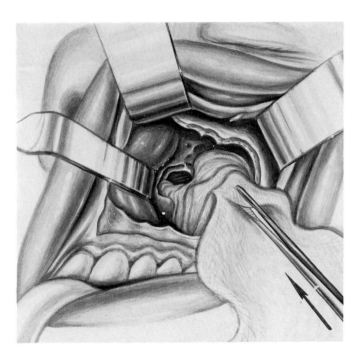

Fig. 10.30

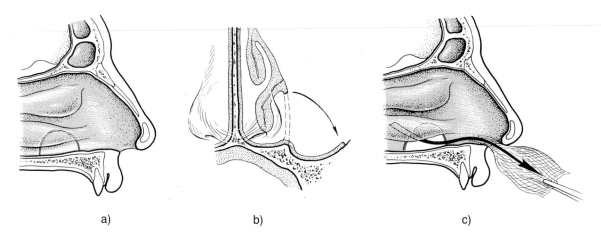

a)   b)   c)

Fig. 10.31

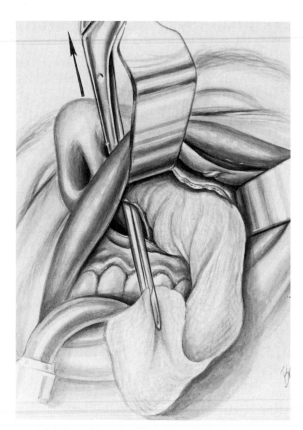

Fig. 10.32

The mucosa of the lateral wall of the nose is now divided in an elliptical shape and the resulting flap is turned down onto the floor of the antral cavity (Fig. 10.31).

The gauze packing is drawn out through the newly created opening in the lateral nasal wall in the inferior meatus, brought out through the nostril and fastened to the cheek (Fig. 10.32).

Next, a finger stall filled with 2 cm wide gauze is introduced through the nose into the antrum (Figs. 10.33, 10.34); packing of the sinuses must be fairly tight.

The incision in the vestibule of the mouth is now closed with nonabsorbable sutures (Fig. 10.35).

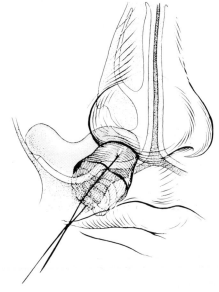

Fig. 10.33

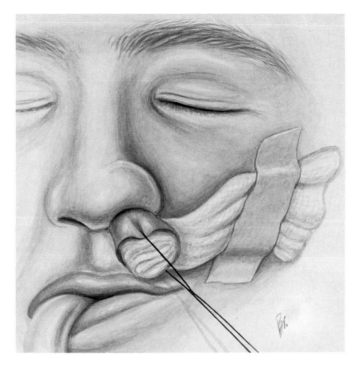

Fig. 10.34

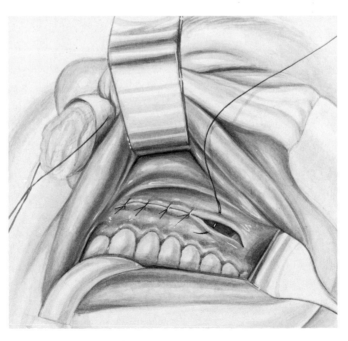

Fig. 10.35

Important Modifications and Surgical Alternatives

1. In patients with a tumor, the above described modifications are necessary.

2. If there is suprasellar extension, a combined transcraniosphenoidal operation is often necessary. Preferably the transsphenoidal operation should be attempted first and, if indicated, the transcranial intervention may be performed three or four weeks later.

3. If doubts should arise concerning the position of the sella, indicators may be applied against the assumed anterior border, and lateral and anteroposterior x-rays are taken with a portable machine. This is especially the case if the pneumatization of the sphenoid sinuses is of the presellar type.

Important Landmarks and Danger Points

● Damage to the *nasolacrimal duct* is prevented by careful removal of the frontal process of the maxilla as far as the lacrimal bone and subluxation of the lateral wall of the nose into the nasal cavity.

● The *sphenopalatine artery,* one of the branches of the internal maxillary artery, runs into the nasal cavity through the sphenopalatine foramen; it can be damaged during resection of the rostrum of the sphenoid. The bleeding can be controlled by diathermy.

● In performing the ethmoidectomy it can be difficult to know when the *base of the skull* has been reached. The base of the skull can generally be recognized by the white, shiny bone which has a characteristic firm consistency on palpation (see also Vol. 1, Chap. 7).

● The opening to the sphenoidal sinus is found at the sphenoethmoidal recess just above the superior concha. It can be identified by introducing a probe along a line which connects the anterior nasal spine with the middle concha. The distance from the nostril to the opening of the sphenoidal sinus is about 6 to 7 cm (see also Vol. 1, Chap. 7).

● In transsphenoidal hypophysectomy attention must be paid to the *intersinus septum* separating the two parts of the sphenoidal cavity and to other bony septa within the sinus. In 20% of patients, the posterior attachment of the intersinus septum is not related to the anterior wall of the sella but lies laterally on the prominence over the internal carotid artery. A strongly developed septum lying lateral to the median plane can be interpreted incorrectly on a radiograph as the intersinus septum. The posterior insertion of this lateral septum is almost always the prominence over the carotid artery. Tomograms in the frontal plane permit differentiation between the two. Only in 25% of the patients is the posterior attachment of the intersinus septum in the midline of the anterior wall of the sella. In these cases the anterior wall of the sella can be 2 to 3 mm thick and consists of cancellous bone. Bleeding from the edges of the bone may present certain problems. A complete transverse septum rarely occurs. The operator must know if such a septum is present since it complicates orientation. Such a transverse septum is usually unilateral so that the operation should then be carried out via the contralateral sinus.

● The structures in immediate relationship to the sella turcica are shown in Fig. 10.36.

● The optic chiasma only rarely lies immediately above or very close to the diaphragma; it usually lies 1 mm superior to it. The arachnoid has been observed bulging into the sella. This condition may be responsible for the appearance of a cerebrospinal fluid leak postoperatively.

● Venous blood from the pituitary gland drains into thin walled vessels in the capsule. Particular attention should be paid to the anterior, inferior and posterior intercavernous sinuses.

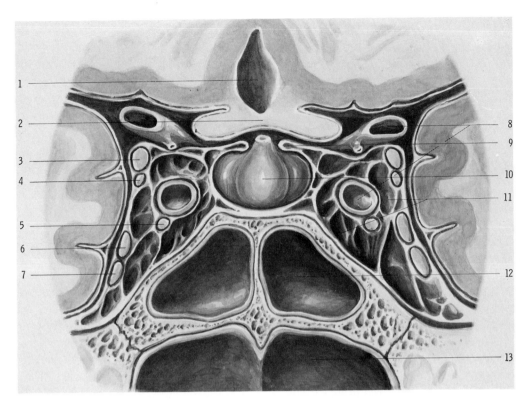

Fig. 10.36   Structures related to the sella turcica.

1. Third ventricle
2. Optic chiasma
3. Oculomotor nerve
4. Trochlear nerve
5. Abducens nerve
6. Ophthalmic division of the trigeminal nerve
7. Maxillary nerve
8. Internal carotid artery
9. Diaphragma sellae
10. Pituitary gland
11. Cavernous sinus
12. Sphenoidal sinus
13. Nasopharynx

Rules, Hints and Typical Errors

● As already stated, the position of the intersinus septum can often cause difficulties. The surgeon can orientate himself by passing an elevator along the nasal septum through the contralateral nasal cavity.

● The diaphragma sellae must always be handled very gently, particularly when there is suprasellar extension of the tumor. The diaphragma bulges down into the sella after removal of the tumor and may pull the chiasma downward.

● The sella must be closed by a muscle graft. This heals and is converted into connective tissue. The technique considerably reduces cerebrospinal fluid leakage and the risk of meningitis.

● The surgeon undertaking hypophysectomy will often encounter difficult situations and must always be prepared to interrupt the operation to allow further radiographs to be taken and then to proceed at a second stage.

Postoperative Care

● The patient is kept in the intensive care unit for 10 days after operation.

● The packing which lies in the transmaxillary sphenoidal access is removed piecemeal between the sixth and ninth day after the operation.

● 1,000,000 I.U of benzyl penicillin and 1 g of sulfamethazine are given 4 times daily intramuscularly for the first 3 days. From the fourth day phenoxymethyl penicillin is given orally in a dose of 0.8 g 4 times a day with 1 g sulfadimethoxine (Madribon) two times a day. This medication is continued for ten days.

● *Cortisone acetate* is given in the following dose:
  1st day   6 × 50 mg
  2nd day   4 × 50 mg
  3rd day   3 × 50 mg
  4th day   4 × 25 mg
  5th day   3 × 25 mg
  6th day   2 × 25 mg,   1 × 12.5 mg
  7th day   1 × 25 mg,   2 × 12.5 mg
  8th day   3 × 12.5 mg

● The dose of antibiotic and cortisone must be increased in the presence of pyrexia, meningitis or postoperative hemorrhage.

● Antidiuretic hormone is given if indicated; usually 1 ml of vasopressin tannate (Pitressin) is necessary if there is a polyuria of more than 2.5 liters per day. Polyuria is usually temporary and decreases during the next few months.

● An intravenous infusion of 5.5% of glucose with 80 mEq of sodium and 40 mEq of potassium/1.000 ml is continued postoperatively until the patient can eat normally again (24 to 48 hours later). Disturbances of sodium balance do not occur during or after the operation since aldosterone production by the adrenal glands is normal. In older patients, serum creatinine should be checked carefully because renal clearance is reduced after hypophysectomy; an elevated serum creatinine is also a symptom of an Addisonian crisis.

● The urethral catheter should remain in place for 24 hours since it facilitates continuous checking of the urinary output. After 24 hours the urinary output is measured daily.

● Diabetic patients require special care. If such a patient has been managed with long acting depot insulin, it should be replaced by standard insulin a few days before the operation. An intravenous infusion of 5.5% glucose is kept running both during and after the operation, and the dose of insulin is given 2 to 3 times a day during the postoperative period, as indicated. The dose is determined by the blood glucose level since these patients are very insulin sensitive after the operation.

● *Postoperative hemorrhage* seldom occurs but may do so when the packing is removed. In such case a new packing is inserted. Sudden postoperative blindness is a rare but serious complication. It requires immediate exploration to determine the cause (usually bleeding into the sella). The treatment consists of evacuation of the hematoma and insertion of a new packing.

● A *postoperative cerebrospinal fluid leak* can occur in some patients after the packing has been removed, but in our cases it has never persisted more than 7 days. If it does so, further exploration of the operated area via the transantrosphenoidal route is necessary.

● *Postoperative meningitis* seldom occurs if the sella is closed with a piece of muscle and the patient is kept isolated after the operation.

Functional Sequelae

● A hypophysectomy which from the surgical point of view appears to have been complete may occasionally have only little or no influence on the endocrine system. In many cases there is a deficiency of only one hormone, for example, *only* ACTH *or* TSH *or* the gonadotropic hormones.

● Ophthalmoneurological and endocrinological investigation is carried out at the end of the second week after operation. At this time the patient usually needs a maintenance dose of 12.5 mg cortisone three times daily.

● A complete endocrinological examination is made 2 months later to detect any endocrine deficits. Replacement therapy must be given with gonadotropins or TSH if the endocrinological examination shows this to be necessary.

Bibliography

Chiari, O.: Über eine Modifikation der Schlofferschen Operation von Tumoren der Hypophyse. Wien. Klin. Wschr. 25: 5, 1912

Denker, A.: Zur Behandlung der Hypophysentumoren. Int. Zbl. Laryng. 19: 97, 1921

Hamberger, C.-A., G. Hammer: Der transnasale Weg der Hypophysektomie. In: Hals-Nasen-Ohren-Heilkunde, Vol. I, ed. by J. Berendes, R. Link, F. Zöllner. Thieme, Stuttgart 1964

Hamberger, C.-A., G. Hammer, G. Norlén, B. Sjögren: Kirurgisk behandling vid akromegali. Nord. Med. 62: 1328, 1959

Hamberger, C.-A., G. Hammer, G. Norlén, B. Sjögren: Surgical treatment of acromegaly. Acta Oto-Laryng. (Stockholm), Suppl. 158: 168, 1960

Hamberger, C.-A., G. Hammer, G. Norlén, B. Sjögren: Transsphenoidal hypophysectomy. Arch. Otolaryng. 74: 2, 1961

Hirsch, O.: Zur endonasalen Operation von Hypophysentumoren. Wien. Med. Wschr. 60: 749, 1910

Lautenschläger, A.: Die permaxilläre Hypophysenoperation. Chirurg. 1: 30, 1928

Luft, R.: Pituitary ablation or destruction in diabetes mellitus. In: Disorders of the Skull Base Region, ed. by C.-A. Hamberger, J. Wersäll. Almqvist & Wiksell, Stockholm 1969

Schloffer, H.: Zur Frage der Operation an der Hypophyse. Beitr. Klin. Chir. 50: 767, 1906

11 Surgery of the Nasopharynx

By E. Nessel and K. Mündnich

Operations for Hyperplasia, Malformations, Tumors and Stenoses of the Nasopharynx

This chapter on operations on the nasopharynx will be confined to illustrating those current operations in which the balance between the risk and the necessity of the operation has been carefully assessed. Heroic operations which have long since been abandoned will not be considered. A complete historical review has been presented by Wilson (1957).

Rather than attempting to give a review of the many different diseases occuring at this site, it is preferable to define clearly the routes of access, the incision and the extension of the operations possible. *Observations on indications* are to be regarded as examples of a specific technique used for an individual disease. The extent, histological nature and radiosensitivity of the particular disease *and* the age, condition and previous treatment of the patient determine the choice of the particular operation.

Preoperative investigation of the nasopharynx is carried out by posterior rhinoscopy (possibly using the palatal retractor) followed, if necessary, by palpation, plain radiographs, tomographs, angiograms and biopsy. These will not be considered further in the rest of the chapter.

Surgical treatment may be possible or necessary for the following pathological conditions of the nasopharynx:

Hyperplasias and Malformations
Adenoidal hyperplasia
Choanal polyp
Choanal atresia
Nasopharyngeal cyst (adenoid retention cyst, pharyngeal bursa)
Teratoma

Benign Tumors
Juvenile nasopharyngeal fibroma
Aberrant salivary gland tumors
Solitary extramedullary plasmocytoma

Potentially Malignant Tumors
Papillomas
Chondromas
Chordomas

Malignant Tumors, possibly recurrent after radiotherapy, possibly needing palliative treatment
Carcinoma of limited extent
Adenoid cystic carcinoma
Fibrosarcoma
Malignant hemangioendothelioma
Leiomyosarcoma
Rhabdomyosarcoma

Peroral Access

(Synonyms: indirect, retropalatal or circumpalatal route)

Indications

- Adenoidectomy for hyperplasia of the adenoids and its sequelae, particularly in children (nasal obstruction, chronic or recurrent obstruction of the eustachian tube, acute otitis media, nasopharyngitis, sinusitis and inflammation of the larynx, trachea and bronchi).

- Adenoidectomy *before* the second year of life is indicated only in very severe developmental disturbances for the above mentioned indications in a persistent suppurative otitis after failure of conservative treatment.

  Removal of the adenoid can exacerbate an open or submucous cleft of the palate which is diagnosed by palpation of the hard palate, especially in the case of a bifid uvula. Indeed adenoidectomy can exacerbate palatal insufficiency or the open component of a mixed rhinolalia. In such cases it should only be carried out for the most urgent otological indications and then only after phoniatric examination and taking into consideration a following palatoplasty.

Peroral operation may be indicated in the following circumstances:

- Choanal polyps;
- Nasopharyngeal cysts;
- Teratomas;
- Possibly for small nasopharyngeal fibromas with a narrow fixed pedicle in the roof or posterior wall of the nasopharynx;
- Possibly for aberrant tumors of the salivary glands;
- Biopsy of the nasopharynx usually using a *palatal retractor*;

- For electrocoagulation of malignant tumors in order to reduce the bulk of such a tumor before radiotherapy (Seiffert 1940);
- For palliative treatment or management of recurrence.

Anesthesia and Position of the Patient in Adenoidectomy

Adenoidectomy under **local anesthesia** in the sitting position should be carried out in adults *only as the exception* and not the rule. The technique is as follows:

Premedication is given and topical anesthesia is then induced using a spray or probes (pernasally and perorally behind the palate). In addition pernasal infiltration anesthesia can be used or transpalatine nerve block (von Gyergyai 1938). Local anesthetic solution (6 ml at most of 1% Xylocaine solution) is injected laterally on both sides into the origin of the soft palate in the direction of the opening of the eustachian tube; the mucosa of the lateral wall of the nasopharynx is also infiltrated.

The swelling of the tissues produced by injection of too much fluid increases the risk of damage to the deeper connective tissue layers and the muscular layers if the ring curette is used.

The standards of modern anesthesia are such that the surgeon must enlist the cooperation of the anesthetist even for such a common and short operation as an adenoidectomy. *Endotracheal anesthesia* must be used with assisted respiration. This is the best way of preventing the main complication of this operation (aspiration) and allows the adenoidectomy to be carried out under vision rather than blind.

After induction of oral endotracheal anesthesia, the patient is placed on the operating table. The head end of the table should be extendable. The patient's shoulders are supported with a pillow and the head is extended (Fig. 11.1). A mouth gag with an anesthetic extension blade, for example, Kilner-Doughty (Fig. 11.2a), Davis-Boyle or McIvor of the appropriate size, is introduced.

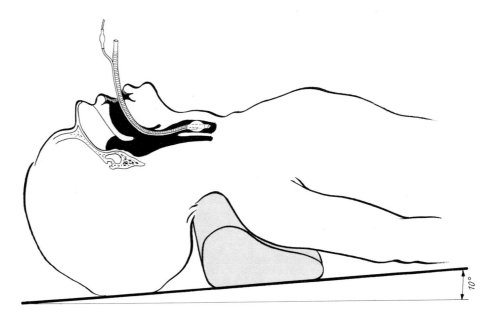

Fig. 11.1   Position for adenoidectomy.

Special Instruments

The special instruments for adenoidectomy are shown in Figure 11.2.

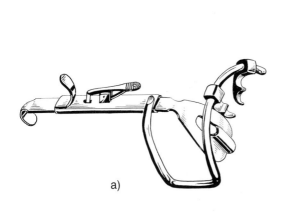

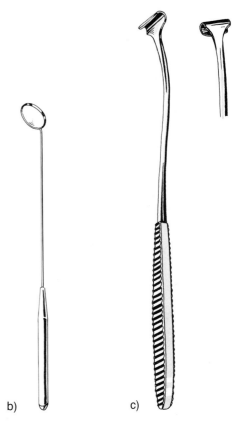

Fig. 11.2   Instruments for adenoidectomy.
a) Mouth gag with Kilner-Doughty blade,
b) Nasopharyngeal mirror,
c) Palatal retractor (Nager's angled pillar retractor),

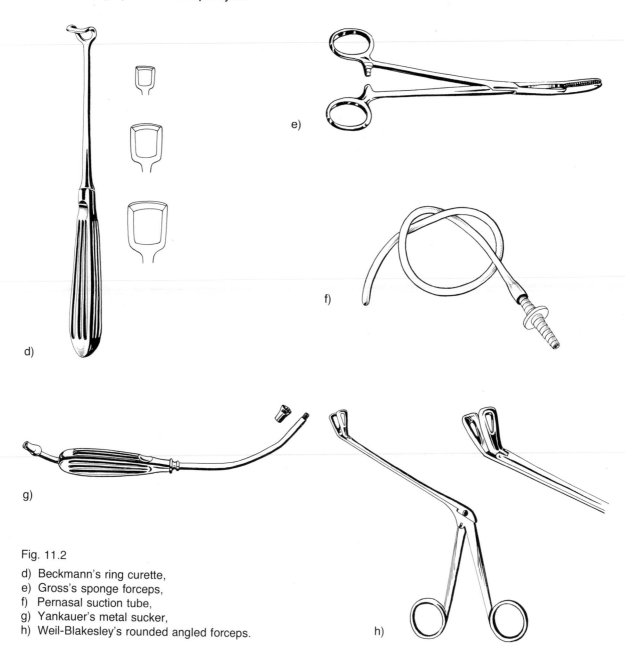

Fig. 11.2

d) Beckmann's ring curette,
e) Gross's sponge forceps,
f) Pernasal suction tube,
g) Yankauer's metal sucker,
h) Weil-Blakesley's rounded angled forceps.

Operative Technique of Adenoidectomy

The nasopharynx is inspected with a postnasal mirror after elevation of the soft palate by a palatal hook. A Beckmann's ring curette of suitable size and curve is introduced with retraction of the soft palate (Fig. 11.3). The ring curette is applied to the superior end of the edge of the vomer, then drawn downward in a continuous movement under moderate pressure without deviating from the midline. Constant contact with the roof and posterior wall of the nasopharynx should be maintained. The tubal recesses are then individually curetted again working strictly in a craniocaudal direction in constant contact with the posterior wall. Movement of the curette in an oblique direction increases the danger of damage to the cartilage of the mouth of the eustachian tube and possibly stricture formation.

The postnasal space is then packed or sucked out with an apparatus introduced through the nose. Posterior rhinoscopy is then repeated with retraction of the palate. If necessary, further curettage, or deliberate removal of adenoidal remnants are carried out with Weil-Blakesley's angled forceps. A mirror should be used to allow direct inspection (Fig. 11.4). Hemostasis is achieved with pledgets or diathermy.

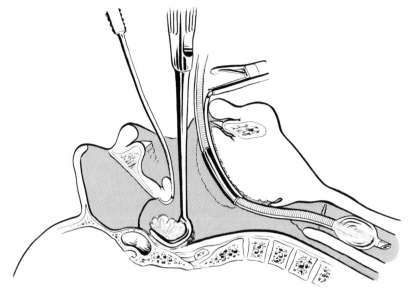

Fig. 11.3

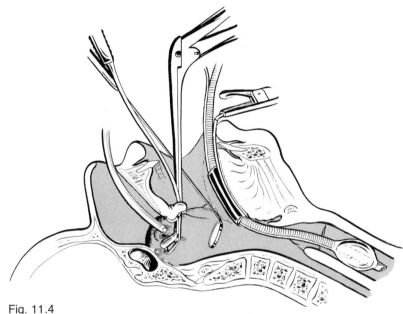

Fig. 11.4

Hemorrhage after Adenoidectomy

Since the most common site of hemorrhage is adenoidal remnants, the first procedure is reoperation.

More severe hemorrhage may be caused by damage to an aberrant vessel, for example, the ascending pharyngeal artery. This should be treated by postnasal packing and possibly ligature of the external carotid artery.

The internal carotid artery can be located close to the nasopharynx if an abnormal loop formation is present (Herrschaft 1969). If the bleeding arises from this vessel, immediate digital compression should be applied to the common carotid artery which should be ligated without delay. A temporary ligature should be applied until angiography has been done (Herrmann 1968).

Pernasal Access

(Synonyms: endonasal, transnasal access).

Indications

A pernasal operation is used in the following circumstances:

- Removal of polypoid lesions with the snare, forceps or hooks, for example, a choanal polyp presenting in the nasopharynx, combined with an operation on the sinuses. Simultaneous peroral finger control of the instruments introduced through the nose is necessary.

- The pernasal route may be suitable for obtaining a biopsy from the nasopharynx, under endoscopic control if possible (posterior rhinoscope with a wide angled telescope).

- The pernasal technique for treatment of a choanal atresia can be regarded as a nasopharyngeal operation but only as far as the operation on the nasopharyngeal mucosa is concerned. It should be discussed in brief since it is close to the nasopharynx particularly in the infant (see p. 113).

After all pernasal operations for choanal atresia there is a considerable degree of recurrence due to scar tissue formation. Such procedures today are restricted to *purely membranous* atresia at any age and as an emergency measure for *bilateral atresia* in a *newborn* with respiratory difficulties.

In these circumstances anesthesia can be omitted, but both sides should be operated on if possible so that one can be used for a feeding tube. This operation is not urgently indicated since, in the immediate postnatal phase, respiratory difficulties can be overcome by means of a Gudel's airway until the operation can be carried out.

Principles of the Operation for Choanal Atresia

In all pernasal operations for atresia, the nasopharynx is approached via the lower part of the nasal cavity. A membranous atresia is incised or divided by the diathermy: a bony atresia is penetrated with a trochar, chisels, curettes, file, hand drill or electrically driven burr (Fig. 11.5). The communication with the nasopharynx is held open by plastic tubes until complete epithelialization has taken place (2 to 5 months). With an accurate technique, accompanied by use of the operating microscope, it may be possible to preserve the nasopharyngeal mucosa, even in the infant, so that bare edges of bone may be covered (Beinfield 1959). Several different methods, instruments and techniques are recommended. There are also several methods recommended for the introduction and anchoring of the tubes (which today should always be made of silicone rubber). Two separate tubes may be introduced on each side in a retrograde direction over a pernasal catheter; or a one-piece U-shaped tube is introduced around the columella with anterior holes for breathing; or a one-piece U-shaped tube is placed around the vomer with posterior holes for breathing, and the ends of the tube are fastened together in front of the columella.

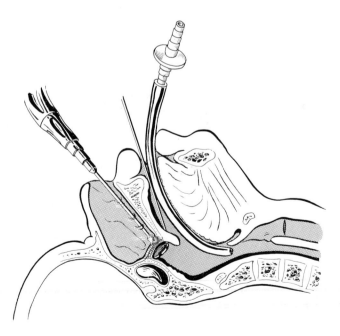

Fig. 11.5   Pernasal penetration of a bony choanal atresia; a retrovelar protector consisting of a nasopharyngeal mirror without its glass and a suction tube in place.

There are so many modifications described in the literature that details and references cannot be given in full here. Bibliographical reviews have been presented by McGovern and Slaughter Fitz-Hugh (1961) and by Masing (1971).

Operative Technique Including Danger Points for Choanal Atresia

Consideration of the anatomical relationships and the risks of the operation are more important than the details of the method. The choanal of an infant should be about 6 mm wide. In a bony atresia of the newborn, the distance from the inferior edge of the nostril to the atretic area is about 32 mm and an additional 12 mm to the posterior wall of the pharynx (Beinfield 1959). Since the base of the skull forms an immediate superior relation to the area of atresia, the atretic area should be pierced at the level of the floor of the nose. The part of the spinal column between the axis and the atlas, however, lies in a direct line of extension of the operative plane. A bony atresia should be pierced by a diamond burr if the surgeon does not wish to introduce a protective plate (for example, a postnasal mirror without its glass [Fig. 11.5] or Beinfield's special protector behind the soft palate). The nasopharynx of the newborn is barely large enough to permit digital inspection. The position, elasticity and diameter of the silicone rubber tube introduced should be checked carefully. Significant cosmetic deformities can arise from necrosis of skin and cartilage produced by pressure, particularly on the columella and on the vestibular surfaces of the upper and lower cartilages.

Transpalatal Access

Indications for and Principles of the Operation

Brunk (1909) was the first to operate via this route for a bony choanal atresia. The modifications and refinements of this method have been reviewed by Masing (1971). Many well known names are associated with different incisions in the mucoperiosteum of the hard palate (Fig. 11.6), but all these modifications are only intended for treatment of choanal atresia.

Wilson (1957) was responsible for popularizing the transpalatal approach for tumor surgery of the nasopharynx. Transpalatal access provides a good view for operations on tumors localized to the nasopharynx such as nasopharyngeal angiofibromas arising from the base of the skull or the tubal area (Coenen 1923, Albrecht 1959) and also for localized nasopharyngeal carcinomas (Burian 1971). Wilson (1957) recommends this method for diagnostic exploration and for taking multiple biopsies (possibly with the use of the microscope) if this area is suspected of being the site of an occult primary tumor. He also described an operation for the creation of a permanent palatal fenestration for follow up after radiotherapy of tumors in this area.

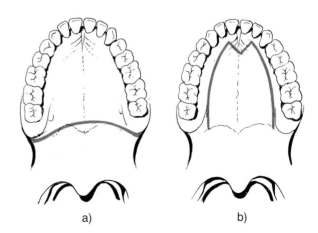

Fig. 11.6a, b Palatal incisions for the transpalatine operation.
a) Přecechtěl's, b) Steinzeug's,

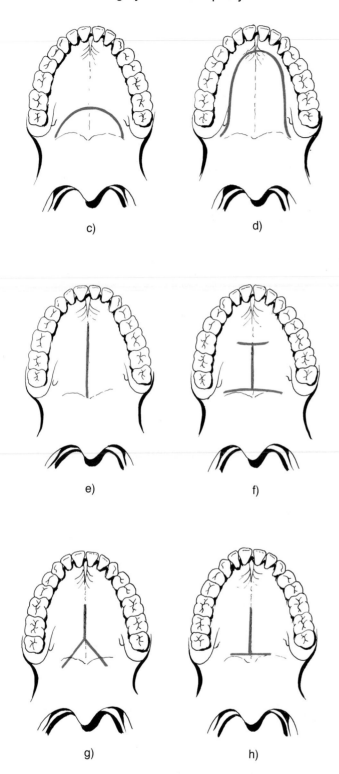

Operative Technique

The position is the same as for the peroral operation (see p. 109). Přecechtěl's curved incision (1938) is used. This incision is convex anteriorly and lies 5 mm anterior to the posterior edge of the hard palate. It is carried down to the bone. This incision was also used by Wilson (1957) rather than the reversed Y-shaped incision ascribed to him. The incision should pass posteromedial to the greater palatine foramen so that the vessels are preserved (Fig. 11.7).

The mucoperiosteum is elevated with a sharp elevator as far as the posterior edge of the hard palate; the posterior nasal spine may be removed with a chisel if necessary. The nasopharynx is opened by dividing the mucosa along the edge of the palatine bone (Fig. 11.8). The soft tissue incision is extended laterally on both sides along the pterygomandibular raphe until the tendon of the tensor palati muscle can be divided close to the pterygoid hamulus. Hemostasis of the posterior palatine vessels is achieved with diathermy or ligature. The mucosal incision is then extended laterally to expose the anterior edge of the eustachian tube. Retraction of the soft palate in a posteroinferior direction brings both eustachian tubes, the fossae of Rosenmüller, the inferior edge of the septum, the choana and the inferior ends of the turbinates into view (Fig. 11.9). The tumor is then removed in accordance with its site and histological type.

The incision in the palate is closed with atraumatic 3 × 0 Mersilene, and postnasal packing is introduced if necessary. If the sutures tear out the wound tends to heal secondarily within 1 week without the formation of a fistula.

Fig. 11.6c-h   Palatal incisions for the transpalatine operation.

c) Ruddy's, d) Owen's, e) Blair's, f) Schweckendieck's, g) Wilson's, h) Meyer's.

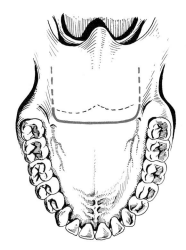

Fig. 11.7

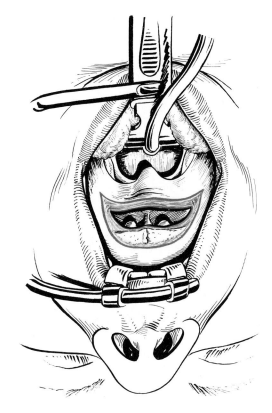

Fig. 11.8

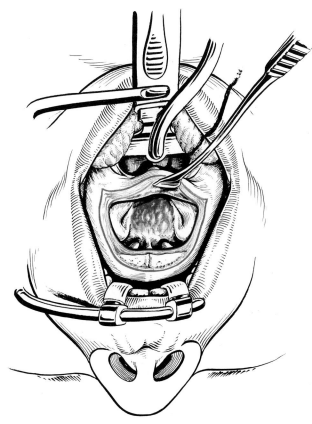

Fig. 11.9

Cryosurgery

Surgery of the nasopharynx has recently been combined with *cryosurgery*. The advantages are decreased bleeding, a smooth granulating surface and less postoperative pain. Barton (1966) uses the cryoprobe transpalatally for all tumors while Work et al. (1966) recommend it for every route of access, especially for nasopharyngeal angiofibromas.

Sublabial Permaxillary Access
(Synonym: endoral transmaxillary route)

Indications for and Principle of the Operation

Denker's method (1905) is the only one of these methods of access to the nasopharynx which is of any value. It allows removal of tumors of the nasopharynx with limited extension into the sphenoid sinus, the inferior part of the ethmoid labyrinth, the inferior and medial part of the antrum or the nasal cavity. This operation is generally used only for benign tumors (e.g., small nasopharyngeal angiofibromas arising from the sphenoethmoidal area).

Since access via the oral cavity is relatively narrow and at a considerable depth, the view into the nasopharynx is often unsatisfactory; the direction of work by this route of access is more toward the sphenoidal area than into the nasopharynx. It is usually difficult to attain accurate hemostasis in the depth of the wound.

Operative Technique

A mucosal incision is made in the buccal sulcus from the second or third molar to the frenulum of the upper lip. The mucoperiosteum of the canine fossa is elevated as far as the piriform aperture. The mucosa is also elevated in the inferior part of the nasal vestibule from the piriform crest.

The anterior wall of the antrum is extensively resected and the bony opening is extended by removing the frontal process of the maxilla (Figs. 11.10, 7.26). The medial wall of the antrum is then removed, if possible preserving the nasolacrimal duct. If possible, the nasal mucosa is also preserved so that it can be used later as a flap. The inferior turbinate must be partially resected if subluxation does not provide sufficient space. Depending on the extent of the tumor, the ethmoid cells are cleared and the antral cavity is opened to provide access to the nasopharynx. The tumor is removed by traction on the surrounding healthy mucosa attached to the tumor. Intermittent packing should be used as required.

Finally the area is packed with iodoform gauze strips brought out through the nose. If necessary, the nasal cavity is packed in layers and posterior nasal packing is introduced. The mucosal incision in the vestibule of the mouth is closed.

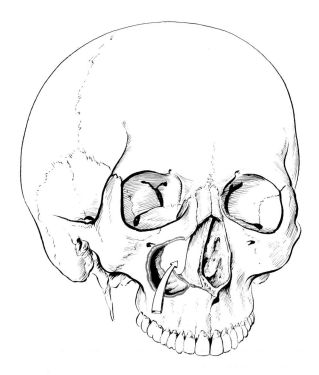

Fig. 11.10   Principle of Denker's operation.

Paranasal Permaxillary Access
(Synonym: paranasal transmaxillary access)

Indications for and Principles of the Operation

Of the methods providing access to the nasopharynx through the central part of the face with elevation of part of the cheek, that of Zange (1950) "should be recognized as the one which guarantees the best view and the greatest adaptability for dealing with all unforseen circumstances" (Albrecht 1959).

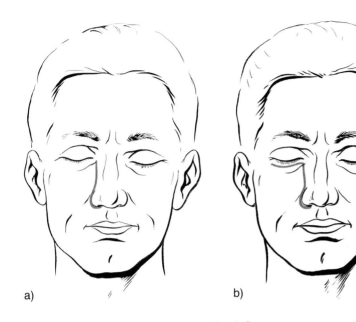

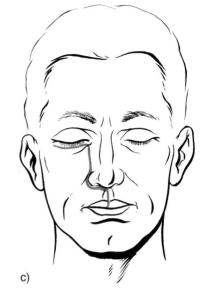

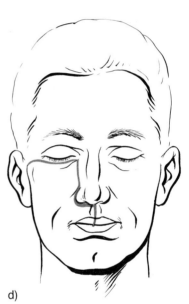

Fig. 11.11   Incisions for creating a cheek flap.
a) Moure's incision,
b) Zange's extension,
c) Heath's extension,
d) Mündnich's extension.

The external incision is based on Moure's paranasal incision (1923) (Fig. 11.11 a) which can be extended, depending on the extent of the tumor, through the edge of the lid (Zange 1950, Zöllner 1956) (Fig. 11.11 b) or by a median incision through the upper lip (Heath 1872) (Fig. 11.11 c).

The cosmetic advantage of this incision is well known. By extending the incision in the lid as far as the center of the zygoma, even the lateral wall of the orbit can be reached and, after division of the zygomatic arch, a more tangential view is obtained of the pterygopalatine fossa and the nasopharynx from the side (Mündnich 1954) (Fig. 11.11 d). This allows surgery of the entire pterygopalatine fossa for advanced nasopharyngeal angiofibromas with extension into the periorbital and maxilloethmoidal regions to be carried out under direct vision. This may also be possible for extensive malignant nasopharyngeal tumors. Surgical removal is limited because tumor invasion is difficult to recognize clinically and during the operation. This invasion may have progressed along lateral pathways to the base of the skull and the intracranial cavity, chiefly along the eustachian tube and the nerve sheaths (Flatmann 1954, Ballantyne et al. 1963).

Preoperative Diagnosis

Radiological estimation of the size of the tumor is indispensable. Angiography to define the vascular supply of the tumor is also valuable in addition to palpation and clinical examination after retraction of the soft palate. Selective embolectomy during preoperative angiography can be useful.

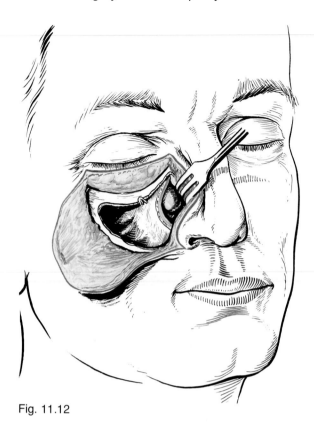

Fig. 11.12

Operative Technique

Moure's skin incision (1923) is made from the medial canthus downward, close to the nasal pyramid. It turns around the ala and ends at the base of the columella (see Fig. 11.11a). Extensions to this incision are shown in Figures 11.11b–d.

Zange's incision, which runs below the eyelashes, is made 1–2 mm from the edge of the lower lid and must divide the orbicularis oculi muscle down to the orbital septum so that the skin and muscles of the lower lid can be elevated in one layer. This is done to preserve the branches of the facial nerve supplying the musculature and to prevent ectropion. At the inner canthus, the skin incision should be several millimeters from the lid margin and should preserve some of the muscle fibers surrounding the nasolacrimal duct (Zöllner 1956) so that the muscle can be reunited at this point at the end of the operation (see also Vol. 1, Figs. 7.142, 7.143).

The cheek flap is elevated from the superomedial angle inferiorly and laterally, and the infraorbital nerve is divided by diathermy (Fig. 11.12).

The operation on the bony facial skeleton then proceeds as in Denker's operation (see p. 116). The antral cavity is exposed widely by resection of its anterior wall together with the frontal process of the maxilla (see Vol. 1, Fig. 7.26). The bone of the medial wall of the antrum is re-moved completely and the soft tissue layers are divided perpendicularly, immediately posterior to the naso lacrimal duct which is sacrificed if necessary. The posterior part of the nasal cavity and the nasopharynx are brought into view by traction on those parts lying anterior to the incision which have now become mobile (nasolacrimal duct, anterior end of the middle turbinate, and inferior turbinate which can possibly be completely preserved) and by temporary displacement of the posterior part of the lateral wall of the nose toward the midline or into the antrum.

The posterior wall of the antrum is removed beginning medially; the internal maxillary artery is exposed and tied (routine tying of this vessel has been found to diminish bleeding more effectively than ligature or temporary clamping of the external carotid artery).

Depending on the extent of the tumor, the pterygo-palatine fossa is exposed further by resection of the posterior wall of the antrum in a lateral direction, resection of the medial pterygoid plate, complete clearance of the ethmoids and opening of the sphenoid sinus as well as resection of the posterior part of the vomer until a view can be obtained of the opposite side of the nasopharynx. This method provides the widest possible access to the nasopharynx, the entire basis of the sphenoid, the eustachian tube, and even the middle cranial fossa (Zöllner 1952). Depending on the type and extent of the tumor, it is removed with a large raspatory or forceps either piecemeal with intermittent packing or in one piece. If necessary, a frozen section is done.

The lateral wall of the nose is replaced in its position. The wound is packed with iodoform gauze brought out through the nose. The nasal cavity is packed in layers and a postnasal packing is introduced if necessary. The facial incision is closed with atraumatic sutures; particular attention should be paid to the inner canthus (see p. 11).

Important Modifications and Surgical Alternatives

Clearance of the orbit may be necessary at the same time; this is dealt with in Vol. 1, Chap. 7. It is generally agreed that a neck dissection should not be carried out as a routine practice for tumors of the nasopharynx (Wustrow 1965). Simultaneous therapeutic neck dissection or neck dissection later when a lymph node metastasis becomes palpable is recommended. In Obregon's experience (1957), prophylactic neck dissection in 100 patients yielded no better results than therapeutic neck dissection when indicated.

The area of lymphatic drainage should be prophylactically included on both sides in any radiation before or after the operation.

Transpterygoid Access

(Synonym: lateral nasopharyngostomy)

Indications for and Principle of the Operation

The anatomy of the pterygopalatine fossa is illustrated in Fig. 11.13. Lateral access to this part of the skull was first described by Kremen (1953), and by Conley (1956). It was further developed by Zehm (1966) and Dingman and Conley (1970). This route provides good access to the entire retromaxillary space, to tumors developing in that space and to tumors of the nasopharynx extending into the space. The ascending ramus of the mandible is divided temporarily (or resected) and is turned upward after the lower lip has been split to provide a good view of this region. Ross and Sukis (1966) have described a very similar technique for a specific approach to the nasopharynx via the retromaxillary space. In their case it was combined with a transpalatal operation.

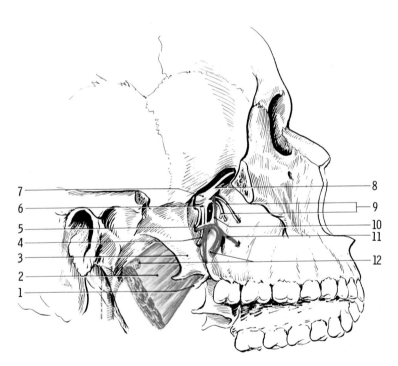

Fig. 11.13   Anatomy of the pterygopalatine fossa.

1. Pterygoid hamulus
2. Medial pterygoid muscle
3. Lateral pterygoid plate
4. Descending palatine artery and vein and the greater palatine nerve in the greater palatine canal
5. Artery and nerve of the pterygoid canal
6. Pterygopalatine nerves and pterygopalatine ganglion

7. Maxillary nerve
8. Infraorbital nerve in the inferior orbital fissure
9. Posterior superior alveolar nerves
10. Infraorbital artery
11. Posterior superior alveolar artery
12. Internal maxillary artery

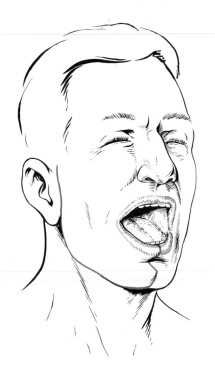

Fig. 11.14   Incision for transpterygoid access.

Diagnostic Preoperative Measures

Tomograms and possibly angiograms are done.

Operative Technique

(Adapted from Ross and Sukis [1966] and Zehm [1966]).

An incision is made in the midline through the lower lip; it is made in the shape of a Z to prevent scar contracture. The incision proceeds downward to the chin, curves posteriorly over the submandibular area and then proceeds upward in front of the ear and finishes in the temporal area (Fig. 11.14).

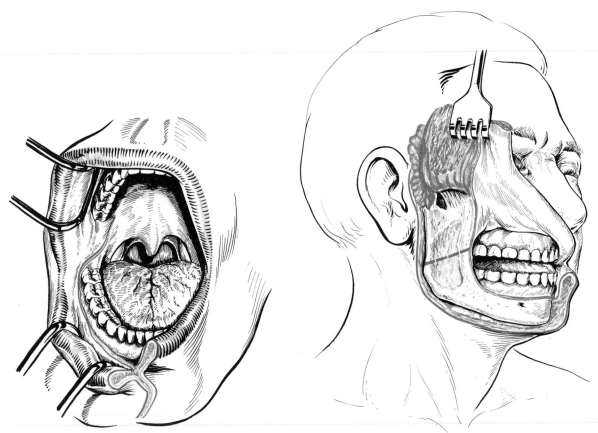

Fig. 11.15   Fig. 11.16

A suprahyoid neck dissection is carried out if indicated. A mucosal incision is made from the corner of the lip incision within the mouth proceeding posteriorly along the lower buccal sulcus; it crosses the ascending ramus of the mandible and finishes close to the pterygoid hamulus (Fig. 11.15).

The flap, consisting of the lower lip and the cheek, is elevated from the mandible in one layer with preservation of the parotid gland, the parotid duct and the branches of the facial nerve within the flap (Fig. 11.16).

The temporalis muscle is divided from the mandible and the mandible is divided at the angle in such a position that the wire or the screws used to fix it can be covered by the masseter muscle (Fig. 11.17).

The ascending ramus of the mandible is turned upward, thereby exposing both lateral parts of the pterygoid muscle and demonstrating the internal maxillary artery which usually runs between them. The lateral pterygoid muscle is separated from the lateral plate of the pterygoid. The internal maxillary artery is divided between double ligatures, deep in the pterygopalatine fossa if possible (Fig. 11.17).

The retromaxillary space has no vessels or nerves in the immediate area; the internal carotid artery and the internal jugular vein lie about 1.5 cm posterolateral to the surgical field.

With the origin of the pterygoid plates and the rounded posterior surface of the maxilla now in good view, the medial pterygoid muscle is divided, and the external and posterior part of the maxilla is removed with a chisel to open the antral cavity (Fig. 11.18). The lateral soft tissue wall of the nasopharynx is exposed by removing the entire origin of the pterygoid plates at their base superiorly (the medial pterygoid plate forms the bony boundary between the retromaxillary space and the nasopharynx).

The nasopharyngeal cavity is opened widely by dividing the exposed surface with diathermy (Fig. 11.17); this area consists of the superior constrictor muscle of the pharynx, the levator and the tensor palati muscles and the nasopharyngeal mucosa. The soft tissue flap, which is pedicled posteriorly, is then turned backward (Fig. 11.18).

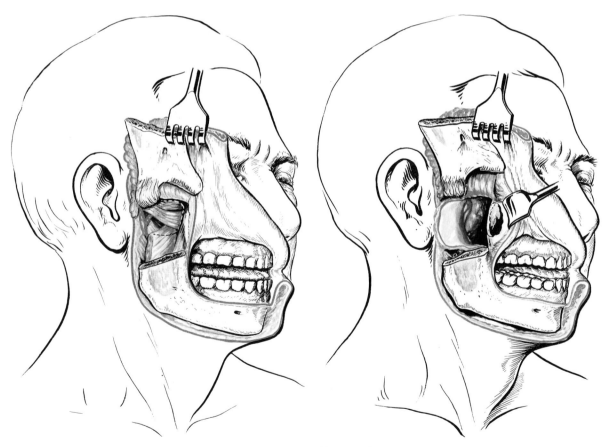

Fig. 11.17   Fig. 11.18

The supplementary transpalatal operation proceeds as follows:

The soft palate is divided in the region of the pterygoid hamulus and, if necessary, a part of the bony palate is removed; the medial wall of the antrum may be opened posteriorly.

The tumor is removed with a margin which depends on the type of the tumor; if necessary, the mandible is disarticulated.

If there has been extensive resection, the defect is covered with free or pedicled fascial flaps or muscle flaps from the temporalis muscle. If not, the pharyngeal wall is reconstructed by replacing the nasopharyngeal flap (Fig. 11.18), suturing the stumps of the pterygoid muscles and fixing the tendon of the temporalis to the coronoid process of the mandible. Intraosseous fixation of the mandible is carried out with 0.8 mm wire introduced in a cross-shape through four burr holes (Fig. 11.19) or by screwing. In the patient with good dentition, this is supplemented by dental cap splints. Submandibular suction drainage is introduced. The wound is closed internally and externally in layers with atraumatic sutures. A nasogastric tube is introduced.

Transzygomatic Access

Indications for and Principles of the Operation

This route of access was described by Mündnich (1954) as an extension of Zange's method; it was also used by McCarten (1963) together with endoral resection of the upper jaw and by Crocket (1963) for exposure of the retromaxillary space. Zehm (1970) recommends this operation combined with resection of the mandible for malignant tumors with involvement of the retromaxillary space and metastases in the retropharyngeal lymph nodes in the region of the internal carotid artery. Denecke (1959) has also described the operative technique.

The transzygomatic method of Samy and Girgis (1965) can only be regarded as original if it is used to expose the nasopharynx after mere temporary resection of the zygomatic arch together with peroral retropalatal access, *specifically for removal of nasopharyngeal fibromas extending into the infratemporal area*. The oblique view from above into the nasopharynx is naturally restricted in that procedure.

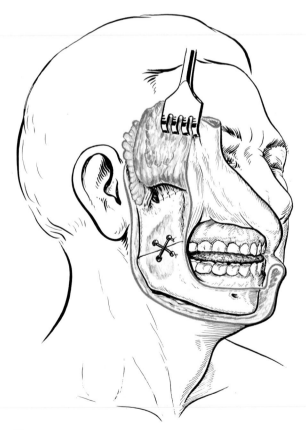

Fig. 11.19

Operative Technique

A horizontal skin incision 12 mm long is made extending forward from the tragus, upward over the zygoma and extending as far as the eyebrow. The skin is elevated superiorly and the temporalis fascia is divided from the zygoma for a distance of 6 mm (Fig. 11.20).

The zygomatic arch is divided at its anterior and posterior ends in such a way that it is wedge-shaped (i.e., shorter inferiorly). In this way it is retained in position by the traction of the masseter when it is replaced at the end of the operation (Fig. 11.20).

The segment of the zygoma is turned downward with the masseter muscle attached to it. The temporalis muscle is dissected forward. The internal maxillary artery is ligated as it lies between the two bellies of the lateral pterygoid muscle, which is elevated superiorly from the infratemporal crest and retracted downward. The infratemporal fossa together with the lateral pterygoid plate and the pharyngobasilar fascia are completely exposed by anterior retraction of the temporalis muscle. This allows unrestricted digital access to the constrictor muscles of the nasopharynx and into the cheek (Fig. 11.21). The tumor can now be mobilized. Temporary packing is carried out with gauze and later with gelatine sponge.

If the base of the tumor is left behind in the nasopharynx, it is dealt with by a peroral retropalatine procedure which can be carried out easier with less blood loss if the transzygomatic operation has been done first. Posterior nasal packing is introduced.

The zygomatic segment is replaced and the bone is sutured with chromic catgut or wire introduced through burr holes. The temporalis fascia is sutured with a tube drain extending below it. The skin is closed with atraumatic sutures.

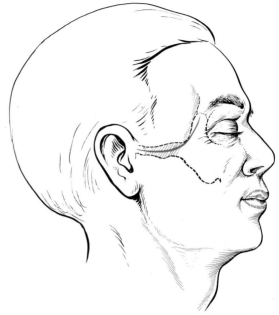

Fig. 11.20

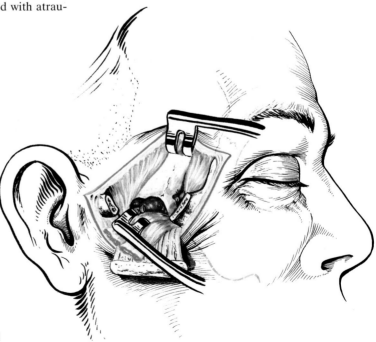

Fig. 11.21

Operations for Stenoses of the Nasopharynx

Diagnostic Preoperative Measures

Acquired adhesions of the palate to the posterior wall of the nasopharynx are now as rare as congenital stenosis in this area. The extensive literature several decades ago indicates the relative frequency of these lesions then. They were caused by infections such as diphtheria, scarlet fever, syphilis, tuberculosis, lupus, rhinoscleroma, occasionally also as a result of chronic pemphigus, glanders, leprosy, cancrum and noma. After about 1930 these infectious diseases were controlled, and iatrogenic and traumatic causes began to predominate in the literature. These were caused by technically inadequate adenotonsillectomies, possibly in patients with a tendency toward keloid of the skin.

The principal symptom of nasopharyngeal stenosis is nasal obstruction with all its sequelae. Patients with this disease also suffer from retention of nasal secretions, disorders of eustachian tube function leading to conductive deafness, disorders of deglutition, disturbances of smell and taste, rhinolalia clausa and inability to blow the nose.

These unmistakable symptoms can be investigated by:

● Radiographic demonstration of the nasopharynx with contrast media,

● Probing,

● Naso-oral inflation with a Politzer balloon,

● Transnasal endoscopy.

This allows the thickness and extent of the scar as well as the extent of the remaining tissue to be determined before the operation. The condition and the blood supply of the mucosa, which determines whether a flap is better pedicled above or below, can be decisive factors in choosing a particular operation.

Principles of the Operation

Illustration of the operative techniques will be limited to operations which have been most frequently used in the last century and which have enjoyed a certain degree of success. Complete historical reviews are provided by Stupka (1928), Denecke and Meyer (1964), Mühler (1967), Stevenson (1969) and Burian (1971).

Simple dilation and division of the adhesions has been completely abandoned because it is only successful on occasion, (for instance with soft congenital adhesions) and seldom prevents inevitable recurrence. The other therapeutic extreme (the techniques described for extensive adhesions by Curtis [1901] and Axhausen [1916]) using a high lateral pharyngotomy and rotation of epidermal flaps into the pharynx do not seem to have found acceptance in the literature.

The following *three principles of management* now appear to be generally accepted:

1. Advancement and rotation flaps of pedicled mucosa appear to have established themselves as the best procedures.

2. Operations using free skin grafts (usually combined with an artificial obturator) have been successful in many cases, although free grafts in the oropharynx are particularly susceptible to infection and do not heal as reliably as mucosal flaps.

3. Operations using the obsolete principle of syndactyly may provide a permanent opening into the nasopharynx. Rings of thread or wire or plastic tubes are used in an attempt to create an epithelialized canal within the scarred adhesions, which is then laid open by sharp dissection.

In a particular case it may not be possible to use a specific method because of the variability of the local conditions. The individual situations may demand variations and combinations of several different techniques. The results are more often unsatisfactory when the operation is carried out for a postinfective stenosis than when it is performed for a traumatic condition.

Obturators used to dilate the stenosis and to carry the graft or protective plates for retention of sutures around the columella should be made of soft silicone rubber (Zühlke 1960) because it causes the least tissue reaction and allows smooth epithelialization along its surface. Silastic (Dow Corning Corporation) appears to be the most useful of the materials available.

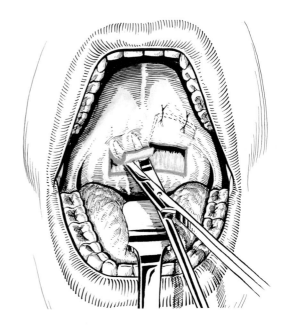

Fig. 11.22

Position and Anesthesia

All the operations about to be described are carried out under oral endotracheal intubation anesthesia with the head extended (see p. 109). A mouth gag with a special anesthetic blade (e.g., the Kilner-Doughty blade) allows a good view of the surgical field.

Operative Technique

Pedicled Mucosal Flaps (Advancement and rotation flaps possibly combined with the use of dilators)

Mackenty's Method

Mackenty's operation type I (1911).

Two flaps are developed from the posterior wall of the nasopharynx on each side of the uvula, pedicled superiorly on the soft palate and divided inferiorly at the level of the lower border of the adhesions. The velopharyngeal adhesions are divided. The flaps are rotated on to the posterior surface of the soft palate to cover the raw surface at that point and are fixed with mattress sutures which pierce the soft palate (Figs. 11.22, 11.23).

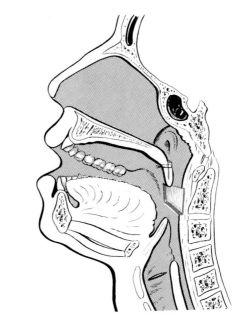

Fig. 11.23

Mackenty's Alternative Method

Mackenty's type II operation (Mackenty, 1927, Rethi, 1957).

A deep vertical incision 2–3 cm long is made in the midline in the region of the uvula. Two horizontal incisions (1.5 cm long) are made proceeding from the inferior end of the vertical incision following the edge of the scarred palate. A triangular mucosal flap is dissected up on each side. The exposed scar tissue of the soft palate is removed. The mucosal triangular flaps are turned posteriorly and sutured to the wound edges of the mucosa of the posterior surface of the soft palate (Figs. 11.24 a, b). This operation ist strongly recommended for very dense scars. Postoperative rhinolalia aperta and dysphagia cannot always be avoided.

Kazanjian-Holmes Method

Reversed Mackenty's type I operation (Kazanjian and Holmes 1946, Kazanjian and Converse 1949, Hamacher 1957).

Two layers are developed from the palatopharyngeal adhesions on each side of the uvula so that each forms an oral flap based inferiorly on the posterior wall of the nasopharynx and a nasal flap based on the soft palate (Figs. 11.25, 11.26). The nasal flap is transposed on to the anterior surface of the soft palate and is fixed in place with mattress sutures which pierce the palate (Fig. 11.27). The oral flaps are transposed posteriorly to cover the wound surface on the posterior wall of the nasopharynx (Fig. 11.27). If necessary, the flaps can be pedicled in reverse.

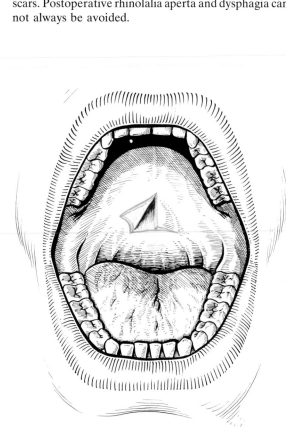

Fig. 11.24 a

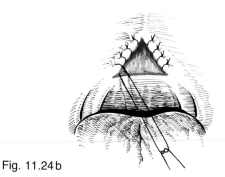

Fig. 11.24 b

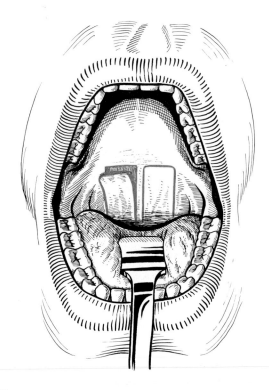

Fig. 11.25

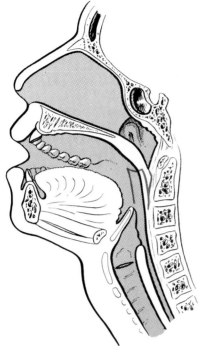

Fig. 11.26

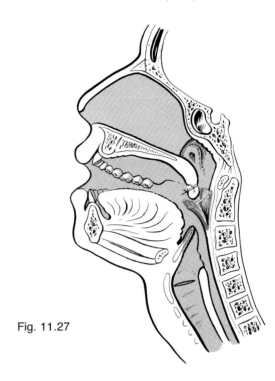

Fig. 11.27

Vaughan's Method
Vaughan (1949)

This procedure consists of a combination of Mackenty's type I operation with the introduction of a dilator behind the soft palate. The dilator consists of two lateral tubes

and one horizontal tube superiorly made of plastic and held loosely together by a suture. The dilator is held in place by means of a suture around the columella (Figs. 11.28, 11.29).

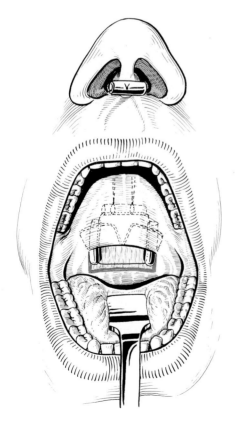

Fig. 11.28

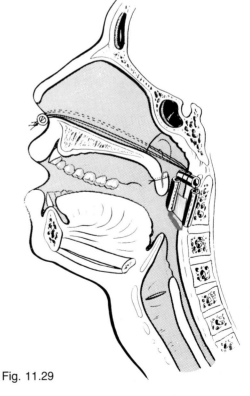

Fig. 11.29

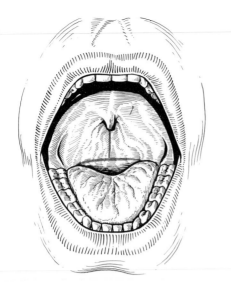

Fig. 11.30

Mühler's Method
Mühler (1969) and Panse (1913)

A vertical incision is made in the midline beginning at the center of the remaining lumen and extending downward to the lower border of the scar tissue. Two horizontal incisions are made perpendicular to the inferior end of the vertical incision (Fig. 11.30). The scar tissue is excised and the triangular mucosal flaps are turned around behind the soft palate or behind the faucial pillars and are fixed with mattress sutures similar to those described by Mackenty (1927) (Figs. 11.31, 11.32). Two further vertical incisions are made through the mucosa and the muscles on both sides through the posterior wall of the nasopharynx, beginning in the scarred area and proceeding downward to the level of the laryngeal inlet. If necessary, Burow's triangles are excised at the base (Fig. 11.33). The inferiorly pedicled flap, which has been freed from the prevertebral fascia, can now be pulled upward so that it completely covers the area previously occupied by the adhesions on the posterior pharyngeal wall (Fig. 11.34). Tension on the flap is distributed by lateral interrupted sutures (Fig. 11.35).

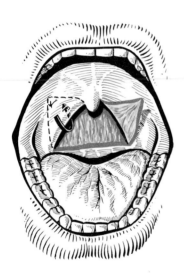

Fig. 11.31

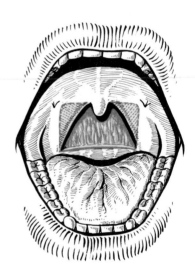

Fig. 11.32

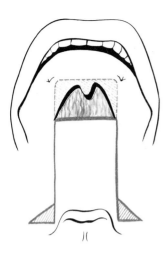

Fig. 11.33

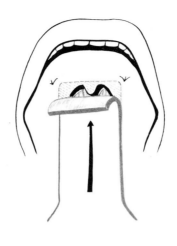

Fig. 11.34

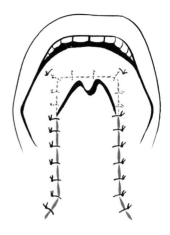

Fig. 11.35

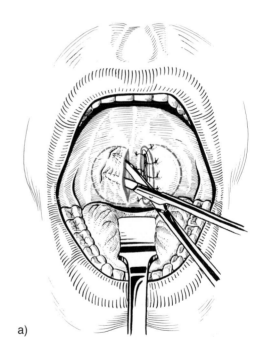

a)

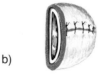

b)

Fig. 11.36

Operations Using Split Skin Grafts

O'Conner's Method
O'Conner (1937), McIndoe (1937) and McLaughlin and Ireland (1950)

Two pockets are created by two perpendicular incisions. The palatopharyngeal adhesions are undermined through these incisions on both sides (Fig. 11.36a). A stent covered with split skin, the subcutaneous surface outward, is introduced into both of these pockets (Fig. 11.36b). The stent, skin graft and mucosa are sutured to the edges of the pocket. The stent is left in place for several weeks.

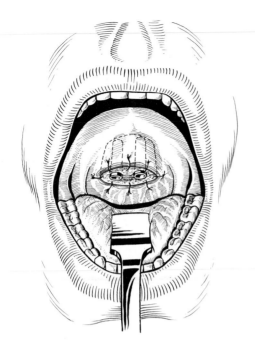

Fig. 11.37

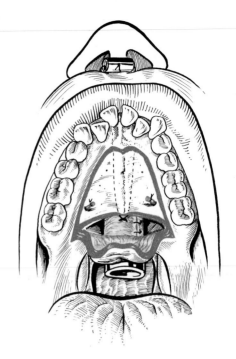

Fig. 11.39

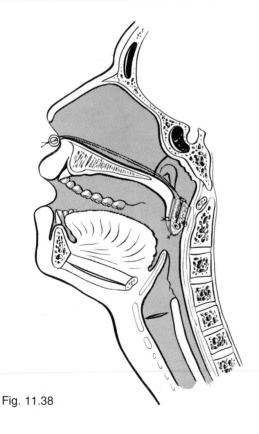

Fig. 11.38

Figi's Method
Figi (1947)

The palatopharyngeal adhesions are divided by sharp dissection and a Silastic sponge obturator covered with split skin and pierced by two plastic tubes is introduced (Fig. 11.37). The dilators are held in place by sutures around the columella (Fig. 11.38). The edge of the split skin is sutured on the oral side to the edges of the scar incision (Fig. 11.38). The dilator is left in place for several weeks.

Herfert's Method
Herfert (1960), Schuchardt (1964)

The transpalatal route is used. Steinzeug's incision is made in the mucosa of the palate (see Fig. 11.6b) and the palatine artery is tied on both sides (Fig. 11.39). The palatopharyngeal adhesions are divided in a naso-oral direction and the scar tissue is excised. A soft, angled plastic tube (Palavit, in Schuchardt's method), covered with split skin is introduced into the wound canal (Fig. 11.39). The soft tissue palatal flap is replaced and sutured in position. The dilator is held in place for 2 to 3 months by a catheter around the columella.

Epithelialization Operations

These operations can only be used for narrow epithelialized ring stenoses of the retropalatal area when the rest of the palate is otherwise free and is covered on both surfaces with mucosa.

Stevenson's Method
Stevenson (1969), Nichols (1896)

Wire loops covered with plastic are introduced from the median lumen through a lateral puncture wound on each side. The wire is knotted, the knot is introduced into the lumen of the tubing and the ring is rotated so that the knot lies behind the palate (Fig. 11.40). The ring is left in place for about 6 weeks. After this time the epithelialized canal which has formed along the tubing is laid open by sharp dissection. The incised edges of the epithelialized canal are sutured to the posterior and anterior mucosal layers of the soft palate or the faucial pillars with fine catgut.

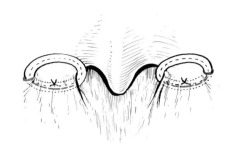

Fig. 11.40

Bibliography

Albrecht, R.: Die Nasenrachentumoren und ihre Behandlung. Arch. Ohren-, Nasen-, Kehlkopfheilk. 175: 34, 1959

Axhausen, G.: Die operative Behandlung der Pharynxstenose, Langenbecks Arch. klin. Chir. 107: 533, 1916

Ballantyne, A. J., A. B. McCarten, M. L. Ibanez: The extension of the head and neck through peripheral nerves. Am. J. Surg. 106: 651, 1963

Barton, R. Th.: Cryosurgical treatment of nasopharyngeal neoplasms. Am. Surg. 32: 744, 1966

Beinfeld, H. H.: Surgery for bilateral bony atresia of the posterior nares in the newborn. Arch. Otolaryng. 70: 1, 1959

Beinfeld, H. H.: Bilateral choanal atresia in the newborn. Arch. Otolaryng. 73: 659, 1961

Blair, V. P.: Congenital atresia or obstruction of air passage. Ann. Otol. 40: 1021, 1931

Brunk, A.: Ein neuer Fall von einseitigem, knöchernem Choanenverschluß. Operationsversuch vom Gaumen aus. Z. Ohrenheilk. 59: 221, 1909

Burian, K.: Die Behandlung der Stenosen des Nasen-Rachen-Raumes. Arch. Klin. Exp. Ohren-, Nasen-, Kehlkopfheilk. 199: 218, 1971

Coenen, H.: Das Basalfibroid. Münch. med. Wochenschr. 70: 829, 1923

Conley, J. J.: The surgical approach to the pterygoid area. Ann. Surg. 144: 39, 1956

Crockett, D. J.: Surgical approach to the back of the maxilla. Brit. J. Surg. 50: 819, 1963

Curtis, B. F.: Cicatricial stricture of pharynx. Ann. Surg. 33: 152, 1901

Denecke, H. J.: Diskussionsbemerkung zum Referat R. Albrecht.

Denecke, H. J., R. Meyer: Korrigierende und rekonstruktive Nasenplastik. In: Plastische Operationen an Kopf und Hals. vol. I. Springer, Berlin 1964

Denker, A.: Zur Radikaloperation des chronischen Kieferhöhlenempyems. Arch. Laryng. 17: 221, 1905

Denker, A.: Die bösartigen Neubildungen der Nase und ihrer Nebenhöhlen. In: Handbuch der Hals-Nasen-Ohren-Heilkunde, vol. I., ed. by A. Denker, O. Kahler. Springer u. Bergmann, Berlin and Munich 1929 (p. 250 ff.)

Dingman, D. L., J. J. Conley: Lateral approach to the pterygoid-maxillary region. Ann. Otol. (St. Louis) 79: 967, 1970

Figi, F. A.: Cicatricial stenosis of the nasopharynx; correction by means of skin graft. Plast. reconstr. Surg. 2: 97, 1947

Flatmann, G. E.: cited in Albrecht 1959

Von Gyergyai, A.: Die vollkommene örtliche Betäubung des Nasen-Rachen-Raumes. Verh. Ges. dtsch. Hals-, Nas.- u. Ohrenärz. 44, 1938

Hamacher, E. N.: Nasopharyngeal stenosis – a method of repair utilizing transposed flaps. Plast. reconstr. Surg. 19: 163, 1957

Heath, Chr.: Diseases and Injuries of the Jaws. London 1872 (p. 275), cited in C. P. Wilson 1957

Herfert, O.: Beitrag zur Therapie der erworbenen Choanalatresie. H.N.O. (Berlin) 8: 335, 1960

Herrmann, A.: Gefahren bei Operationen an Hals, Ohr und Gesicht und die Korrektur fehlerhafter Eingriffe. Springer, Berlin 1968

Herrschaft, H.: Abnorme Schlingenbildung der A. carotis interna und ihre klinische Bedeutung bei Operationen im Halsbereich. Z. Laryngol. Rhinol. 48: 85, 1969

Kazanjian, V. H., J. M. Converse: The surgical treatment of facial injuries. Williams & Wilkins, Baltimore 1949 (p. 467)

Kazanjian, V. H., E. M. Holmes: Stenosis of the nasopharynx and its correction. Arch. Otolaryng. 44: 261, 1946

Kremen, A. J.: Surgical management of angiofibroma of the nasopharynx. Ann. Surg. 138: 672, 1953

Mackenty, J. E.: Three new plastic operations on the nose and throat. Med. Rec. (N.Y.) 80: 1071, 1911

Mackenty, J. E.: Nasopharyngeal atresia. Arch. Otolaryng. 6: 1, 1927

Masing, H.: Die Behandlung der Stenosen der Nase. Arch. Klin. Exp. Ohren-, Nasen-, Kehlkopfheilk. 199: 173, 1971

McCarten, A. B.: The combined transzygomatic approach in resection of the maxilla. Amer. J. Surg. 106: 696, 1963

McGovern, F. H., G. Slaughter Fitz-Hugh: Surgical management of congenital choanal atresia. Arch. Otolaryng. 73: 627, 1961

McIndoe, A. H.: Applications of cavity grafting. Am. J. Surg. 1: 535, 1937

McLaughlin, C. R., V. E. Ireland: Nasopharyngeal atresia. Plast. reconstr. Surg. 6: 301, 1950

Meyer, R.: Transpalatinaler Operationsweg. In: Plastische Operationen an Kopf und Hals, vol. I, ed. by H. J. Denecke, R. Meyer. Springer, Berlin 1964 (p. 268–276)

Moure, E. J.: Des fibromes dits nasopharyngiens. Bull. et. Mém. Soc. Franç. d'Ophtalm. Paris 1923

Mühler, G.: Die velopharyngealen Synechien und ihre Behandlung. H.N.O. (Berlin) 15: 6, 1967

Mündnich, K.: Zur Röntgendiagnostik und Operation maligner Oberkiefer- und Flügelgaumengrubentumoren. Z. Laryngol. Rhinol. 33: 125, 1954

Nichols, J. E. H.: The sequelae of syphilis in the pharynx and their treatment. N.Y. Med. J. 64: 418, 1896

Obregon, G.: A study of hundred cases of neck dissection. Arch. Otolaryng. Chicago 66: 54, 1957

O'Conner, G. B.: Pharyngeal reconstruction. Ann. Otol. (St. Louis) 46: 376, 1937

Owens, H.: Observations in treating seven cases of choanal atresia by the transpalatine approach. Laryngoscope (St. Louis) 61: 304, 1951

Panse, R.: Zur Behandlung der Verwachsungen des Gaumens mit der Rachenwand. Verhandl. d. Vereins Dtsch. Laryngologen 172, 1913

Přecechtěl, L.: Transpalatine operation of choanal atresia. Ann. Oto-laryng. (Paris) 1014: 187, 1938

Réthi, A.: Operative Lösung der velopharyngealen narbigen Verwachsungen. Z. Laryngol. Rhinol. 36: 465, 1957

Ross, D. E., A. E. Sukis: Nasopharyngeal tumors. A new surgical approach. Am. J. Surg. 111: 524, 1966

Ruddy, L. W.: A transpalatine operation for congenital atresia of the choanae in the small child or in the infant. Arch. Otolaryng. 41: 432, 1945

Samy, L. L., I. H. Girgis: Transzygomatic approach for nasopharyngeal fibromata with extrapharyngeal extension. J. Laryng. 79: 782, 1965

Schuchardt, K.: Zur chirurgischen Behandlung der Atresie des Epipharynx und Mesopharynx. Langenbecks Arch. Klin. Chir. 306: 66, 1964

Schweckendiek, H.: Transpalatine Behandlung angeborener Choanalatresien. Z. Hals-, Nasen- u. Ohrenheilk. 42: 367, 1937

Seiffert, A.: Zur Behandlung maligner Nasenrachentumoren. Arch. Ohren-, Nasen-, Kehlkopfheilk. 148: 246, 1940

Steinzeug, A.: Ein neues Operationsverfahren zur Beseitigung der Choanenverwachsungen. Arch. Ohren-, Nasen-, Kehlkopfheilk. 137: 364, 1933

Stevenson, E. W.: Cicatricial stenosis of the nasopharynx. A comprehensive review. Larnygoscope (St. Louis) 79: 2035, 1969

Stupka, W.: Die Verwachsungen des Rachens und des Mundes. In: Handbuch der Hals-Nasen-Ohren-Heilkunde, Vol. III, ed. by A. Denker, O. Kahler. Springer u. Bergmann, Berlin and Munich 1928 (p. 1025 ff.)

Vaughan, H. S.: Nasopharyngeal stenosis. Plast. Reconstr. Surg. 4: 522, 1949

Wilson, C. P.: Observations on the surgery of the nasopharynx. Ann. Otol. (St. Louis) 66: 5, 1957

Work, W. P., R. Boles, R. D. Nichols: Angiofibromas: Diagnosis and treatment including cryosurgery. Trans. Am. Acad. Ophthal. Otolaryng. 70: 922, 1966

Wustrow, F.: Die Tumoren des Gesichtsschädels. Topographie, Pathologie und Klinik. Urban and Schwarzenberg, München 1965

Zange, J.: Operationen der Nase und ihrer Nebenhöhlen. In: Ophthalmologische Operationslehre, Vol. 4, ed. by R. Thiel. Thieme, Leipzig 1950

Zehm, S.: Die Topographie des retromaxillären Raumes in chirurgischer Sicht. Habil.-Schrift, Würzburg 1966

Zehm, S.: Der retromaxilläre Raum. Eine Darstellung aus klinischer, röntgenologischer und chirurgischer Sicht. Thieme, Stuttgart 1970

Zöllner, F.: Die Grenzen der Operabilität der Geschwülste des Nasenrachens. Z. Laryng. Rhinol. 31: 1, 1952

Zöllner, F.: Der Lidrandschnitt nach Zange. Acta Otolaryng. (Stockholm) 46: 462, 1956

Zühlke, D.: Weiche, elastische Kunststoffe in der H.N.O.-Heilkunde. Pract. Oto-rhino-laryng. (Basel) 22: 99, 1960

12 Surgery of the Jaws

By B. Spiessl and H. M. Tschopp

Surgery of Malignant Tumors Affecting the Mandible

More than 95% of all malignant tumors affecting the mandible are carcinomas. The rest consists of sarcomas and odontogenic tumors.

TNM Classification*

For the following sites and subsites:

1. Lower alveolus and gingiva
2. Tongue
   a) Dorsal surface and lateral borders anterior to vallate papillae (anterior two-thirds)
   b) Inferior surface
3. Floor of mouth.

Rules for Classification

The classification applies only to carcinoma.

There must be histological or cytological verification of the disease. The following are the minimum requirements for assessment of the T, N, and M categories. If these cannot be met, the symbol TX, NX, or MX will be used.

T categories: Clinical examination and radiography.

N categories: Clinical examination and radiography.

M categories: Clinical examination and radiography.

---

* 3rd Edition of the TNM Classification of Malignant Tumours by the International Union against Cancer (UICC), Oct. 1978

TNM Pretreatment Clinical Classification

T – Primary Tumor

TIS Preinvasive carcinoma (carcinoma in situ).

T0 No evidence of primary tumor.

T1 Tumor 2 cm or less in its greatest dimension.

T2 Tumor more than 2 cm but not more than 4 cm in its greatest dimension.

T3 Tumor more than 4 cm in its greatest dimension and with superficial extension.

T4 Tumor with extension to bone, muscle, skin, antrum, neck, etc.

TX The minimum requirements to assess fully the extent of the primary tumor cannot be met.

N – Regional Lymph Nodes

N0 Regional lymph nodes not palpable.

N1 Movable homolateral nodes.
N1a Nodes not considered to contain growth.
N1b Nodes considered to contain growth.

N2 Movable contralateral or bilateral nodes.
N2a Nodes not considered to contain growth.
N2b Nodes considered to contain growth.

N3 Fixed nodes.

NX The minimum requirements to assess the regional lymph nodes cannot be met.

M – Distant Metastases

M0 No evidence of distant metastases.

M1 Distant metastases present.

MX The minimum requirements to assess the presence of distant metastases cannot be met.

p. TNM Postsurgical Histopathological Classification

pT **Primary Tumor**
The pT categories correspond to the T categories.

pN **Regional Lymph Nodes**
The pN categories correspond to the N categories.

pM **Distant Metastases**
The pM categories correspond to the M categories.

Stage Grouping

Stage I	T1	N0	M0
Stage II	T2	N0	M0
Stage III	T3	N0	M0
	T1, T2, T3	N1	M0
Stage IV	T4	N0, N1	M0
	Any T	N2 or N3	M0
	Any T	Any N	M1

Scheme of Indications for Functional and Classical Neck Dissection

N	T	Treatment
N0	T1	No treatment
	T2	
N0	T3	Functional or classical neck dissection
N1	T1	Functional or classical neck dissection
N1	T2	Classical neck dissection
	T3	
	T4	
N2	T1	Classical neck dissection
	T2	(If bilateral neck dissection
	T3	is carried out, usually there should
	T4	be an interval of 3 weeks)
N3	T1	Radiotherapy, followed by
	T2	classical neck dissection if there
	T3	is a significant diminution and
	T4	delineation of the lymph nodes after application of 4000 R

Site of origin of sarcomas: Undifferentiated and differentiated sarcomas may develop from mesodermal elements of any part of the jaws. They occur most frequently in the angle of the mandible and the ascending ramus. They originate from the embryonic tissue of the mandibular growth centers which contain a cartilaginous type of tissue.

The most frequently occurring sarcomas are osteogenic sarcomas, fibrosarcomas, reticulum cell sarcomas, and, in certain geographical areas, Burkitt's sarcoma.

Sarcomas of the mandible rarely metastasize to the lymph nodes (out of 43 of our cases, this occurred only in 3 patients; in 2 cases the disease was already generalized).

Tissue of origin of the ameloblastoma: This is an odontogenic tumor arising from the enamel organ and rarely from a reticular or follicular cyst of the mandible. The sites of predilection are the angle of the jaw and the ascending ramus.

Diagnostic Preoperative Measures

● History and intraoral and extraoral examination;

● Classification of the tumor by the TNM system;

● Determination of the risks of operation;

● Measurement of the blood pressure, hematocrit, full blood count, ESR, chest radiographs and an ECG. Pulmonary function tests are optional. If distant metastases are suspected, liver function tests and a skeletal series should be done.

Special Radiographs

If the primary tumor is localized in the precanine area:

● Occipitomental contact views of the mandible;

● Lateral views of the mandible, centered on the chin;

● Occlusal views of the mandible;

● Dentosubmental views of the mandible.

If the primary tumor is localized in the postcanine area:

- Posteroanterior views of the skull;
- Mandibular views of each half of the mandible;
- Mandibular views centered on the chin.

If the primary tumor is localized in the retromolar area:

- Posteroanterior skull views;
- Mandibular views of each half of the mandible;
- Rösli's transbuccal view of the ascending ramus;
- Parma's laterolateral contact view of the temporomandibular joint, with the mouth open.

Biopsy

Most carcinomas of the oral cavity can be diagnosed by the expert on the basis of their macroscopic appearance. It is preferable to verify the histological nature of the tumor during the operation with a frozen section because of the danger of tumor dissemination and secondary infection.

If a biopsy is absolutely necessary, a piece of tissue (1 cm long and 0.5 cm wide) is taken from the edge of the tumor in such a way that a piece of healthy mucosa is included. Immediately after the specimen has been removed, the wound surface is cauterized.

The preoperative and intraoperative histological examination is difficult for sarcomas of the mandible and odontogenic tumors, which may be ectodermal, mesodermal or of mixed origin. The biopsy often indicates a diagnosis different from that acquired by the histological examination of the operative specimen. For this reason, the whole clinical picture (history as well as local radiographic and laboratory findings) should be communicated to the pathologist to ensure a reliable diagnosis.

Indication

Due to the particular difficulties involved in radiological treatment of these tumors, surgery is the treatment of choice for malignant tumors affecting the mandible. "A therapeutic dose often produces extensive bone necrosis with severe pain and prolonged sequestra formation" (Berven 1931). In spite of the introduction of new sources of

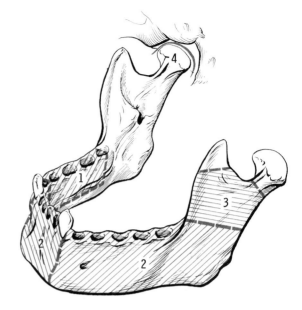

Fig. 12.1   Types of jaw resection
1 = Partial
2 = Segmental
3 = High
4 = Disarticulation

radiation and new techniques of radiotherapy, this dictum is still valid today. Depending on the extent of the tumor, one of the following procedures is indicated:

- A partial resection,
- A full-thickness or segmental resection,
- A high resection,
- A disarticulation (Fig. 12.1).

Resection of the affected segment of the mandible is also indicated in ameloblastomas and chondromas due to the danger of recurrence from local invasion of the tumor.

Partial resection with preservation of the lower border of the mandible suffices in many cases for small tumors confined to the alveolus (T1), with or without palpable lymph nodes (N0 or N1a). In doubtful cases a full-thickness resection should be carried out.

More advanced carcinomas (T2 and T3) in the region of the front teeth require resection of the arch of the chin with simultaneous functional neck dissection (N0, N1a and N2a) or classical neck dissec-

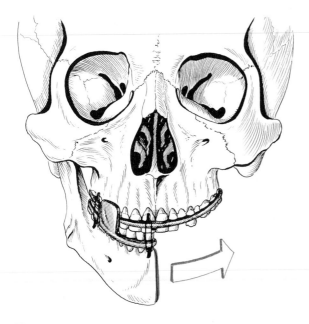

Fig. 12.2   Intermaxillary fixation of jaw segment with rubber bands and training flange. Fixation maintained for 6–8 weeks and training flange 6–8 weeks more.

tion if positive lymph nodes are present (N1 b, N2 b and N3). When the primary tumor is localized in the lateral part of the mandible, an en bloc operation is usually carried out.

Disarticulation is indicated if the angle of the jaw is involved, but in some of these cases a high resection will suffice.

Localized sarcomas can be managed with good results by resection and disarticulation. If the sarcoma extends into the surrounding tissue, resection is not indicated. Some sarcomas of the mandible are very radiosensitive, particularly the reticulum cell sarcoma.

Principles of the Operation

The operation consists of two parts:

● Radical removal of the local tumor and the regional metastases, usually en bloc.

● Prevention of significant disturbance of the masticatory function by intermaxillary fixation

of the remaining parts of the mandible or by temporary replacement of the supportive and mobile functions of the lower jaw by means of grafts or implants.

Preparation for Surgery

Prosthetic procedures. Certain prosthetic procedures are indicated to prevent deviation and displacement of the remaining segments of the mandible and to restore support to the soft tissues. The principle of these procedures, which should be carried out before the operation, is that the tissues are put at rest in the first postoperative phase and mobilized during the second phase.

Immobilization by intermaxillary fixation should be continued for at least 6 weeks. After this time the scarring process is complete. The opening and closing movements of the remaining fragments are controlled by intermaxillary fixation with rubbber bands. In more severe degrees of deviation, the splint is supplemented by a training flange. This flange fits against the buccal surface of the upper teeth and extends over 3 or 4 teeth (Fig. 12.2). The gliding surface, which brings the segments into correct occlusion, is applied at the same time as the splints in a planned resection of the lateral part of the mandible or of the chin.

The splint is removed only after scar contracture has fully formed and after the patient is able to bring the mandibular segment into correct occlusion with the help of the training flange.

An existing denture or a baseplate made on a model is used if dentition is poor or if the patient is edentulous. The mandibular prosthesis is shortened to correspond to the probable length of the remaining fragment. Occlusion rims are fashioned on the baseplate from plastic material; they fit together exactly when the mouth is closed.

The real problem in such cases is to provide intermaxillary fixation. The plates or modified dentures can only be fixed to the alveolus by circumferential wiring. Since the wire loop is not securely fixed and it also communicates with the oral cavity, the surrounding soft tissue usually becomes infected within 3 to 4 weeks. Prophylactic administration of antibiotics is hardly justifiable here. Every movement, e.g., during suction of the nasogastric tube or the mouth, causes pain from this unstable fixation wire and often produces more discomfort than the actual operative trauma. For this reason we prefer fixation of the remaining fragments with a plate screwed into position, with or without bone grafts, if the site, the extent and the malignancy of the tumor as well as the general condition of the patient permit.

Premedication. For high risk cases, we use neuroleptanalgesia (Hofstedt), which selectively acts on the thalamus, the hypothalamus, the reticular system and the gamma neurones. The following scheme of premedication is used:

One-half to one hour before the beginning of the operation, the following intramuscular injection is given: 2.5–5 mg dehydrobenzperidol (droperidol), 0.05–0.1 mg fentanyl and 0.25 mg atropine. At the time of induction of the neuroleptanalgesia, an additional 20–30 mg of dehydrobenzperidol (droperidol) and 0.2–06 mg fentanyl are administered.

Position. For lateral resection or disarticulation with en bloc neck dissection, the head and cervical spine are extended. At the same time, the head is turned toward the opposite side.

For a chin resection, the head is extended in the midline position but otherwise the position is as described above.

Superficial sterilization. The teeth and the alveolus are swabbed 3 times with 0.5% cetrimide solution on a cotton swab. Next, the oral cavity is sprayed for 3 minutes with a cetrimide spray. The skin of the face and neck are also sterilized with 80% alcohol (applied 3 times) and with 2% cetrimide (applied 3 times also).

If removal of a bone graft from the iliac crest is planned, alcohol dressings are applied overnight and the usual skin sterilization is carried out immediately before the operation.

Location of the surgical team. The surgeon stands on the side of the resection or the neck dissection (Fig. 12.3).

Fig. 12.3   Position of the surgical team

1 = Surgeon
2 = Assistant
3 = Assistant
4 = Anesthesiologist
5 = Nurse

A = Anesthesia machine
B = Mayo stand
C = I-V stand
D = Electrocoagulator
E = Microspraymatic
F = Back table
G = Surgical stand for iliac bone grafts.

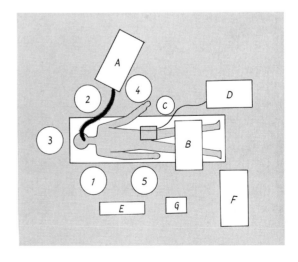

Special Instruments

The necessary instruments are illustrated in Fig.
12.4 a–g.

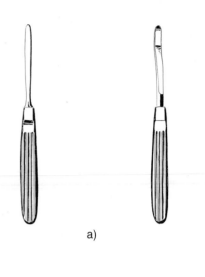

a)

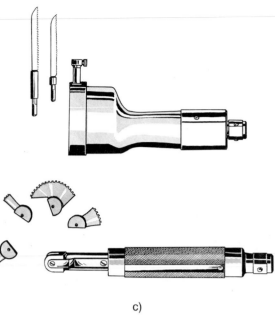

c)

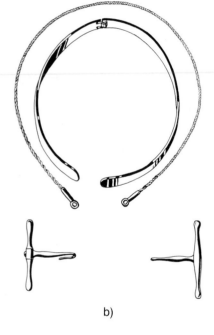

b)

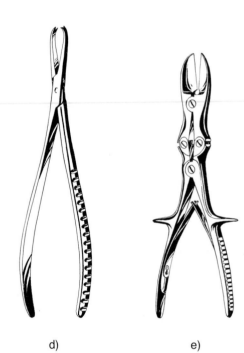

d)

e)

Fig. 12.4   Special instruments
a) Rasps
b) Gigli saw
c) Stryker saw, with special blades
d) Bone forceps
e) Bone cutter
f) AO plate
g) Various bone forceps.

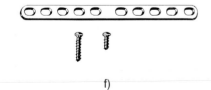

f)

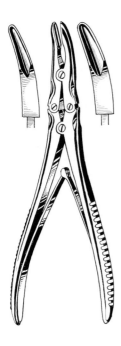

Fig. 12.4g

Anesthesia

Intubation anesthesia must be used.

Selection of the Route of Intubation

A nasal endotracheal tube is to be preferred irrespective of the location of the tumor within the mouth. The anesthetic tube is led away from the head and is fixed in such a way that it is not disturbed by intraoral and extraoral manipulation. Furthermore, pernasal intubation facilitates introduction of the tube into the trachea in patients with trismus.

Tracheostomy

A tracheostomy causes severe psychological and physical disturbance for the patient. A prophylactic tracheostomy is not necessary in a jaw resection if sufficient trained nurses are available. A preopera-

tive tracheostomy is indicated only in extensive operations such as resection of the entire mandible.

Hypotension

Induced hypotension has been shown to be useful in certain cases. It should be remembered that lowering the blood pressure too much and for too long is dangerous. The systolic blood pressure should, therefore, not be reduced below 80 mm Hg. Reduction of intraoperative blood loss is determined more by the loss of vascular tone than by the degree of blood pressure reduction.

A practical method which does not carry the danger of reactionary hemorrhage is the easily reversible hypotension achieved by the use of ganglion blockers plus lowering the patient's legs.

In most cases the use of ganglion blockers is superfluous. Careful induction of anesthesia can limit bleeding to some extent. With the reversed Trendelenburg position orthostatic forces can affect the circulation in such a way that the blood pressure is effectively reduced.

Blood and Fluid Replacement

Blood loss with a disarticulation may be extensive. On average the intraoperative and postoperative blood loss in this operation is 600–1500 ml. The amount of blood replaced should correspond to the amount of blood lost.

Since the operation is not carried out in an opened body cavity, the fluid and electrolyte loss is relatively small. It is, therefore, only necessary to prevent shock. For a resection of the mandible alone (e.g., for an adamantinoma), a colloid-free infusion (e.g., Ringer's lactate) or 10% low molecular weight dextran (e.g., Rheomacrodex) is used. Resection of the mandible with a neck dissection requires the transfusion of 500–1000 ml of blood which, if possible, should be given only toward the end of the operation.

The best protection against shock is careful hemostasis. The use of diathermy considerably reduces the formation of a seroma later.

Principles for the Incision and Exposure of the Operative Field

In *planning the incision,* the following should be taken into account:

- The extent of the operation: is mandibulectomy to be carried out alone or is it to be combined with a neck dissection?

- Primary cover of the defect in the presence of fixed lymph nodes.

- Impairment of the skin by previous radiation. In such a case, there should be no sharp angles and no suture lines over the carotid system.

One fundamental question arises during *exposure of the operative field:* Should the platysma be preserved as part of the subcutaneous tissue on the skin flap or should it be removed?

In favor of preservation of the platysma, it has been argued that the lymphatic vessels of this thin layer of muscle are involved only when the lymph nodes are fixed. If the lymph nodes are mobile, it can, therefore, be preserved.

The objections are as follows:

First, the median group of submandibular lymph nodes lies lateral to the mandible more frequently than inferior to it and, therefore, is closely related to the platysma. Elevation of the platysma thus compromises the radicality of the operation.

Second, superficial lymph glands occasionally lie between the fibers of the platysma. When the platysma is preserved, a lymph node may be overlooked.

The submandibular flap is elevated as far as the origin of the buccinator muscle at the center, to the risorius, the depressor angulae oris and depressor labii inferioris muscles anteriorly as well as to the tail of the parotid gland and the origin of the sternomastoid muscle posteriorly.

Resection of the Center of the Mandible (Chin Resection)

Operative Technique

The operation starts with the removal of a piece of bone from the iliac crest (see p. 178).

Splitting the Center of the Lower Lip, Circumscribing the Tumor in the Vestibule

Resection begins with the extraction of a tooth on each side of the point where the division of the mandible is planned. The tumor is circumscribed with a cautery knife in the vestibule of the mouth, leaving a margin of 1.5 cm from its border, without penetrating in depth.

Before the lip is split in the midline, the vermilion border is marked on both sides of the midline with the point of a cannula dipped in methylene blue (Fig. 12.5 a). The lip is held with a Sadinski clamp on both sides and is stretched in the center (Fig. 12.5 b). It is divided in layers between the clamps to form a Blair-Brown flap within the vermilion. The incision is extended on both sides along the submandibular area as far as the mastoid process (see above, with elevation of the submandibular skin flaps).

After splitting the lip, the circumscribing incision is encountered within the vestibule; a gaping wound is formed which allows the submucous and subcutaneous extent of the tumor to be both seen and felt.

According to the extent of invasion, parts of the muscle inserted into the bone may be left in place. The periosteum is elevated on each side of the site of resection, both on the vestibular and on the lingual sides.

To permit visual inspection, the mandible is not yet exposed on its lingual side. On the vestibular side, however, the lateral part of the lower border of the mandible including the angle is freed in preparation for the later screwing into position of the plate.

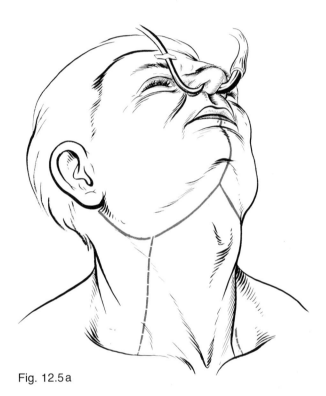

Fig. 12.5 a

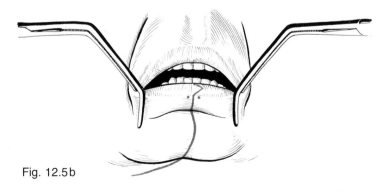

Fig. 12.5 b

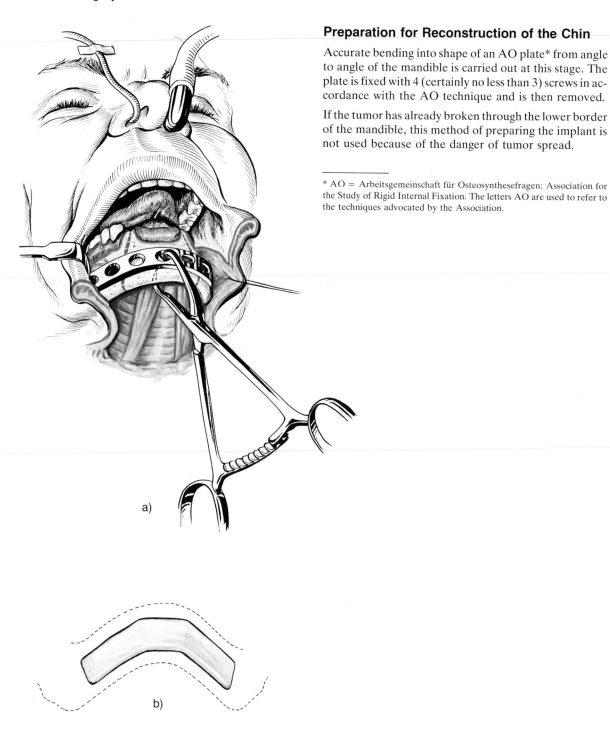

a)

Preparation for Reconstruction of the Chin

Accurate bending into shape of an AO plate* from angle to angle of the mandible is carried out at this stage. The plate is fixed with 4 (certainly no less than 3) screws in accordance with the AO technique and is then removed.

If the tumor has already broken through the lower border of the mandible, this method of preparing the implant is not used because of the danger of tumor spread.

---

* AO = Arbeitsgemeinschaft für Osteosynthesefragen: Association for the Study of Rigid Internal Fixation. The letters AO are used to refer to the techniques advocated by the Association.

b)

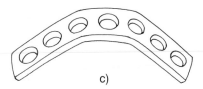

c)

Fig. 12.6   a) Shows the AO plate in place (before resection) to achieve exact and stable fixation of the stumps of the jaw. Holes have already been drilled in the jaw. The plate is screwed into position and is then removed. b) Shows a lead template for modeling the steel or titanium plate. c) Shows a 7-hole titanium plate. which conforms to the original form of the mandible.

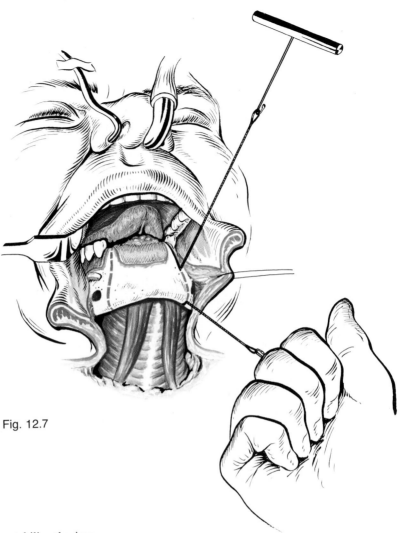

Fig. 12.7

Division of the Bone

A mouth gag is introduced laterally to stabilize the jaw with the mouth wide open. A Gigli saw is introduced around the mandible from the floor of the mouth at the point of division (Fig. 12.7). A Lindemann drill or a Stryker saw may also be used. To facilitate division on the opposite side, the bone is not yet completely divided. The bone is first divided completely on the opposite side and the cut is completed on the first side.

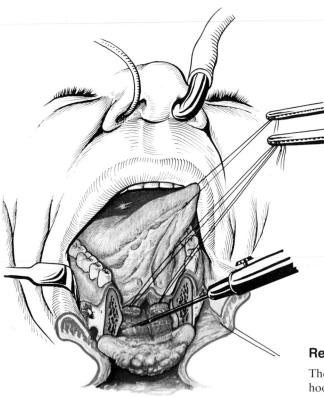

Fig. 12.8

Removal of the Specimen

The specimen is retracted forward with bone forceps or a hook while an assistant draws the tip of the tongue upward and forward. This maneuver brings the sublingual region into view, and the tumor can be circumscribed on this side under vision, 1.5 cm from its edges. No consideration is given to the duct of the submandibular gland.

The genioglossus and the geniohyoid muscles are dissected out with forceps. Each is fixed with a 3 × 0 Mersilene suture and the muscles are then divided with the cautery knife on the tumor side of the sutures (Fig. 12.8). The specimen can now be displaced forward. In this way the view into the wound is preserved in spite of the fact that the operative area is highly vascular. The mylohyoid muscle, which is under tension, is now held with an additional suture and divided on the side of the tumor. This is repeated with the digastric muscles. The specimen is now divided at its edges, in a clockwise direction from within outward, and is sent for frozen section.

Reconstruction of the Mandibular Arch in the Presence of a Small Mucosal Defect

While the specimen is being examined histologically, the stumps of the mandible are fixed in their original position by srewing the AO* plate in place (see p. 187) (Fig. 12.9). A lead template of the size of the specimen is made, and the graft is shaped using this template. Four holes are drilled in the middle of the graft and stay sutures are introduced through them to reinsert the muscles of the floor of the mouth. The graft is fixed under pressure with several screws (Fig. 12.10).

---

* Adjustable compression plate.

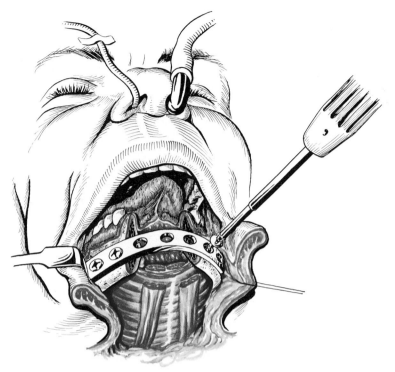

Fig. 12.9

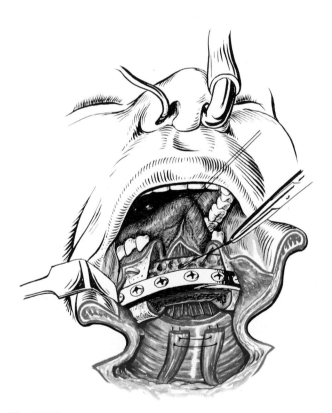

Fig. 12.10

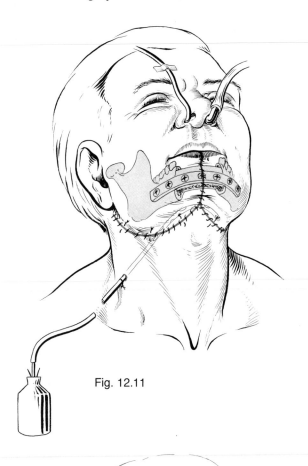

Fig. 12.11

Soft Tissue Repair

This is carried out from within outward. The mucosal defect can be closed with local tissue. Sometimes a flap must be formed, pedicled lingually, turned in the labial direction and stitched to the edges of the horizontal part of the wound. The tip of the tongue can be mobilized again with an epithelial inlay in a later operation. The labial mucosa is sutured with a continuous suture of atraumatic 4×0 Supramid as far as the Blair-Brown flap. The orbicularis oris muscle is then sutured with 4×0 polyglycolic acid (Dexon). The vermilion border is then sutured accurately using the intracutaneous points marked with methylene blue. The wound edges are adapted with 6–8 vertical mattress sutures on each side and a continuous skin suture (4×0 or 5×0 Supramid) (Fig. 12.11).

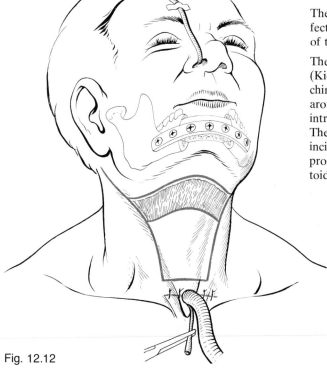

Fig. 12.12

Reconstruction of the Mandibular Arch in the Presence of a Large Mucosal Defect

The problem here is primary cover of a large mucosal defect following radical removal of an extensive carcinoma of the anterior part of the jaw.

The apron-flap method appears to be a useful method (Kiehn and Desprez 1964). A skin flap pedicled on the chin is created from the central region of the neck, turned around the newly created mandibular arch and sutured intraorally to the remaining mucosa of the oral cavity. The incision is shown in Figure 12.12. A submandibular incision is made on both sides beginning at the mastoid process and is continued along the line of the sternomastoid muscle down to the sternoclavicular joint.

Both incisions are joined in the suprasternal notch to form an apron flap pedicled on the submental and submandibular areas. It should be long enough to be drawn without tension through the incision into the mouth (Fig. 12.13). The flap serves to cover the graft lying between the two mandibular fragments. To allow reinsertion of the muscles of the floor of the mouth on the inner side of the reconstructed mandibular arch, the epithelium is re-

moved from the flap in the appropriate area (Figs. 12.12, 12.14). The resulting island flap is sutured with a continuous suture of 4×0 Supramid to the free edges of the wound of the oral cavity, the tongue and the alveolus. The graft bed is drained on both sides with a suction drain. The defect in the center of the neck is covered with a free split-skin graft.

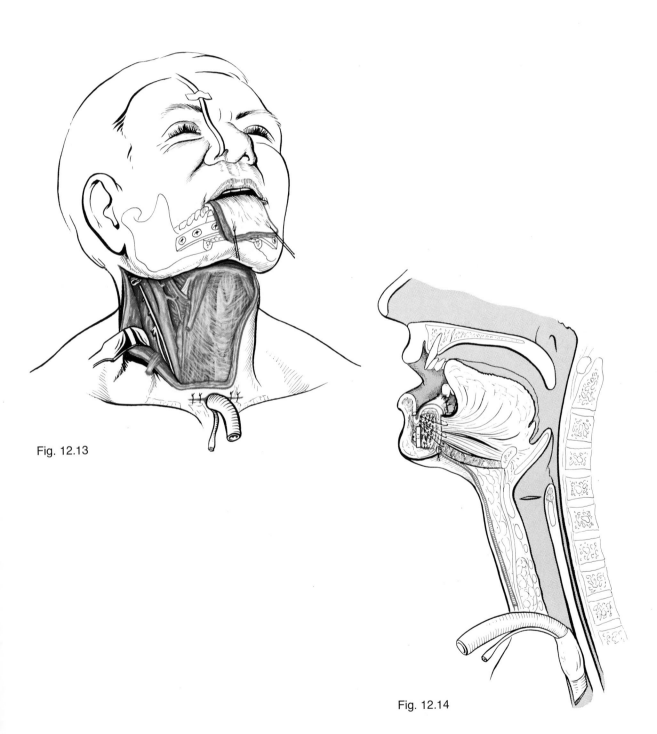

Fig. 12.13

Fig. 12.14

Extended Chin Resection

In principle this operation is the same as that described above. Primary bone grafting, however, cannot always be recommended. The decision is largely dependent on the size of the defect to be bridged. Immediate replacement of large parts of the mandible is not advisable. The overriding consideration is that permanent healing is more important than reconstruction. Consequently, the mandibular stumps are fixed in the manner described above, but without the insertion of a graft. Here the stability of the implant is important. In our experience all prefabricated steel frameworks, wires and metal plates are too weak in terms of anchorage and stability. A loosening of the implant which in turn causes rarefaction and infection of the bony stumps occurs at the latest with mobilization (removal of intermaxillary fixation) and most certainly with function. Steel implants in the shape of a gutter filled with bone chips are recommended to reduce this danger. The bone chips are, however, resorbed; what remains in the metal gutter is, at the most, calcified scar tissue.

Fixation of the mandibular stumps by means of an implant is a biomechanical problem. An implant used as a replacement for the mandibular arch can resist strong traction only if the implant *and* its anchorage are absolutely stable. The small, adjustable AO plates do not fulfil these requirements. We now use the dynamic compression plate (used in surgery of the extremities). This plate has 10 symmetrically placed holes and is composed of 99% technically pure titanium. Since the tension caused by bending and pressure around the points of anchorage is considerable because of the high leverage forces and since the depth of the screws in the mandible is relatively shallow (between 12 and 16 mm), at least 3 screws should be used on each side to guarantee the necessary frictional adhesion between the plate and the bone. Our experience indicates that, because of the stable connection and the good tissue tolerance exhibited by titanium, healing occurs even after preoperative radiotherapy up to doses of 4000–5000 R.

The great advantage of this method is that, since intraoral and extraoral fixation are no longer necessary, the mouth may be opened immediately. This considerably facilitates postoperative nursing care and oral hygiene.

Lateral Resection of the Mandible

(with preservation of the chin and the ascending ramus)

Operative Technique

For carcinomas of types T1 and T2 or where the tumor is located posterior to the canine teeth the resection can be carried out by a submandibular approach without splitting the lip. If resection of the mandible through the canine tooth or anterior to it is necessitated because of the extent of the tumor, elevation of the overlying soft tissues as far as the midline is advisable (Fig. 12.15). After the lip has been split, the submandibular incision is made, beginning at the chin and proceeding backward along the inferior edge of the mandible and then turning upward. The cheek is then dissected free from the tumor on the oral side.

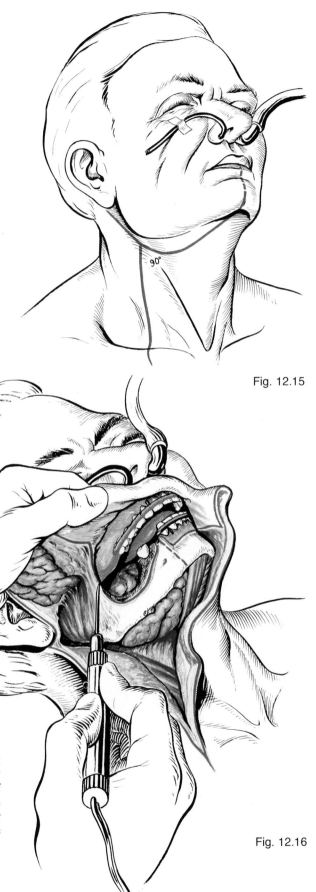

Fig. 12.15

Without doubt this method of exposure allows the best view. If necessary, the mandible can be exposed widely without endangering the marginal mandibular branch of the facial nerve. The masseter muscle is dissected free from anteriorly and above rather than from the inferior edge of the mandible if the site and extension of the tumor permit (Fig. 12.16).

Fig. 12.16

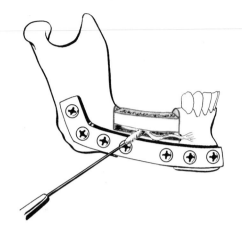

Fig. 12.17

The resection is carried out with the Lindemann drill; the cortex is divided on the lingual side with Liston scissors. The advantage of this technique is that, since the lingual side remains completely intact up to this step, hemorrhage is slight. Furthermore, the specimen can be drawn outward so that the tumor can be cut around along the floor of the mouth under good vision. Finally, this technique facilitates preservation of the inferior dental nerve. This nerve is preserved in certain cases, for example with an ameloblastic fibroma (benign odontogenic mixed tumor). Figure 12.17 shows primary reconstruction of the mandible by means of an iliac-crest graft following removal of a benign tumor. The illustrations show replacement of the preserved inferior dental nerve within the graft.

In such cases primary reconstruction with a transplanted iliac-crest graft using a stable form of fixation is a most important part of the operation (Fig. 12.17). If the angle between the body of the mandible and the ascending ramus must be replaced, angled plates of varying lengths are used (Fig. 12.18).

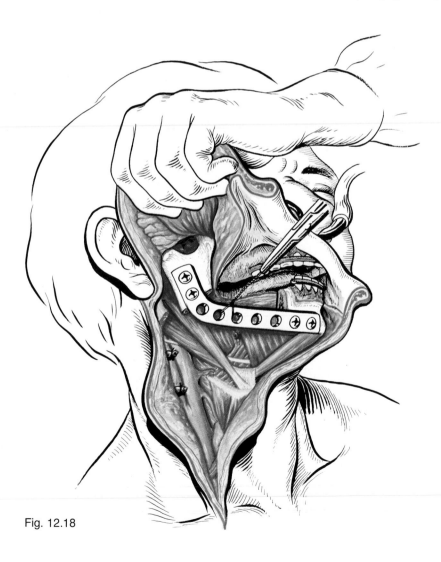

Fig. 12.18

If such a plate is not available, a piece of rib is fixed in place using dynamic compression plates (from the AO mandibular set – Spiessl 1972) positioned proximally and distally (see Fig. 12.63). Figure 12.18 demonstrates stable fixation of the mandibular stumps with an AO angled plate following lateral resection. The remaining soft tissues are fixed to the plate with steel wires to prevent contracture. The plate is shortened by cutting at both ends in accordance with the extent of the defect.

Stable fixation of a rib graft with compression plates (DCP's) rather than unstable wires is shown in Figure 12.19. The musculature of the floor of the mouth and of the tongue is reinserted to the graft to prevent contracture and to improve revascularization of the graft. Figure 12.20 shows the final results following lateral resection of the mandible. Intermaxillary fixation is necessary in this case because the short stump of the condyle cannot be fixed rigidly to the graft (only 1 screw can be used rather than the recommended minimum of 3). If a simultaneous radical neck dissection is carried out, 3 suction drains (Redon drains) should be introduced.

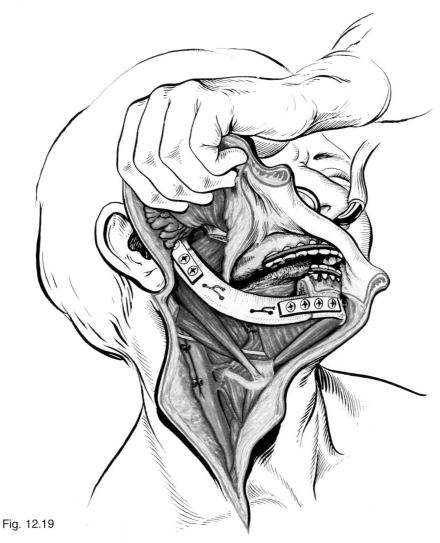

Fig. 12.19

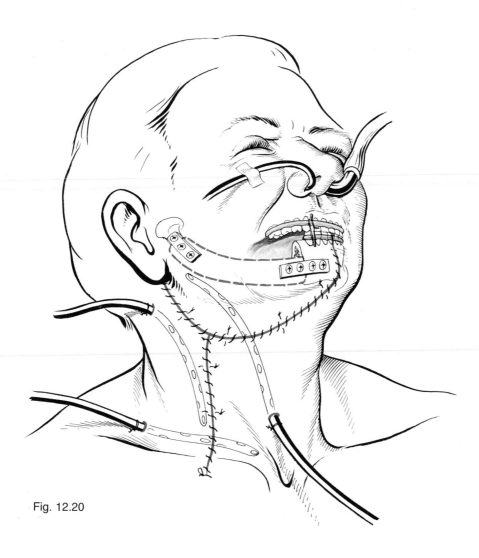

Fig. 12.20

Disarticulation

This is indicated for adamantinomas and other primary tumors of the ascending ramus because preservation of the articular process and the muscles can easily lead to recurrence. The muscles inserted into the ascending ramus direct the recurrence toward the base of the skull or the temporal fossa. If resection has not been radical enough, the recurrence then develops at a most unfavorable site.

In patients with a carcinoma, the necessity for disarticulation is determined by the intraosseous extent of the tumor. Usually there is a sharply demarcated, semicircular zone of destruction in the postcanine area. Radiologically, the tumor is therefore confined to the horizontal ramus. In this case a high resection rather than disarticulation suffices; division is carried out at the lower part of the neck of the mandible. This procedure saves time in a commando operation (which is important), since the condyle stump is extremely useful for reconstruction (Fig. 12.21, see also 12.20).

The other form of extension of a carcinoma into the mandible is in an axial direction along the mandibular canal. The radiograph shows a continuous area of destruction along the horizontal and ascending ramus. Here disarticulation is strongly indicated, as is generally the case when the angle of the mandible is involved.

Operative Technique

Skin Incision and Lateral Exposure of the Mandible

It is advisable to split the lower lip for disarticulation. The incision proceeds along a skin crease in the neck and the flap so delineated is raised (see p. 149). The lip and the soft tissues of the cheek are retracted laterally so that the site and extent of the tumor can be easily seen. The soft tissues of the cheek are dissected off parallel to the external surface of the mandible leaving a margin of at least 1.5 cm around the tumor.

If the carcinoma extends into the alveolobuccal sulcus, the cheek is often swollen, partly as a result of secondary infection and partly as a result of tumor infiltration. Correct assessment of such swelling of the cheek is difficult, particularly when there has been previous radiotherapy. In this case a frozen section of the deeper parts of the wound edges is essential.

The soft tissues surrounding the site of origin of the tumor as well as the masseter and its tendon are divided successively with a cautery knife; the external surface of the mandible is then exposed up to the mandibular notch (see Fig. 12.16).

First step: The mandible is divided anteriorly (see p. 149) and the attachments of the floor of the mouth are detached. The first assistant retracts the tongue to the midline, putting the floor of the mouth under tension, while the freed jaw segment is retracted with a single hook. The cautery knife is applied to the buccinator crest, then brought forward along the posterior part of the floor of the mouth parallel to the mandible to open the sublingual space by dividing the lingual sulcus. The mylohyoid muscle is detached.

Second step: The faucial isthmus is separated from the mandible, the temporal muscle is separated from the coronoid process and the pterygoid muscle is exposed (see Fig. 12.21). The pterygomandibular ligament is divided from the buccinator crest externally so that the insertion of the temporalis muscle can be divided easily with the cautery knife on the inner side of the coronoid process. Strong scissors can be helpful at the point of origin of the coronoid process. The specimen can now be retracted inferiorly and externally so that the coronoid process can be freed from beneath the zygomatic arch. If the condyle itself is invaded by tumor, the zygomatic arch may need to be resected.

Next, the head of the mandible is retracted externally so that access to the pterygomandibular space is considerably facilitated (Fig. 12.21). The medial pterygoid muscle can now be either dissected off or divided from in front, depending on the extent of the tumor. The advantage of this method is that, while access exclusively from the lower border of the mandible (i.e., from inferiorly and posteriorly) does not permit an anatomical dissection, division of the pterygoid muscles can be carried out under vision since the inner side of the mandible is exposed (see Fig. 12.21). In this way structures such as the lingual nerve and the maxillary artery can be protected from unnecessary damage. The neurovascular bundle leaving the mandibular foramen is grasped with a hemostat and divided.

Third step: Opening of the joint. The insertion of the pterygoid muscles (see Fig. 12.21) is divided, the capsule is opened and the specimen is removed from the joint. The remaining muscular and capsular attachments are divided with Metzenbaum scissors.

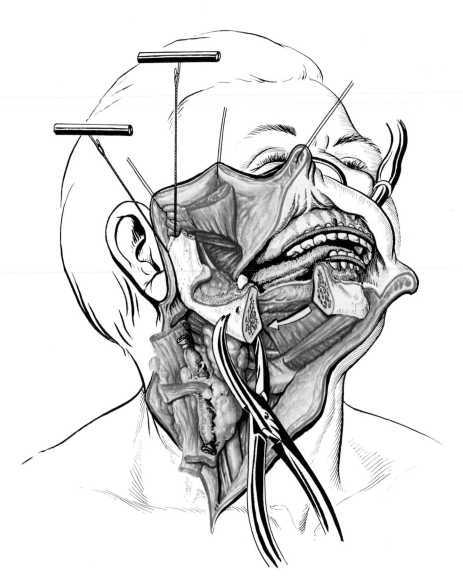

Fig. 12.21   External rotation of the part of the mandible to be resected in a high resection (the same procedure is carried out for disarticulation).

The purpose of this step is to provide access under vision to the anatomical structures of the floor of the mouth and to the pterygomandibular space. In a high resection with division of the base of the condylar and coronoid processes and in disarticulation, intermaxillary fixation by splinting of the remaining mandible is necessary. Grafts of artificial condylar heads have not been completely successful.

Simultaneous Intra-operative Prostheses and Free Grafts

Prostheses after disarticulation and implants of an artificial mandibular head have proved to be completely unsatisfactory. Resorption and fistulas at the site of fixation regularly occur following the emplacement of an implant, because the latter does not provide satisfactory support during opening and closing of the jaw. It is not advisable to attempt such forms of reconstruction. In the first postoperative weeks, it is important to maintain the remaining part of the mandible in normal occlusion with a splint. Later, opening and correct closure of the jaw should be possible without a splint. This is achieved by employing a training flange which is fastened to a wire-Palavit splint (a splint consisting of the previously prepared body with transverse bars, wire ligatures and self-hardening plastic), a denture or hinged plate depending on the dentition of the remaining part of the mandible (see p. 136). If the remaining segment is edentulous, an upper plate with the guiding flange attached by polymerization is used for a period (Fig. 12.22).

Such procedures cannot, of course, be carried out if the upper and lower jaws are edentulous. In this case daily exercises are done for 1 to 2 hours, beginning 3 weeks after the operation. The exercises are performed in front of a mirror; the hand is used to grasp the chin and guide the jaw. The left hand is used for the right stump; the right hand, for the left stump.

Wound closure. The wound is closed from within outward. The floor of the mouth as well as the mucous membrane of the tongue and cheek are sutured with continuous atraumatic sutures. (4 × 0 Supramid). Three suction drains are introduced in the submandibular, nuchal and supraclavicular positions.

Skin closure. Skin closure is carried out as described on page 146.

Important Modifications and Surgical Alternatives

Mandibulectomy, including disarticulation, has undergone no major modifications since the exemplary description given by Dieffenbach. Whether the mandible is divided with a Gigli saw, a Lindemann drill or an oscillating saw is unimportant. The division of the lip is a more important question. When only the lateral part of the body of the mandible between the canine tooth and the angle or the angle itself is to be resected, the lip should not be divided provided that the tumor is small (T1 and T2) or is of low-grade malignancy (e.g., adamantinoma). In this regard the question of whether the described access allows a sufficiently radical operation will always be crucial. Generally, we also prefer to divide the lip in order to exteriorize the intraoral part of the operation. Functionally and cosmetically, there is little difference between dividing the soft tissues of the lip and chin in the midline or in a curved line in the creases.

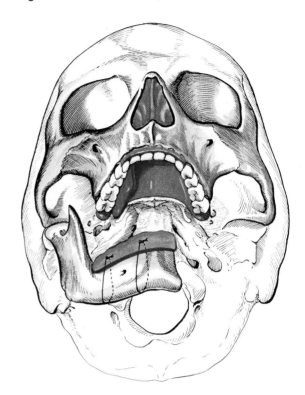

Fig. 12.22   Orthodontic management after disarticulation of an edentulous mandible. The remaining stump is provided with a base plate fixed with two wire loops and the upper jaw with a palatal plate to which the training flange and the artificial teeth are attached by polymerization.

Landmarks and Danger Points

The following **anatomical landmarks** are critical for resection and disarticulation of the mandible:

● For the incision: The center of the lower lip, the hyoid bone (natural neck crease) and the mastoid process.

● For the exposure: The lower border of the mandible, the external surface of the platysma, the angle of the jaw, the buccinator crest, the notch, the capsule of the parotid gland and the cervical fascia.

● For the resection: The tooth sockets or the gap between the teeth; the mandibular canal in benign tumors.

● For disarticulation: The buccinator crest, the pterygomandibular ligament, the notch, the coronoid process, the neck of the mandible and the capsule of the temporomandibular joint.

Danger points. There are two dangerous moments during disarticulation:

1. During freeing or resection of the pterygoid muscle,

2. During freeing of the mandibular head.

Sites of Hemorrhage

These include:

● The mandibular vessels in the pterygomandibular fossa or the posterior facial vein which is formed by the union of the superficial temporal vein and the maxillary veins (for example, during division of the medial pterygoid muscle from the lower border of the mandible).

● The maxillary artery which runs medial to the neck of the mandible between the 2 heads of the lateral pterygoid muscle in the direction of the pterygopalatine fossa (see Fig. 12.21). Since the muscles are inserted into the ascending ramus and the disc, they can be freed without danger of brisk hemorrhage only by exposing the inner surface of the mandible or by cutting very closely along the bone. In tumors of the mandibular head, exposure of the medial side can be achieved only after prior resection of the root of the zygoma or of the entire zygomatic arch.

● The pterygoid plexus is another source of hemorrhage. If brisk venous bleeding occurs from this area, the muscular tissue must not be damaged by excessive use of the cautery knife. It is preferable to pack the entire area for 5 to 10 minutes with a warm saline pack. The pack is removed gradually allowing the bleeding points to be found and sutured or possibly covered with muscle tissue.

● Bleeding from the superficial temporal and buccal arteries is easily controlled.

Nerve Damage

If the inferior dental artery and nerve are not clamped and divided exactly at the lingula, there is a danger that the lingual nerve and the chorda tympani which run parallel to them will be damaged or divided.

During disarticulation of a tumor-invaded mandibular head when it has been invaded by tumor, the auriculotemporal nerve can be damaged.

There are few reports of damage to the branches of the facial nerve during disarticulation. However, such damage may occur if, in order to achieve complete removal of the tumor, the masseter muscle must be included in the resection. Involvement of the parotid gland is unusual and generally indicates inoperability if the site of origin of the primary tumor is in the mouth. In such cases the main branch should be sought and the most important of the resected branches should be replaced by a nerve graft.

Peripheral resection of the mandible has no particular danger points.

Rules, Hints and Typical Errors

● The incision should be planned carefully. The malignancy of the tumor, its staging, previous treatment (in particular radiotherapy), the extent of the operation (if lymph nodes are clinically enlarged an en bloc operation is always carried out) and primary or secondary reconstruction should be taken into consideration.

● A good view of the operative field should be obtained using one of the following techniques:

1. Exteriorization of the area of origin of the tumor by splitting the lower lip (e.g., in T2 and T3 tumors):
   a) Exposure of the external surface of the mandible;
   b) Extension of the incision around the primary tumor in the vestibule;
   c) Division in continuity;
   d) Extension of the incision on the lingual side around the primary tumor;
   e) Exposure of the inner surface of the mandible with the attached muscles and the neighboring soft tissues.

2. A combination of the intraoral and extraoral technique for small tumors (e.g., T1 and T2):
   a) Circumscription of the primary tumor within the oral cavity;
   b) Resection of the mandible in the area of the intraoral incision with an external approach.

3. Extraoral technique (usually without opening the oral mucosa), e.g., for odontogenic tumors of low-grade malignancy, central giant cell tumors and fibrous dysplasia.

● Permanent healing is the overriding consideration rather than reconstruction. There are 4 reasons for this:

1. Early recognition of a recurrence is made considerably more difficult by the presence of a graft or an implant.

2. Primary reconstruction in this area of the mouth often fails.

3. Reconstruction can prolong the operation to unacceptable limits.

4. Follow-up shows that the vast majority of patients are satisfied with the conditions after resection of the mandible so that there is little interest in further reconstructive measures.

In summary, primary reconstruction should only be carried out when it is absolutely necessary for the prevention of postoperative complications and for cosmetically unacceptable results.

Hints

● In chin resection, the individual muscle bundles of the floor of the mouth should be fixed with retention sutures before they are divided.

● Liston scissors should be used for the resection.

● In disarticulation, the specimen should be rotated externally and the internal surface of the mandible should be freed from in front backward (i.e., not beginning at the lower border of the mandible and proceeding internally and upward).

● If the head of the mandible is expanded due to tumor invasion, the zygomatic arch should be temporarily resected.

● If the masseter muscle is invaded by tumor and the parotid gland is involved, the preauricular incision should be extended as is the case for a parotidectomy. The facial nerve trunk and the marginal mandibular and buccal branches of the facial nerve should be exposed *before* the mandible is skeletonized.

● The wound should be intermittently irrigated with Ringer's solution.

Typical Errors

Minimizing the presumed degree of mutilation at the cost of radicality (e.g., failing to split the lip when the primary tumor is in an unfavorable position or carrying out a primary repair of the bone in spite of a large mucosal defect and a poor bed for the graft).

Postoperative Care

Prophylactic antibiotic therapy is not a routine procedure if the operation lasts less than 2 hours. With operations of longer duration, postoperative prophylactic antibiotic therapy may be administered under certain circumstances such as secondary infection of the tumor and extensive en bloc resection, introduction of a graft or an implant. In general, penicillin (20–40 million I.U. per day) combined with streptomycin (1 gram per day) is administered by continuous intravenous infusion.

Important: The optimal antibiotic level should be achieved before surgery is begun.

In the first few hours after surgery:

After chin resection, disarticulation and extensive en bloc operations, the patient is attended constantly by a nurse. Oxygen is insufflated pernasally through a nasopharyngeal tube.

In the days following surgery:

Replacement of metabolic and fluid balance by feeding via a nasogastric tube. The following is an example of the composition of a fluid diet:

Spiessl's diet: (This diet does not contain starches: starch tends to adhere to the suture and, thereby, encourages wound infection).

7:00 a.m. Coffee with 200 g milk
Mixture of:
    1   egg
    100 g banana
    100 g fruit juice
    10 g sugar

9:00 a.m. Tea with 10 g sugar
Yoghurt mixture consisting of:
    180 g yoghurt
    Nescafe or powdered cocoa
    100 g milk
    10 g sugar

12:00 a.m. Cream of vegetable soup consisting of:
    200 g broth
    50 g vegetable purée (e.g., asparagus)
    5   g butter
    10 g cream
    200 g carrot juice

Mixture of:
    1   egg
    100 g banana
    100 g orange juice
    20 g cream

Cottage cheese dish consisting of:
    100 g cottage cheese
    Spices, (e.g., salt, paprika, curry, tomato ketchup or Worcestershire sauce broth)
    20 g cream

4:00 p.m. Tea with 10 g sugar

6:00 p.m. Broth with one egg
    200 g tomato juice

Mixture of:
    1   egg
    100 g banana
    100 g grape juice
    20 g cream

Yoghurt mixture of:
    100 g yoghurt
    100 g pineapple juice
    20 g honey

This daily amount contains:
    72 g protein
    94 g fat
    224 g carbohydrate
    2388 calories.

Intravenous hyperalimentation should be considered for patients in poor nutritional and general condition. It may be necessary in either extensive ulcerating carcinomas affecting the mandible or a recurrence when postoperative radiotherapy must be given as soon as possible after a subtotal resection. Radiotherapy can often not be given because of the poor healing properties, particularly in those patients who have difficulties eating after surgery.

In order to convert the existing catabolism to anabolism and to improve the nutritional status within a reasonable time, hypertonic solutions of protein hydrolysate and glucose are given by the *central venous route*.

Recently, intravenous hyperalimentation has been carried out by a central venous catheter. This has replaced the intravenous route since it allows the necessary rapid dilution of concentrated solutions in the blood. If the catheter is introduced into the vena cava, thrombosis develops less frequently than if it lies in the subclavian vein. Certain general complications, however, must always be expected since relatively large quantities of fluid are being given to a patient whose regulatory mechanisms are impaired. Furthermore, a central venous catheter can provide a means of access for infection, particularly since the highly concentrated solutions provide an ideal culture medium for bacteria. These complications occur less often in such patients because hyperalimentation is employed for only 2 to 3 weeks at the most, during which time the patient's condition improves remarkably.

We have repeatedly observed that infection of the resected area and of a pedicled flap in a marasmic patient is brought under control within 2 weeks by hyperalimentation and intensive irrigation.

The initial improvement in the general condition of the patient and, therefore, in wound healing and the resistance to infection is achieved by administering protein hydrolysate or amino acids in a ratio of 100–150 calories per gram of nitrogen. Calories must be given at the same time to ensure that the infused amino acids are not converted primarily into energy. Glucose may be used since it releases insulin and stimulates protein synthesis. Fat emulsion prepared from soya oil reduces the osmotic load by replacing the hypertonic glucose solution with an isotonic fat emulsion, which reduces the danger of hyperglycemia. Furthermore, the fat emulsions contain the essential fatty acids. Regular clinical and laboratory controls should be carried out by a specialist in this field in order to prevent complications such as fluid retention, electrolyte imbalance and metabolic acidosis. Since this method is both costly and time consuming, it should be used only for very strict indications regardless of how desirable it may be to conduct postoperative hypercaloric therapy in all patients with extensive mouth cancer. Tube feeding should be resumed as soon as possible in patients being fed intravenously so that adequate nutrition is continued.

Venous thrombosis is prevented by early mobilization. The patient is allowed to sit up and to get up for 1–2 hours on the first postoperative day. Anticoagulants are not usually necessary.

The patient must expectorate secretions to *prevent palmonary complications*. Repeated suction of the mouth and throat is necessary, especially in patients with intraoral splints.

Additional measures: Inhalations should be administered.

The *bottle on the suction drain should be changed* 3 times daily for the first few days after surgery.

Functional Sequelae

Limitation or persistent disturbances of mastication are produced by displacement of the remaining stumps as a result of muscle traction and wound contracture. These disturbances are more pronounced in the edentulous mandible.

The provision of dentures is difficult, even with the best bone repairs, since the alveolar crest is not present to act as a base for the denture. An additional operation on the bone and the soft tissues of the vestibule is required to provide such a base. The operation is justifiable only in exceptional cases (e.g., a mixed odontogenic tumor or a locally invasive adamantinoma) since further operations in the area of resection make aftercare difficult.

A functionally and esthetically acceptable denture can be fitted in patients with a good dentition of the remaining fragments. The prerequisite is metallic blocking of the remaining teeth.

Although swallowing is only slightly disturbed after lateral resection or disarticulation, a fairly long interval is necessary for the loss of the muscles of the floor of the mouth to be compensated for after resection of the center of the mandible.

The feeding tube is left in place for several weeks. During this period, at the latest 3 weeks after the operation, the patient practices drinking tea with a spoon. The exercises are initially supervised by a nurse who must suck out the mouth and throat if the patient coughs.

Speech is difficult for a period of time but there is no permanent serious impairment.

Corrective Surgery of the Jaws

Introduction

The purpose of orthopedic operations on the jaws is to correct deformed bone, bony fragments which have healed in displacement, and anomalies of occlusion. In general, corrective operations are referred to as osteotomies.

Types of Osteotomy

The following types must be differentiated:

● According to the way in which the bone is divided:

Transverse (Fig. 12.23),
Sagittal (Fig. 12.24),
Wedge-shaped (Fig. 12.25),
Stepped (Fig. 12.26).

● The purpose of the operation:

Shortening (Figs. 12.23a, 12.24a, 12.26a),
Lengthening (Figs. 12.23b, 12.24b, 12.26b),
Rotation (Figs. 12.25, 12.27),
Displacement (Figs. 12.28).

● According to the method:

Displacement osteotomy:

Shortening or lengthening by formation of fragments with large surfaces (Fig. 12.24),

Resection osteotomy:

Shortening by resection of a transverse segment (Fig. 12.23a),

Lengthening osteotomy:

Lengthening by interposition of a bone graft (Fig. 12.23).

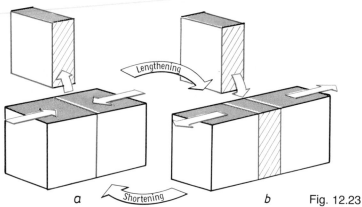

a   Shortening   b

Fig. 12.23
Transverse osteotomy
Shortening osteotomy
Resection osteotomy
Lengthening osteotomy
and bone graft.

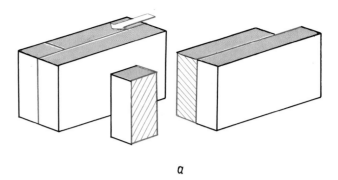

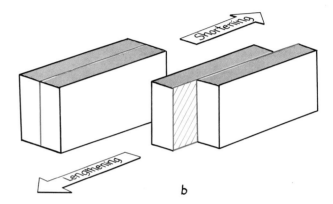

Fig. 12.24
Sagittal osteotomy
Shortening osteotomy (relative shortening by
retroposition of one half)
Lengthening osteotomy (true lengthening by
anteropositioning of the other half)
Displacement osteotomy.

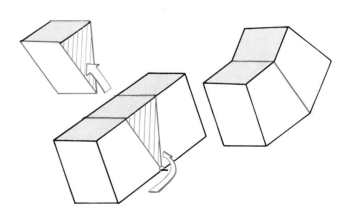

Fig. 12.25
Wedge osteotomy
Rotation osteotomy.

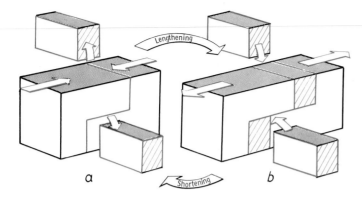

Fig. 12.26
Stepped osteotomy
Shortening osteotomy
Lengthening osteotomy and bone graft.

Fig. 12.27   Rotation osteotomy.

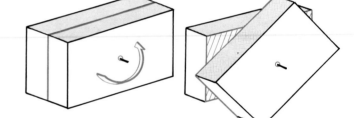

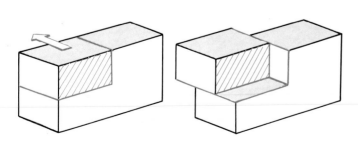

Fig. 12.28   Displacement osteotomy.

Fixation

Fixation is as important as the execution of the osteotomy. External, internal or combined fixation is used depending on the site and type of osteotomy in order to ensure the precision of the osteotomy until bony bealing has occurred (see. p. 181).

Bone grafting (see p. 176), in many cases is an integral part of the displacement osteotomy and of certain operations for improving the contours of the face. It is indicated in secondary bony defects and for correction of the profile of the lower part of the face, e.g., building up the prominence of the chin.

Osteoplasty also serves to wedge the fragments in the desired position, and prevents, for example, relapse of the position of the fragments in a Le Fort I or Le Fort III osteotomy.

Indications

Surgical procedures are indicated if the possibilities of orthodontic management have been exhausted. This generally applies to patients over the age of eighteen with failure of skeletal development or with posttraumatic jaw deformities.

Functional disturbances are a crucial indication, but in certain cases esthetic considerations are also important. Operations for improving masticatory function are, therefore, often combined with a procedure to improve the shape of the face.

Diagnostic Preoperative Measures: Aesthetic and Functional Analysis

The jaw deformity is measured before each operation by means of radiographs and photographs. The facial skeleton is divided for this purpose into 3 sections of equal height (Leonardo da Vinci):

Upper part of the face or forehead third,
Middle part of the face or nasal third,
Lower part of the face or the mandibular third.

This ratio is largely theoretical. For example, the lower part of the face in many individuals is 5 to 10 millimeters longer than the middle part and this in no way distorts the balance of the face.

The sharp division between the middle and lower parts of the face is also not really possible since the upper third of the lower part of the face (base of the maxilla with the dental arch) determines the form of the middle third of the face. For this reason the upper third of the lower part of the face is included in the middle third.

Division of the face into 3 segments of equal height is, however, a useful method of confirming whether one segment of the face is underdeveloped or overdeveloped compared to another segment. The basic types illustrated in Figures 12.30–12.35 are used as orientation aids for determining the disproportion of the lower and middle parts of the face (Köle 1968) based on division of the face into 3 parts and a vertical profile line (Fig. 12.29).

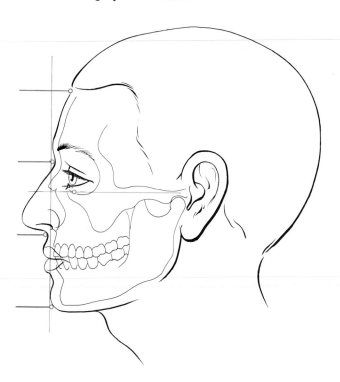

Fig. 12.29 A well proportioned profile: the lower, nasal and temporal thirds are of equal size, and the positioning is orthognathic, i.e., the upper jaw is in an approximately vertical relationship to the profile of the facial skeleton when the skull is orientated on the Frankfurt horizontal plane.

Textbooks provide an approximate indication of the natural dimensions which may be regarded as well proportioned. In practice it is advisable to adapt one standard (e.g., Leonardo da Vinci).

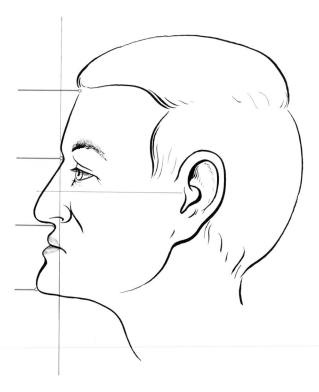

Fig. 12.30 Overdeveloped lower third of the face.

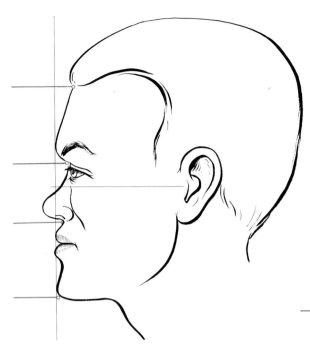

Fig. 12.31   Underdeveloped middle third of the face.

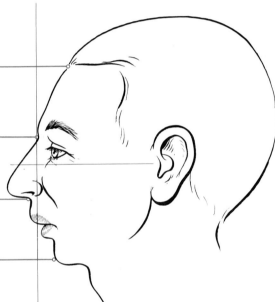

Fig. 12.32   Underdeveloped lower third of the face.

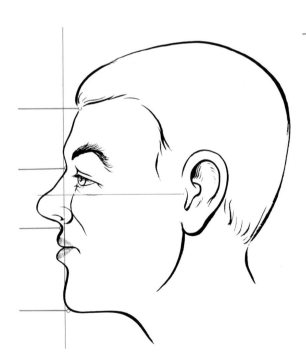

Fig. 12.33   High lower third of the face.

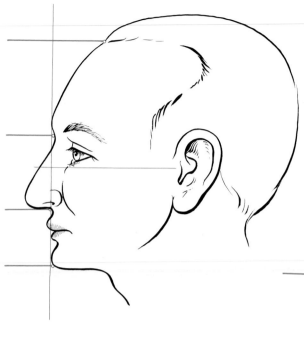

Fig. 12.34   Shallow lower third of the face.

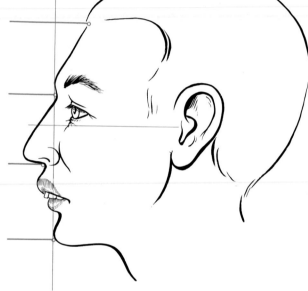

Fig. 12.35   Overdeveloped middle third of the face.

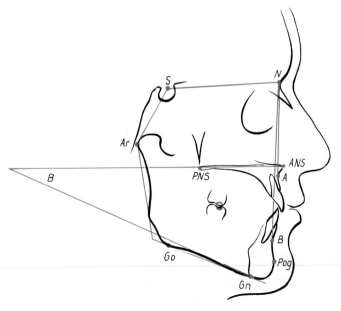

Fig. 12.36

Teleroentgenograms (Cephalic Views)

The soft tissue contours can be as equally well recognized as the bony contours on radiographs of the profile. One particular method of radiographic analysis of teleroentgenograms has been developed which is a prerequisite for determining the correct indications for and planning of an orthopedic jaw operation intended to improve the profile.

The *purpose of the radiographic analysis* is to determine and localize a preexisting developmental defect or to isolate a particular skeletal area within the facial skeleton. Cephalometry is used in the individual case to determine:

● Relationships between the facial skeleton and the skull as a whole;
● Dentoalveolar and skeletal developmental disturbances.

Radiographic technique. The teleroentgenogram taken in a straight lateral skull view with an anode-film distance of 1.5 to 4 meters. The photograph must be neither enlarged nor distorted. The head must be fixed in a headrest so that the center of the beam passes through the central point between the 2 external auditory meatuses to strike the film.

Interpretation of the teleroentgenograms is based on certain landmarks and lines which allow both *linear* and *angular* interpretation.

A standardized cephalometric examination with a simplified system of reference points suffices for practical purposes.

The *points of reference* may be divided into anatomic, anthropologic and radiographic. The latter are formed by the superimposition of two shadows. In addition to bony points, there are also soft tissue points which may be central or bilateral. The central points occur in the midline while the bilateral points are produced by the superimposition of two existing bilateral points.

The following points are noted (Fig. 12.36):

A   – Anterior end of the superior alveolus
ANS – Anterior nasal spine
Ar   – Point of intersection of the posterior edge of the articular process with the temporal bone
B   – Anterior end of the inferior alveolus

Gn   – Gnathion (most inferior and anterior point of the lower border of the mandible)
Go   – Gonion (apex of the angle of the jaw which lies at the most posterior, inferior and external point)
N   – Nasion (point of intersection of the naso-frontal suture with the median plane)
PNS – Posterior nasal spine (point of intersection between the hard and soft palates)
Pog – Progonion (anterior projecting point of the chin)
S   – Sella (sella turcica)

The *reference lines* are constructed with the help of the reference points, as shown in Figure 12.36.

Linear assessment of the teleroentgenograms is made on the basis of the following measurements:

N-S   – Horizontal part of the anterior base of the skull; mean: 71 mm
S-Ar   – Vertical part of the base of the skull; mean: 35 mm
ANS-PNS – Base of the upper jaw; mean: 47 mm
Ar-Go   – Length of the ascending ramus; mean: 44 mm
Go-Gn   – Length of the lower border of the mandible; mean: 71 mm

Angular assessment is made on the basis of the following angle measurements:

N-S-Ar   – Lateral angle of the base of the skull; mean: 123°
S-Ar-Go – Joint angle; mean: 143°
S-N-A   – Basal prognathism of the upper jaw; mean: 80°
S-N-B   – Alveolar prognathism of the lower jaw; mean: 78°
S-N-Pog – Basal prognathism of the mandible; mean: 79°
Angle B – Angle between the bases of the upper and lower jaws; mean: 25°
Angle Go – Angle of the jaw between Ar-Go and Go-Gn; mean: 123°

Interpretation of the linear relationships. Using the above values for the lengths and angles, the skeletal and dentoalveolar anomalies of the facial skeleton can be classified as one of the individual types of overdevelopment or underdevelopment of the skeleton of the jaws.

In *overdevelopment of the lower part of the face*, the lengths of the lower border of the mandible and of the ascending ramus are increased; the angles of the base of the skull (N-S-Ar) and the joint angle (S-Ar-Go) are decreased; the basal angle (B), the jaw angle (Ar-Go-Gn) and the basal prognathic angle of the mandible (S-N-Pog) are increased (Fig. 12.37).

In *underdevelopment of the middle third of the face*, the base of the upper jaw (ANS-PNS) and the basal prognathism of the upper jaw (S-N-A) are decreased (Fig. 12.38).

In *underdevelopment of the lower part of the face*, the lower border of the mandible (Go-Gn) as well as the alveolar (S-N-B) and basal prognathism (S-N-Pog) of the mandible are decreased while the angle of the base of the skull (N-S-Ar) and the joint angle (S-Ar-Go) are large (Fig. 12.39).

If the *lower third of the face is high*, the basic angle (B) and the jaw angle (Ar-Go-Gn) are increased while the length of the ascending ramus is decreased. If the ascending ramus is long as in the case above, there is a high-standing joint of Fig. 12.40.

In *overdevelopment of the middle third of the face*, the size of the base of the upper jaw (PNS-ANS) and the angle of the basal prognathism of the upper jaw (S-N-A) are increased; the upper incisor teeth are more than 4 mm in front of the N-Pog line (Fig. 12.41).

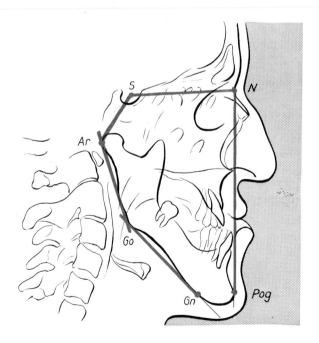

Fig. 12.37   Overdeveloped lower third of the face.

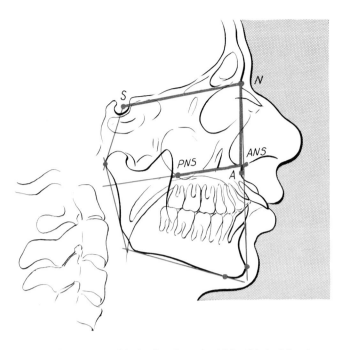

Fig. 12.38   Underdeveloped middle third of the face.

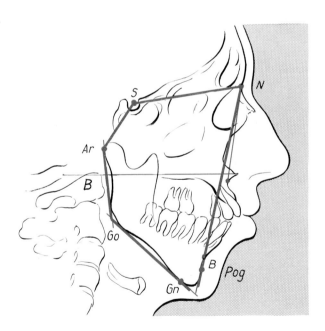

Fig. 12.39   Underdeveloped lower third of the face.

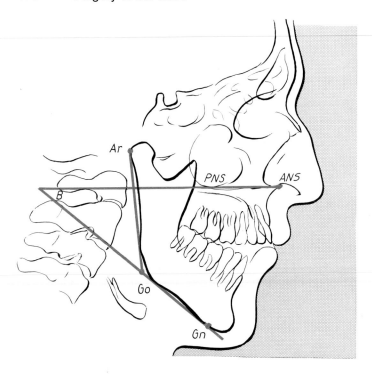

Fig. 12.40   High lower third of the face.

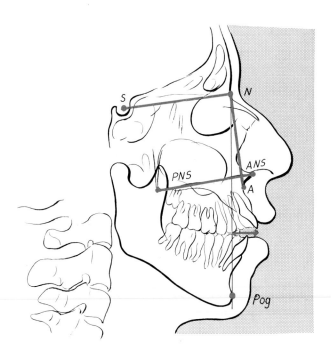

Fig. 12.41   Overdeveloped middle third of the face.

Complexity of the anomaly. In the above-mentioned anomalies, a complex integration of disordered form and function is present. Here the skeletal component principally determines dysproportion and the dentoalveolar component, dysfunction. Both must be taken into account when planning treatment.

Malocclusion is the principal feature for assessing dentoalveolar relationships. A simple diagnostic method is to assess the position of the incisors in relation to the N-Pog line (see Fig. 12.36). Normally, the upper incisor is 4 mm and the lower incisor 2 mm anterior to this line. As a rule of thumb, it can be said that incisor teeth more than 4 mm anterior to this line should be set back and those lying posterior to the line should be brought forward.

The position of the first molar should be assessed in the same way. Normally, the mesiobuccal cusp of the upper molar engages the mesiobuccal fissure of the lower molar (Fig. 12.42).

Using this normal type of occlusion (neutral or Class I bite) as a basis, Angle has classified the more common types of malocclusion as follows:

Class II: *Distocclusion* (distal bite, posterior bite, retrognathia) is often accompanied by a small or receding chin (Fig. 12.43).

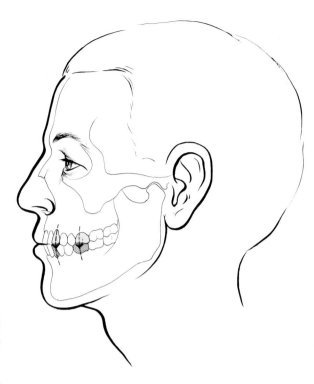

Fig. 12.42   Neutral bite (Class I).

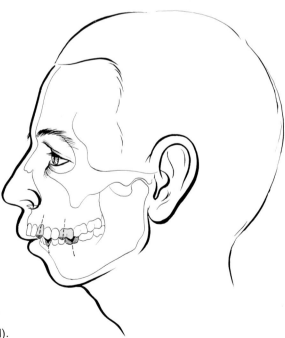

Fig. 12.43   Distocclusion (Class II).

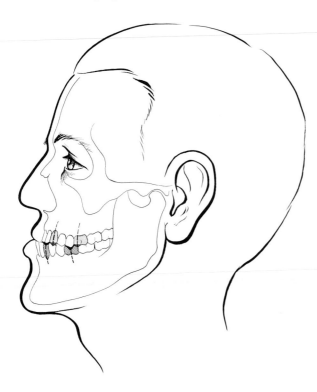

Fig. 12.44   Mesiocclusion (Class III).

Class III: *Mesiocclusion* (anterior open bite, mandibular prognathism) is accompanied by pronounced anterior protrusion of the chin (Fig. 12.44).

Additional disturbances of occlusion are characterized according to their principal feature such as open bite, complete overbite, deep overbite, crossbite and anterior overbite. They can occur in isolation but are usually an important part of a complex anomaly of the skeleton of the jaw.

The type of operation indicated depends fundamentally on these main features. The classification of anomalies is expanded on the basis of the principal gnathic or dentoalveolar features.

Classification of the Anomalies Based on the Main Features

1. *Overdevelopment of the lower third of the face*
   Main features:
   True prognathism (hyperplasia of the mandible: skeletal)
   Alveolar mandibular protrusion (dentoalveolar)

2. *Underdevelopment of the middle third of the face*
   Main features:
   Pseudoprognathism (hypoplasia of the maxilla: gnathic)
   Dish face (skeletal)

3. *Underdevelopment of the lower third of the face*
   Main features:
   Distal bite (dentoalveolar)
   Micrognathia and retrognathia (skeletal)

4. *High lower third of the face*
   Main features:
   Anterior open bite (dentoalveolar)
   Prognathism (skeletal)

5. *Shallow lower third of the face*
   Main features:
   Complete overbite and deep bite (dentoalveolar)
   Micrognathia (skeletal)

6. *Overdeveloped middle third of the face*
   Main features:
   Maxillary prognathism (skeletal)
   Protrusion with a narrow dental arch (dentoalveolar)

7. *Asymmetric face*
   Main features:
   Laterognathia (skeletal)

Profile photographs. A profile photograph is insufficient for determining the jaw profile exactly. In addition to inaccurate localization and the smallness of the usual format, the Frankfurt horizontal plane can only be approximately assessed on the photo because the superior point of the external auditory meatus cannot be clearly defined. Profile photographs are, therefore, more useful for clinical documentation.

Planning of Correction of the Dentoalveolar and Skeletal Components

Classification according to underdevelopment or overdevelopment of the skeleton of the jaws as well as the orientation according to "main features" (e.g., a prognathic bite) facilitates treatment planning. Treatment can be difficult, particularly with the common complex anomalies.

A complex anomaly is the integration of a skeletal and a dentoalveolar disturbance of development. In these cases both the model and teleroentgenogram are important accessories for the accurate determination of the individual treatment program. The purpose of planning on the model is to produce a replica of the patient's jaws by means of an anatomical model on which the various operations can be practiced and the best solution found.

In simple dentoalveolar anomalies such as alveolar protrusion of the upper jaw and in simple skeletal anomalies such as prognathism, occlusal models suffice on which practice operations or displacement osteotomies can be carried out in a simulator (Barrow and Dingman 1950, Obwegeser 1965).

Caldwell and Lettermann (1954), Ginestet and Merville (1966), Rowe (1960) and others plan the operation on the teleroentgenograms. They determine the most favorable site for the operation, the type of operation and the amount of bone to be resected by using a paper template.

The value of such templates is limited. Apart from the absence of spatial dimensions, complex anomalies requiring complicated operations on the bone at several sites cannot be planned in detail.

Trauner (1971) attempted to overcome this disadvantage by combining planning on the teleroentgenogram with geometric principles which he himself worked out. The fragment is not displaced in a bi-axial coordinate system as is usually the case. Rather, its movement at the desired point is regarded as "*rotation* in a circular system, the central point of which is easy to determine diagrammatically on the teleroentgenogram".

Practical application of this system is limited and, in part, inaccurate. The fixed points, the incisor point and the buccal cusp of the second molar are seldom shown exactly on the teleroentgenogram. In practice this method does not allow the stereoscopic assessment required for the more difficult types of correction. Finally, not only aesthetic and anatomical factors but also functional (articulation) and biomechanical (fixation) factors must be taken into account. The correction of a complex anomaly (e.g., overdevelopment of the mandible with prognathism, simultaneous underdevelopment of the upper jaw and bilateral crossbite (see Fig. 12.37) demands as complete a simulation as possible of the possible operations, including external and internal fixation, since consolidation of the fragments is as important as mobilization. Our aim, therefore, is to obtain as plastic an idea as possible of the entire operation in terms of procedure and postoperative results.

For several patients Schmuziger (1961) used models made from teleroentgenograms and plaster-of-Paris casts.

We found it advisable to make this a routine procedure, particularly as the production of the simulator, after the surgical tactics have been decided, is the job of the technicians. The main difficulty is the construction of the actual model of the mandible. The following procedure should be employed: An alginate impression of the mandible is made from ivory colored plastic with a consistency similar to that of bone. The following mixture should be used:

To 100 g Araldite 554 (Ciba-Geigy AG, Basel) are added:

    20 g hardener
    50 g whitener
     3 g marble cement.

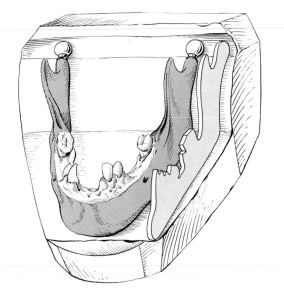

Fig. 12.45 Construction of the basic shape: Lateral part of the mandible is constructed according to the radiographs using a paper template.

When the model has hardened, the dental arch is sawed off the alveolus. The cardboard template of the mandible is cut out using the radiograph as a model (1:1 ratio), and a modeling stand is prepared from plaster of Paris on which the technician copies the lateral parts of the rami of the mandible in wax (Fig. 12.45). Preparation of the model is completed on the basis of measurements taken directly from the patient according to a fixed plan (Fig. 12.46).

The sawed-off dental arch is fixed on the wax mandible and a silicone pattern is constructed from the prepared model. At least 10 artificial mandibles can be produced in this way. The condyles of the mandible are not copied but rather are replaced by brass spheres. A form is prepared directly from the plaster-of-Paris model of the upper jaw and is cast in plastic.

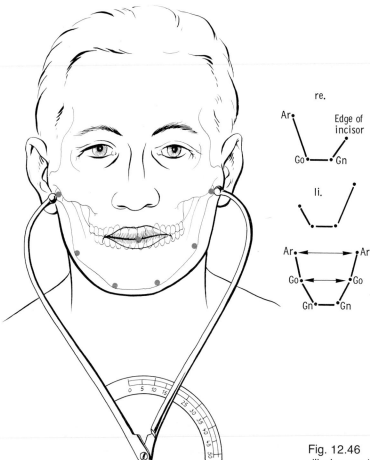

Fig. 12.46 Data for construction of an individual mandibular model (see p. 167 for the abbreviations).

The anatomical model is adjusted on a simulator (Fig. 12.47).

The simulator is constructed in the shape of a cross. The crossbar includes a socket in which the ball-shaped condyles of the mandible are held in such a way that they can be moved. A T-shaped, perpendicular, adjustable harness engages the sigmoid notch and maintains the ascending ramus in its original position after the mandible has been divided. This allows assessment of the form and extent of the osteotomy on the ascending ramus as well as the shape of the new angle of the jaw on the attenuated mandible.

The perpendicular beam of the simulator is provided with a harness to which the model of the upper jaw is fastened in a moveable position.

The unique advantage of the simulation technique with this apparatus is that the dentoalveolar and skeletal components of the operation, including fixation of the fragments, can be practiced on the model. All details of the optimal solution can be exactly presented.

There are some individual cases of complex anomalies in which it is advisable to include orthodontic preoperative management in the simulation. For example, frontal crowding of the upper jaw may be present in addition to prognathism. This excludes ideal operative adjustment of the occlusion without previous orthodontic management.

Expansion of the dental arch is simulated with the use of the apparatus described above. This can be done with a wax model, the deformed dental arch of which is composed of reproductions of each individual tooth. The teeth are made of acrylate and are provided with brackets on the fixed orthodontic apparatus so that they can be moved into a natural position within the wax alveolus.

The results of orthodontic simulation can thus be confirmed beforehand on the model and can be taken into account during the planning of the operation.

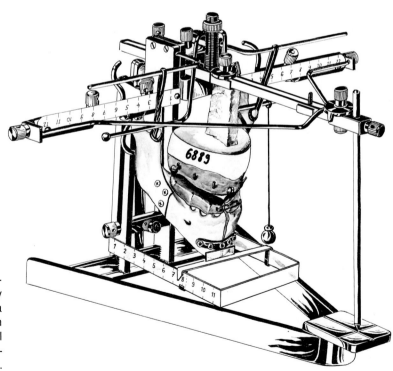

Fig. 12.47
Simulator. Simulated osteotomy, fixation and alteration of the intermaxillary relationships for later treatment with a complete denture. The original situation is extreme prognathism with bilateral crossbite resulting from simultaneously existing hypoplasia of the upper jaw.

Removal of Bone for Grafting

The bone graft is taken either from a rib, from the iliac crest or from the greater trochanter depending on the size of the required graft. Removal of a section of *rib* is indicated in those cases in which a large defect must be bridged immediately without great expenditure of time and material (e.g., after mandibulectomy and neck dissection).

If a graft of cortical cancellous bone is required, the *iliac crest* is used as the donor site. The *greater trochanter* is required as a donor site only if a large amount of cancellous bone chips is required.

● To prevent infection, removal of bone is carried out before the operation.

● The size of the required bone graft is determined by measurements made before the operation on the simulator.

● It is advisable to take more bone than initially appears necessary since further correction is often necessary during the operation. The excess bony material can then be kept for use later.

● After sterilizing the skin with alcohol and cetrimide, the operative area is covered with a sterile drape.

Taking a Rib Graft

The anterior quarter of the sixth and seventh ribs is usually used for a rib graft; the periosteal covering is preserved. The rib can be used as it stands to bridge the defect or it can be introduced into the defect after having been split sagittally and with one cortical surface laid upon the other.

Position. The patient is placed in the supine position with the right side of the chest elevated (Fig. 12.48).

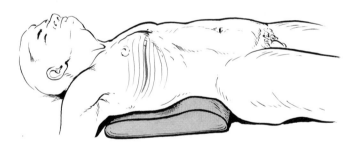

Fig. 12.48   Removal of a segment of a rib: Position of the patient in a slightly left lateral position with a small pad beneath the right side of the chest and the shoulder.

Special instruments. Doyen's raspatory, a rib raspatory, Liston's scissors and special rib shears.

Operative Technique

The external oblique muscle of the abdomen and part of the serratus anterior muscle are divided through a 5–6 cm long skin incision parallel to the sixth or seventh rib. The periosteum of the rib to be removed is exposed. The periosteum is divided lengthwise directly over the rib, and the extent of the rib to be removed is marked with 2 periosteal incisions. The periosteum is elevated from the external surface of the rib with an ordinary periosteal elevator and then on its medial surface with a Doyen's raspatory (Fig. 12.49). The rib is divided at its junction with the cartilage. The free end is elevated with bone forceps and, after the required length has been measured, the posterior part is divided. The periosteum is closed with individual 3 × 0 Dexon (polyglycolic acid) sutures and a suction drain is introduced. The muscle layers are closed and the skin is sutured with continuous 4 × 0 Supramid sutures.

Danger Points

● Damage to the pleura (pneumothorax). In order not to overlook such a complication, sterile saline solution is poured into the defect after the bone has been removed; the anesthetist hyperventilates the patient temporarily. If bubbles appear in the fluid, the perforation must be sought and closed with individual Dexon (polyglycolic acid) sutures. When tightening the last suture, a suction cannula is placed through the hole in the pleura and accumulated blood and air are suctioned out. Under maximal aspiration the pleura is closed tightly with the last suture, which requires the cooperation of the anesthetist. An underwater seal is usually not necessary.

● Damage to the intercostal arteries or nerves.

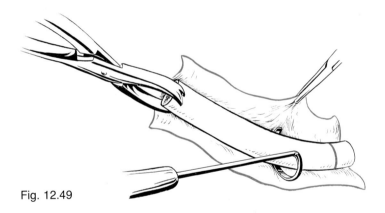

Fig. 12.49

Taking a Bone Graft from the Iliac Crest

Cancellous bone chips can be removed from a small hole in the cortex or a large block of cortical bone with cancellous bone attached must be used. The entire iliac crest is seldom needed (see also Vol. 1, Chap. 5).

Position. The patient is placed in the supine position with the right hip elevated (Fig. 12.50).

Special instruments. Osteotomes, curettes and Stryker saw.

Operative Technique

The skin incision lies parallel to the iliac crest and 2 to 3 fingerbreadths below it (Fig. 12.51). This prevents the scar from lying directly on the iliac crest. Dissection is carried down to the bony iliac crest, preserving the lateral cutaneous branch of the iliohypogastric nerve. The incision is made along its lateral edge through the attached muscles and fascia. Anteriorly and posteriorly, the iliac crest is divided transversely with an osteotome to a depth of about 5 mm. On the lateral side, the bone is now di-

vided with an osteotome so that the crest remains pedicled medially on the periosteum and can be turned aside to reveal the cancellous bone underneath. Cortical material can then be removed with a chisel or a sharp curette via this access (Fig. 12.52).

If more material is needed, the periosteum of the outer cortex and the site of insertion of the gluteus medius muscle must be elevated from the bone over the area through which the bone is to be removed by means of an osteotome or a Stryker saw (Fig. 12.53).

The wound is closed by turning the crest back and stitching the muscular insertions with 3 × 0 Dexon (polyglycolic acid) sutures. A suction drain is introduced and the skin is closed with continuous 4 × 0 Supramid sutures.

Danger Points

● Division of the cutaneous branches of the iliohypogastric nerve producing anesthesia in the area of distribution (inguinal region and lateral part of the thigh).

● Perforation of the abdominal cavity if the medial part of the cortex must also be removed.

● Disturbances of growth of the iliac crest in children if the growth center is damaged.

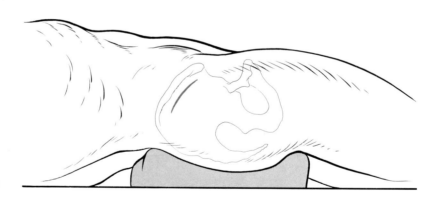

Fig. 12.50

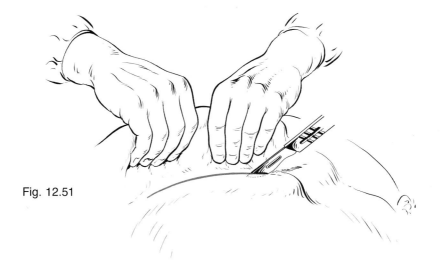

Fig. 12.51

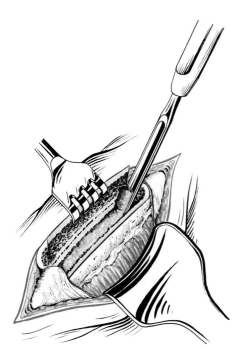

Fig. 12.52

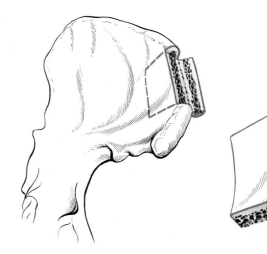

Fig. 12.53

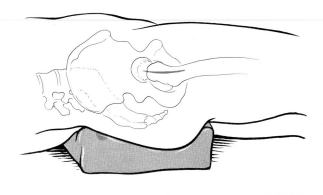

Fig. 12.54

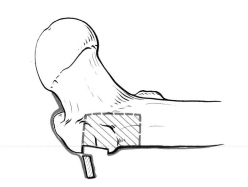

Fig. 12.55 a

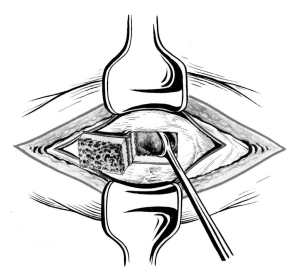

Fig. 12.55 b

Removal of Bone from the Greater Trochanter

If more cancellous material is required than usual, the greater trochanter is used as the donor site.

Position. The patient is placed in the lateral position with the right buttock elevated (Fig. 12.54).

Instruments. Chisel, hammer and a sharp curette.

Operative Technique

A 5 cm skin incision is made over the greater trochanter on the right side (Fig. 12.54). The tensor fascia lata is split longitudinally. After elevating the gluteus medius and maximus muscles, the greater trochanter is exposed. A cortical flap is formed which is pedicled on the periosteum (Fig. 12.55 a) and the cancellous bone is removed with a sharp curette (Fig. 12.55 b).

The cavity is closed by returning the bony flap. The periosteum and muscles are closed with 3 × 0 Dexon (polyglycolic acid) sutures, a suction drain is introduced and the skin is closed with continuous 4 × 0 Supramid sutures.

Danger points. None.

Fixation of the Bony Fragments

In addition to the precise correction of the mal-occlusion (dysgnathia) the bony fragments must be fixed exactly in the desired position. Basically 2 methods are available:

1. External fixation,
2. Internal fixation.

External fixation. This is accomplished with an *undivided* or *divided* splint fastened to the teeth and is usually fitted before surgery. Maintenance of the fragments in central occlusion is often supplemented by intermaxillary wiring. It is important that the splint be such that it can be applied without technical help, that it be rigid enough and thus will remain fixed. Schuchardt's wire-Palavit splint meets these requirements.

The splint consists of the previously prepared body with transverse bars, wire (0.35 mm) and self-hardening plastic.

The technique of splinting is shown in Figures 12.56, 12.57, 12.58, 12.59, 12.60 and is also described in Chapter 9.

The *duration of fixation* is at least 4 and at most 12 weeks, depending on the type and extent of the osteotomy. If the postoperative period is free of complications, intermaxillary fixation for 6 to 8 weeks suffices. To be absolutely certain, however, the splints should be left in place for an additional period of 2 weeks.

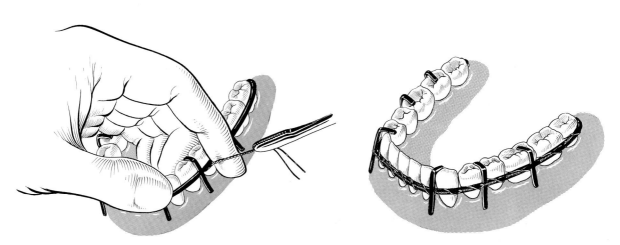

Fig. 12.56   Fixing the body of the archbar by tightening both shanks of the wire with Pean's forceps. The index finger is used to check when the ligature has been tightened maximally without exceeding the limits of elasticity.

Fig. 12.57   The position of the body of the archbar fixed with wire ligatures (0.35 mm) on the outer circumference of the dental arch. The hooks bent over the occlusal surfaces prevent sliding of the splint downward onto the gingiva.

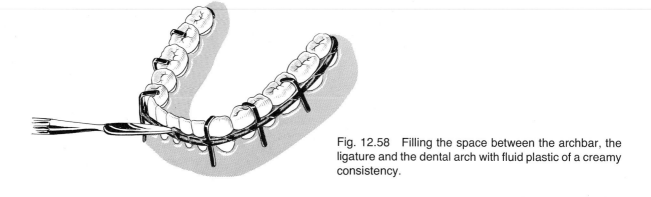

Fig. 12.58   Filling the space between the archbar, the ligature and the dental arch with fluid plastic of a creamy consistency.

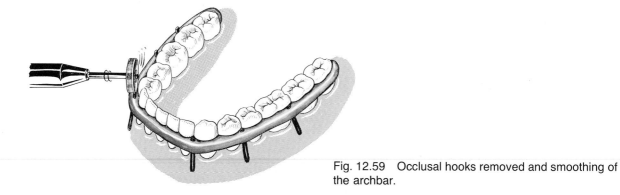

Fig. 12.59   Occlusal hooks removed and smoothing of the archbar.

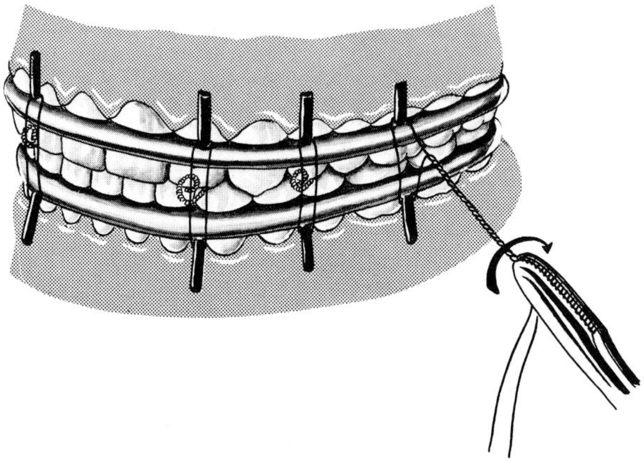

Fig. 12.60   Intermaxillary fixation. The ends of the wire ligatures are rolled up in a spiral and pushed between the teeth and the ligature.

Internal fixation. Internal fixation allows early resumption of chewing as well as fixation of the bony fragments. The main principle is to shorten the period of fixation. This goal is based on the following concepts:

1. The fastest possible healing of the bone is achieved by direct *bridging* of the osteotomy gap without an intermediate stage of a callous tissue (primary bone healing).

2. Direct penetration of the osteotomy gap occurs only if the blood supply is good and if the fragments are rigidly fixed.

3. Absolute fixation of the fragments is achieved only by fixing the divided parts of the bone under compression (pressure fixation).

Since the upper jaw has a static function and the lower jaw has a dynamic function, different types of interfragmentary fixation must be distinguished. These are achieved either *with* or *without compression* of the individual bone fragments against each other.

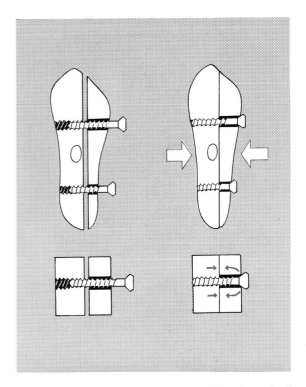

Fig. 12.61   Interfragmentary compression of a sagittally split mandible (in cross section) using a lag screw. Left: In the left fragment there is a thread hole and in the right fragment a gliding hole. Right: Engagement of the screw head and tightening of the screw to produce interfragmentary compression.

Interfragmentary Fixation by Compression

Compression fixation is used after certain forms of mandibular osteotomy. Three possibilities are available:

1. Lag screw,

2. Compression plate (DCP = dynamic compression plate),

3. Tension band.

Principle of the Traction Screw

This can be carried out only with an osteotomy which is similar to an ideal oblique fracture such as, for example, sagittal splitting of the ascending ramus (see p. 190). A thread hole is made in one fragment and a gliding hole is made in the overlying fragment (Fig. 12.61, left). The screw engages the screw hole and moves through the gliding hole until the head of the screw engages the bone; the last turns of the screw then bring both fragments together (Fig. 12.61, right).

Principle of the Compression Plate

This type of compression plate is used when bridging of the fragments can be carried out only from the periphery of the bone. In such cases a compression plate is used in which the opening of the screw holes is designed according to the principle of the inclined plane (Fig. 12.62). If a screw is introduced at the upper point of the inclined plane through an elliptical opening in the plate, the head of the screw slides downward on the inclined plane and the last turns of the screw close the fracture or osteotomy line. Since the screw is fastened firmly to the bone, the bone moves in relation to the plate. If inclined planes pointing in opposite directions are provided on both sides, tightening the screw leads to compression of the bony fragments (Fig. 12.62, below). The special technique for the application of such plates is presented below.

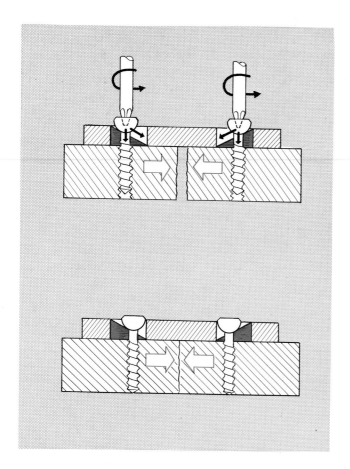

Fig. 12.62
Axial compression by means of a dynamic compression plate (DCP). Above: The adaptation phase (approximation of the fragments). The head of the screw lies on the inclined plane of the screw hole. When the screw is tightened, the head moves on the inclined plane so that underneath the plate, the fragments move in the direction of the arrows. Below: The compression phase when the second screw is tightened.

AO Technique

Instruments (see Fig. 12.63)

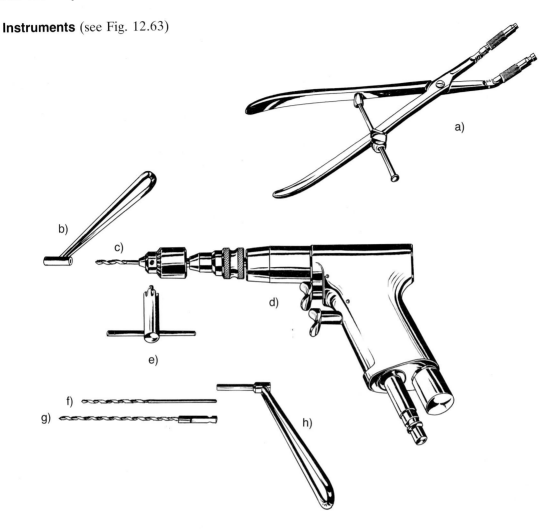

Fig. 12.63   Instruments (Continued on page 186)
a) Repositioning and fixation forceps
b) Tap sleeve
c) 2.7 mm spiral drill for boring th gliding hole
d) Small AO drill
e) Chuck key

f) 1.4 mm spiral drill (for making the thread hole for the cortical screw, 2.0 mm)
g) 2 mm spiral drill (for making the 2.7 mm gliding hole for the cortical screw)
h) Drill guide

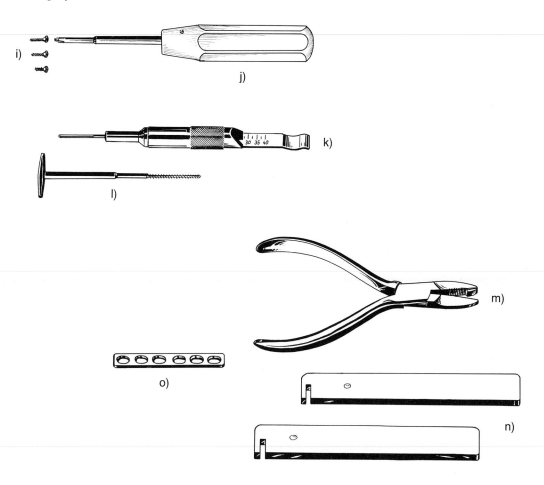

Fig. 12.63   (Continued)

i) Cortical screws (external diameter: 2.7 mm; thread
   core diameter: 2.0 mm; length: 6–24 mm)
   These screws are particularly suitable for the strong
   cortex of the mandible
j) Phillips screwdriver

k) Depth gauge
l) Thread cutter, 2.7 mm
m) Pliers
n) Bending irons
o) Mandibular plate (dynamic compression plate).

Application of the dynamic compression plate (DCP). The size of the plate must be such that at least 2 screws engage the bony fragments of each side. The plate is adapted to the surface of the bone using a bending iron or bending pliers (Figs. 12.64, 12.65).

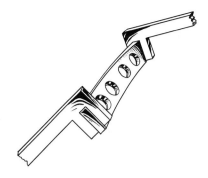

Fig. 12.64   Bending a compression plate (titanium) with a bending iron.

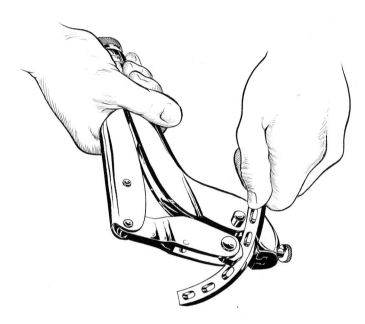

Fig. 12.65   Bending a compression plate (titanium) with a bending pliers.

It is advantageous to "overbend" the plate so that the bone is not distracted on the lingual side when it is screwed into place (Figs. 12.66, 12.67). The compression plate is fixed along the inferior edge of the mandible (below the course of the canal of the mandible) over the site of the osteotomy. The first hole is made near the osteotomy gap on the most easily accessible side, a thread is cut in the bone and the first screw is introduced. The second screw is introduced in the same way near the osteotomy gap on the opposite fragment. In accordance with the principle of the compression plate, the screw must be placed at one edge of the hemicylindrical slope of the screw hole at the uppermost point of the inclined plane.

Adaptation of the fragments. Introduction of the screws on both sides of the osteotomy gap causes both bony fragments to move toward the gap. The remaining screws are introduced in a similar manner before these 2 screws are tightened (see Fig. 12.62, above).

Compression of the fragments. Compression of both bony fragments is complete when all the screws have been tightened in the correct sequence (see Fig. 12.62, below).

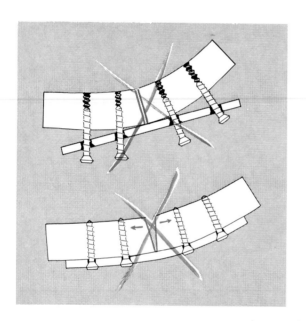

Fig. 12.66   Incorrect fixation as a result of incomplete bending of the plate. Result: Distraction of the fragments on the lingual side.

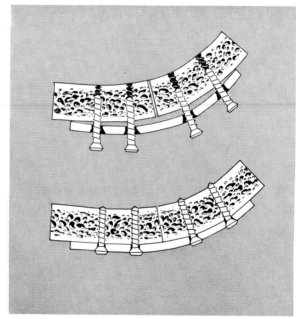

Fig. 12.67   Plate fixation taking into consideration the curve of the mandible; the slightly overbent plate produces compression on the lingual side of the fragments.

Tension-Band Splinting

The plate should be screwed only into the lower half of the body of the mandible in order to avoid damaging the nerves and the roots of the teeth. Applying the pressure plate to only one side causes distraction of the fragments on the other side (Fig. 12.68a, b); the result is malocclusion. To prevent this complication, either a tension-band splint made of wire-Palavit (see p. 181) is applied to toothbearing fragments (Fig. 12.69a) or a tension-band plate is applied to the oval side of edentulous fragments (Fig. 12.69b).

Interfragmentary Fixation Without Compression

This type of bony fixation is carried out on the upper jaw by means of interosseous wires or wire-Palavit splints. Healing following such osteosynthesis is by fibrous union (see also Chap. 9).

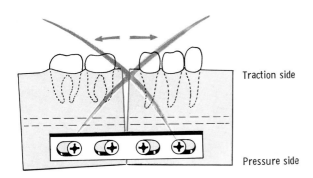

Fig. 12.68 a   Incorrect fixation with a compression plate; eccentric compression of the lower border of the mandible (pressure side) and distraction of the teeth row (traction side).

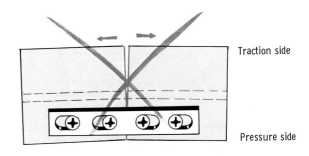

Fig. 12.68 b   Analogous process in edentulous fragments.

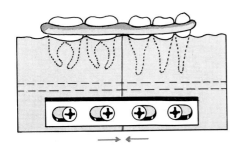

Fig. 12.69 a   Correct fixation with a compression plate and a tension-band splint consisting of a rigid wire-Palavit archbar on both tooth bearing fragments. There is no interfragmentary gap but rather axial compression.

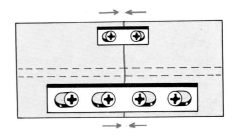

Fig. 12.69 b   Similar axial compression of edentulous fragments.

Mandibular Osteotomies

Displacement Osteotomies of the Ascending Ramus

Sagittal Shortening Osteotomy

Principles of the Operation

Sagittal splitting of the ascending ramus (Trauner and Obwegeser 1957) including the angle of the jaw (Dal Pont 1958) guarantees the maximal surface area of the bony section. This permits full displacement of the bone segments, in the anterior as well as the posterior direction (shortening or lengthening).

The advantages of this method are:

● Minimal risk of recurrence and pseudoarthrosis,

● No visible scar,

● Traction screws can be used for stable fixation of the fragments.

Indications

The sagittal split as a shortening osteotomy is indicated in the following circumstances:

● Overdeveloped lower third of the face; main feature: *true mandibular prognathism.*

● Unilateral overdevelopment of the mandible; main features: *asymmetry of the face, mandibular prognathism* and *lateral deviation of the chin.*

● Underdeveloped middle third of the face; main feature: pseudoprognathism.

True prognathism is partially hereditary and partially functional (macroglossia). Occasionally it is due to an endocrine disturbance (acromegaly). The main characteristics are:

● Abnormally long body of the mandible,

● Abnormally long ascending ramus,

● Shallow angle of the jaw.

Unilateral overdevelopment of the mandible (condylar hypertrophy) results from hyperplasia of the temporomandibular joint, or of the entire half of the mandible of unknown origin (Fig. 12.70). Unilateral localized gigantism leads to unilateral prognathism and displacement of the chin toward the healthy side.

The main characteristics are:

● Displaced midline.

● The angle of the jaw is lower and more anterior on one side,

● Open bite on the affected side,

● Crossbite on the opposite side.

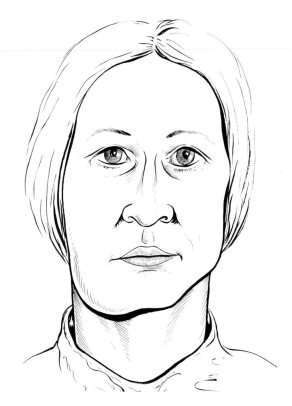

Fig. 12.70   Unilateral prognathism: Hyperplasia of the right temporomandibular joint, anterior displacement of the chin and displacement of the midline to the healthy side.

Pseudoprognathism is characterized by hypoplasia of the upper jaw in the presence of a normally developed mandible (apparent prognathism). It occurs most frequently in patients with the cleft lip-palate syndrome. Occasionally, it occurs with premature loss of teeth or is produced by a lack of dental development in the upper jaw or by a central middle third fracture of the face which has healed in displacement (dish face).

In such cases the operation usually indicated is a sagittal split since posterior displacement of the lower jaw is achieved more easily than anterior displacement of the upper jaw. The profile line vertical to the forehead is crucial for the decision as to whether maxillotomy, which is frequently used today, is indicated. A corrective operation on the mandible is usually preferred if the central middle third of the face does not lie conspicuously posterior.

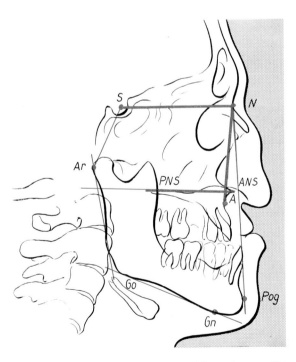

Fig. 12.71 Pseudoprognathism: Normal mandible (normal length and angle) with underdevelopment of the maxilla: ANS-PNS and S-N-A are small.

Preoperative Diagnosis

An *intraoral* examination is performed; the vestibule is exposed and the patient is asked to appose his jaws. With the teeth clenched and the masticatory muscles tensioned, the position of the upper and lower teeth in occlusion can be ascertained.

The bite anomaly is characterized by a typical occlusal pattern. We refer to the following basic types of occlusal disturbances in the diagnosis:

Reverse anterior overbite: *prognathism* or *pseudoprognathism*. The **teleroentgenogram** is determinative. To facilitate analysis the typical patterns are demonstrated:

● In true prognathism (see Fig. 12.37),

● In pseudoprognathism (Fig. 12.71).

Routine Radiography

This includes: Eccentric skull view: suboccipitofrontal (posteroanterior);

Mandibular view of the right and left half of the mandible, separately;

Orthopantomograms of the mandible or dental views.

The following factors must be evaluated:

● The strength of the ascending ramus (skull view);

● The status of the wisdom teeth, particularly whether they are erupted or displaced (separate films of the mandible);

● The status of the apices of the teeth, particularly periapical inflammation, cysts or other intraosseous processes, (orthopantomogram or film of the anterior part of the mandible).

The *plaster-of-Paris model* is also helpful. The type of dentoalveolar and skeletal disturbance is documented. At the same time it documents the preoperative findings as a basis for comparison with the results of the operation, later.

A *profile film* contributes considerably to preoperative documentation.

Preparation for Surgery

Out-Patient Preparation

Simulation. As already mentioned. Dal Pont's extended incision is considered for every simulation since it allows stable fixation with traction screws.

If the size of the angle of the jaw is within normal limits, a simple plaster-of-Paris model without a simulator usually suffices. In assessing the optimal occlusion, the mandible is set back far enough to achieve satisfactory occlusion, provided sagittal symmetry of both dental arches is present. This adjustment should result in a perfect alignment of the molar teeth and a normal frontal overbite. Disturbing cusps and edges are ground down and the resulting grinding surfaces are marked with a black felt-tip pen. Corresponding to these marks, the individual teeth are carefully ground on the day before the operation.

In most cases of extreme prognathism, the angle of the jaw is enlarged. If the body of the mandible protrudes excessively, a deep or open bite is also present.

Simulation on the replica (p. 175) is preferable since, in addition to altering the angle of the jaw, the body of the mandible must be sagittally repositioned as well as elevated or lowered.

The advantage is that after simulated division the ascending rami can be fixed in their original position. Only the body of the mandible with its dental arch is displaced until ideal occlusion is achieved. This produces an angulation of both ascending rami with optimal functional and esthetic results. The extent to which the end of the posteriorly displaced body of the mandible should be shortened so that it can be exactly reunited to the ascending rami can be ascertained with a centimeter rule (see Fig. 12.47). This measurement is one of the most important pieces of information for the retention or modification of the angle of the jaw in this operation.

In-Patient Preparation

On the day before the operation: The upper and lower dental arches are provided with a wire-Palavit splint. If necessary, individual teeth are ground down to conform to the model. When fitting the splints, care should be taken that they do not have a disturbing effect during the intraoperative adjustment of occlusion.

On the day of the operation (in the preparation room): The patient is placed with the head in normal position. The oral cavity is sprayed thoroughly with cetrimide solution. The lips are smeared with Vaseline.

Special Instruments

The required instruments are shown in Figure 12.72. It is essential that drills be used which allow atraumatic work (low speed burrs or drills with high penetrability and intensive cooling). In cooperation with A. Kühner AG of Basel, we have developed the "Microspraymatic" on this basis (Fig. 12.73). Its advantages consist of automatic cooling of the cutting instrument and irrigation of the bone with a sterile air-fluid mixture (isotonic saline or Ringer's solution). This allows the work to be carried out under direct vision, particularly at sites which are difficult to reach.

Anesthesia

Nasal endotracheal intubation is used. The hypopharynx is packed with Vaseline – or paraffin – impregnated gauze, with a holding thread attached to its end. The patient's eyes are held shut with nonirritant adhesive tape and protected with large pledgets.

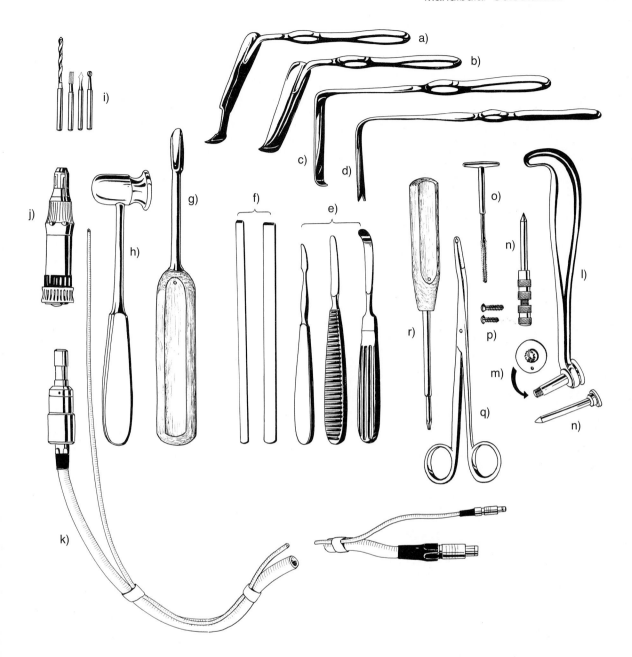

Fig. 12.72 Instruments:

(A newly composed set is available from Synthes Ltd., 4437 Waldenburg, Switzerland, or from their representatives at your location).

a, b) Metz-Schuchardt's prognathism retractors
c) Langenbeck's retractors
d) Swallow tail retractors
e) Raspatories
f) Osteotomes
g) Rounded chisel
h) Hammer
i) Lindemann drill, fissure, cutting and arrow-head bits
j) Handpiece

k) Cable for the Microspraymatic (see Fig. 12.73) and the tube for the water jet
l) Trocar with hand grip
m) Drill guide which can be screwed in place and which, at the same time, acts as a retractor for the soft tissues of the cheek
n) Trocar
o) Thread cutter
p) 2.7 mm cortical screws
q) Holding forceps for the drill guide
r) Phillips screw driver.

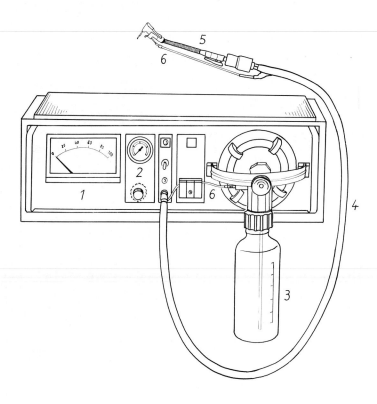

Fig. 12.73   Microspraymatic

1 = Rotation counter
2 = Above: Working air pressure manometer
    Below: Air pressure reducing valve

3 = Spray reducing valve
    Below: Glass for 1 liter of irrigating solution (Ringer's solution)
4 = Cable
5 = Hand piece
6 = Fluid line.

Operative Technique

A lateral mouth gag holds the mouth open as far as possible. The intermaxillary incision begins at the first lower molar and ends lateral to the maxillary tuberosity (Fig. 12.74).

The anterior edge of the ascending ramus is exposed in two stages so that bone contact is not lost. The mucosa and the periosteum are first divided along the oblique line as far as the origin of the buccinator muscle, and the tendon of the masseter muscle is freed down to the inferior edge of the mandible. The incision is then continued under tension on the mucosa along the oblique line as far as the coronoid process.

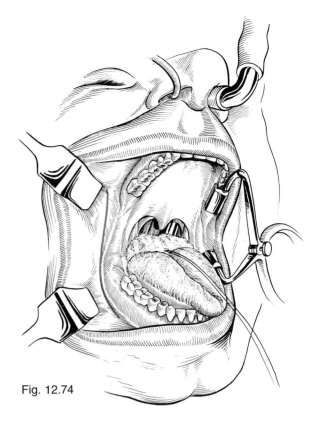

Fig. 12.74

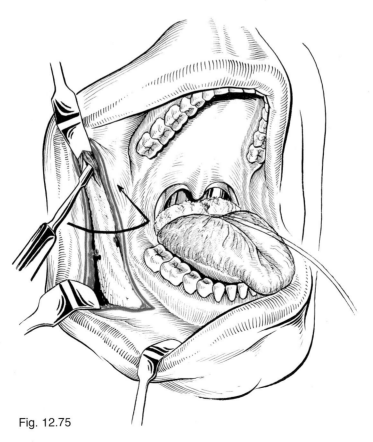

Fig. 12.75

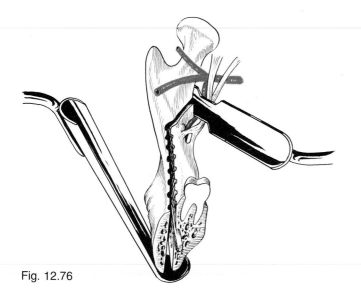

Fig. 12.76

The swallow-tail retractor is introduced around the exposed edge of the bone (Fig. 12.75). The mandibular notch is sought with a raspatory, and the neurovascular bundle is elevated as far as the posterior edge of the ascending ramus. If the elevation is generous, the chance of preserving the vessels and nerves in the connective tissue plane (maxillary artery and inferior alveolar nerve) is greater. Figure 12.76 shows an anatomical model of sagittal splitting. The narrow prognathism retractor protects the neurovascular bundle and the structures of the parotid gland. The broad prognathism retractor supports the angle of the jaw while the osteotomy is being performed.

The narrow prognathism retractor is introduced in such a way that it grasps the posterior edge of the ascending ramus and, at the same time, protects the neurovascular bundle by drawing it to one side; the swallow-tail retractor retracts the soft tissues and the tendons inserted into the coronoid process. With the operative field exposed in this way, the ascending ramus is divided in its entire width including the posterior edge down to the boundary layer of the external cortex. The incision is begun 1 cm below the notch and is continued parallel to the occlusal surfaces of the lower teeth.

The second incision is made anterior to the angle of the jaw, this time perpendicular to the occlusal surface, and through the lateral part of the cortex only.

Both incisions are joined together along the oblique line with a groove (Fig. 12.77). This determines the direction and position of the sagittal split. The split is carried out with specially ground osteotomes of various widths and is begun in front of the angle parallel to the inferior incision. Figure 12.78 shows the splitting of the horizontal part of the angle of the mandible. The prognathism retractor provides a firm support during this maneuver (see Fig. 12.76).

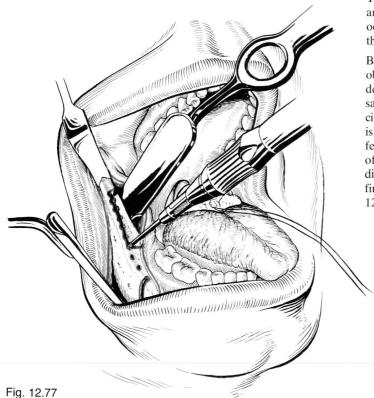

Fig. 12.77

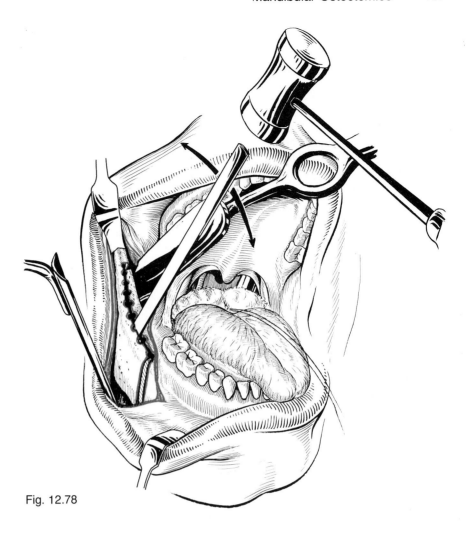

Fig. 12.78

The cortex is split successively as far as the angle of the
jaw; special attention should be paid to the superficial
curve of the bone. This area represents the "safety" zone
in which the nerve is unlikely to be damaged since the
canal at this point runs in the lingual edge. Figure 12.79
shows the topography of the sagittal splitting made in
front of the angle. The mandibular canal lies on the *lingual* side. Between the buccal cortex and the lateral wall
of the canal, there is a cancellous layer which is as wide as
the enclosing cortex (a = a'). Therefore, if splitting is carried out along the inner side of the cortex, there is no
danger of damaging the nerve.

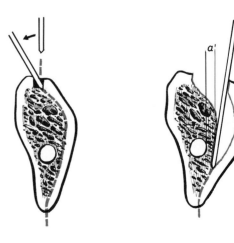

Fig. 12.79

The correct depth for carrying out an atraumatic osteotomy is ascertained by studying the transverse sections of the mandible; the osteotomy must be carried out within the *lateral* part of the border zone. In view of the danger of nerve damage, the lateral border zone is divided into *preangular* (1), *angular* (2) and *postangular* (3) areas. Figure 12.80 shows the position of the nerve canal relative to the lateral cortex in these 3 areas. In the angular and postangular areas, there is almost no cancellous bone between the wall of the canal and the lateral cortex (sections c and d).

The most difficult point is in the postangular area. Postangular splitting is begun here directly at the superior end of the bony incision. A 5 mm osteotome is introduced obliquely in the direction of a line joining the center of the mandible with the oblique line (Fig. 12.81 shows sagittal splitting in the postangular area). The initial direction of the osteotomy is 30° to the external surface of the ascending ramus. The osteotome crosses the midline of the mandible. After the osteotome has been introduced 1.5 cm, it is gradually turned outward toward the corner of the mouth. Quick, light taps with the hammer force the osteotome as far as the boundary zone of the cortex. When this layer has been reached the osteotome is turned into the sagittal plane, parallel to the external surface of the ascending ramus. The osteotome is carefully pushed deeper. Finally the bone of the posterior edge of the mandible is split. At this point the osteotome strikes the metal of the prognathism retractor.

The osteotome is left in place and the splitting is continued immediately beneath it at the angle of the jaw; *a narrow area in the immediate vicinity of the point of entry of the nerve should be preserved.* These last connections are carefully loosened by separating movements with a chisel with a wooden handle.

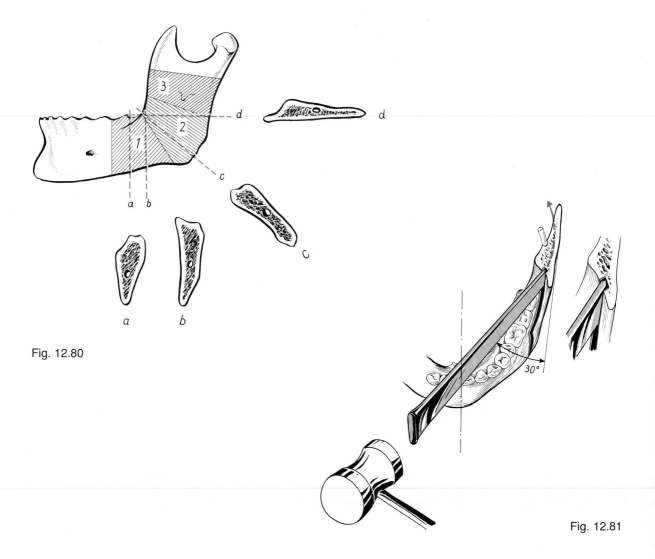

Fig. 12.80

Fig. 12.81

Fixation

After splitting has been carried out on the other side, the now completely mobile body of the mandible is repositioned and fixed in the desired occlusal position with intermaxillary fixation (Fig. 12.82).

The shortening of the proximal fragment corresponds to the posterior displacement of the distal fragment (see simulation, p. 192). The simulated model is consulted during shortening of the fragments, particularly for an excessively protruding angle of the jaw and for a closed bite deformity.

Traditionally, (unstable) fixation is provided by a wire ligature (Fig. 12.83 a) or circummandibular wiring (Ob-

wegeser 1971) (Fig. 12.83 b). The instability of the wire fixation requires intermaxillary fixation for at least 6 weeks (not 3 weeks as is sometimes stated). Shorter intervals carry the risk of infection and relapse.

The aim must be to use a secure and practical method of fixation which provides:

● Guaranteed positioning of the fragments,

● Primary bone healing,

● Immediate mobilization.

The method which we have worked out is based on the principle of interfragmentary compression with lag screws (see p. 183). The procedure is described below.

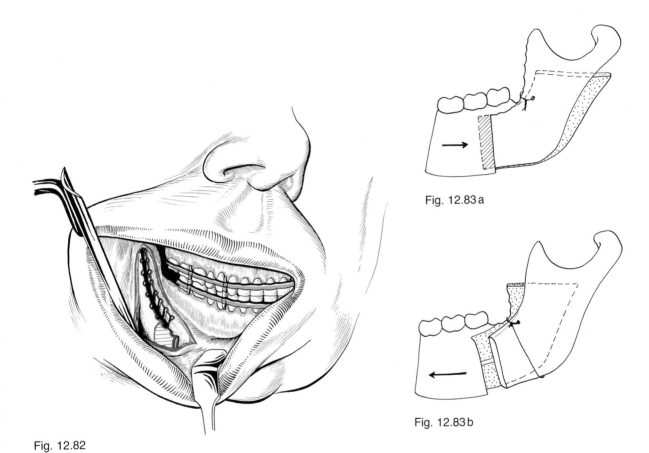

Fig. 12.83 a

Fig. 12.83 b

Fig. 12.82

After the horizontal ramus has been fixed by intermaxillary fixation in the desired occlusal position by means of either Ernst ligatures or wire-Palavit splints and the shortened ascending ramus is in the correct upright position, a stab incision is made over the angle of the jaw along a skin crease. The subcutaneous soft tissues are separated with fine scissors parallel to the direction of the marginal mandibular branch of the facial nerve until the site of the osteotomy is reached (Fig. 12.84). A trocar with a handle is introduced. Holes are drilled through the trocar in the fragments perpendicular to the bone surface. A screw thread is then made in the hole of the medial fragment. Figure 12.85 shows the sleeve of the trocar in situ serving as protection for the soft tissues of the face while the burr holes are drilled perpendicular to the external bony surface. The fragments are fixed exactly (a) by intermaxillary wiring and (b) by retention forceps.

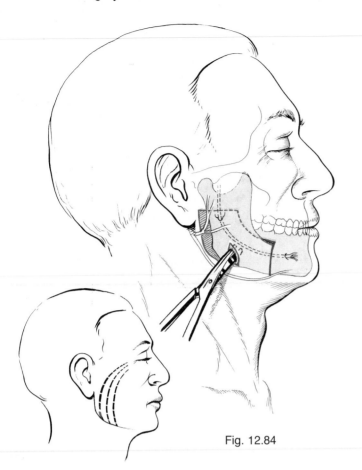

Fig. 12.84

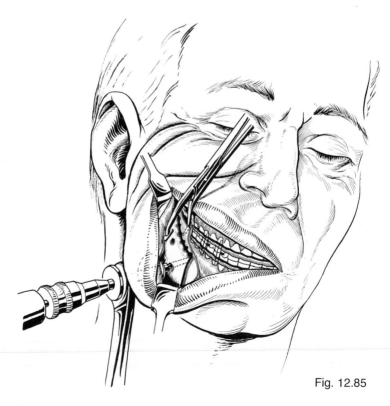

Fig. 12.85

There is a screw thread located on the free end of the trocar, and with a special forceps a drill guide is introduced from within the mouth and screwed to this thread. The drill guide serves not only as a sighting mechanism but also as a soft tissue retractor (see Fig. 12.72).

A gliding hole is bored into the lateral lamella by means of a 2.7 mm spiral bit. Drilling is continued in the same direction with a 2 mm bit; the traction hole in the medial part of the lamella of the horizontal ramus is made in this way. A thread for a 2.7 mm cortical screw is cut into this hole. After the burr hole has been irrigated a lag screw is introduced through the trocar. The screw is then tightened.

The procedure is repeated for the second and third screws where the end of the trocar is shifted in relation to the position of the mandibular canal. (Fig. 12.86 shows stable fixation of the fragments by introducing 3 traction screws. Then the intermaxillary fixation is removed.) A diagram for the location of the screws is shown in Figure 12.91.

Before the trocar is removed, a suction drain is inserted from intraorally through the soft tissues over the angle of the jaw. The intermaxillary ligatures are then removed.

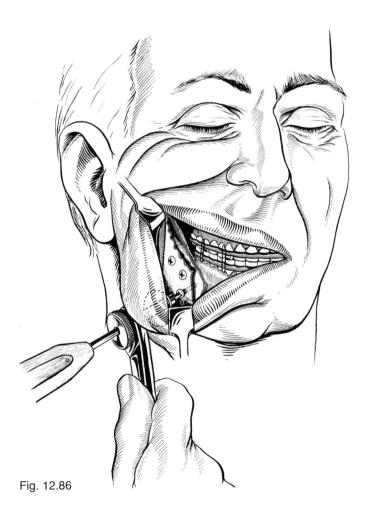

Fig. 12.86

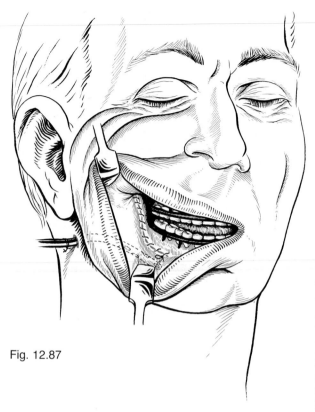

Fig. 12.87

The wound is closed with continuous 4 × 0 Supramid sutures (Fig. 12.87). The suction drain is fixed externally and the stab incision is closed with 5 × 0 Supramid sutures (Fig. 12.88).

Before extubation passive opening and closing movements are carried out as a final test to see whether the required occlusion and articulation have been achieved. If the third screw could not be applied, the jaw is immobilized for 3 to 4 weeks.

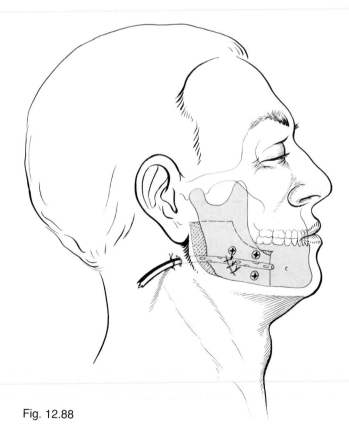

Fig. 12.88

Correction of Unilateral Prognathism

(Asymmetry of the face, prognathism, lateral curvature of the chin; see p. 190).

Three variants of the sagittal osteotomy can be considered:

- Homolateral,
- Bilateral,
- Contralateral, with simultaneous resection osteotomy on the hyperplastic side.

If hyperplasia of the head of the mandible and the condylar process is accompanied by functional disturbances in opening of the mouth, particularly trismus, a *condylectomy* is indicated (see p. 260 for operative technique).

The indications for *homolateral displacement* osteotomy are demonstrated with the help of the simulation model. This model must allow satisfactory adjustment of the occlusion. If minimal displacement of the mandible toward the midline is adequate for optimal improvement of the occlusion, the slight rotation of the axis of the joint on the healthy side does not cause a functional disturbance. The operative procedure and the type of fixation are, in principle, the same as those described above.

A *bilateral displacement* osteotomy is indicated in hyperplasia of the entire half of the mandible. The hyperplastic side is displaced posteriorly which automatically results in anterior displacement of the normal side. It is important that the angle of the jaw on the healthy side remain unaltered. The ascending ramus, therefore, is fixed in its original position with an adjustable clamp (Figs. 12.89, 12.90).

This provides an opportunity for comparison while adjusting the angle of the jaw on the hyperplastic side, and an accurate assessment of the amount of shortening required for the fragment near the joint is possible.

In extreme hyperplasia and disfiguration of the angle of the jaw, it is still possible to carry out a resection osteotomy on the hyperplastic side and a ramisection on the contralateral (normal) side. The resection osteotomy is performed either with Trauner's operation (see p. 224) or with a simple preangular transverse osteotomy (see p. 225). We

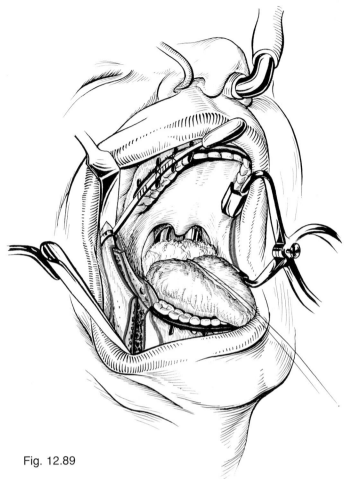

Fig. 12.89

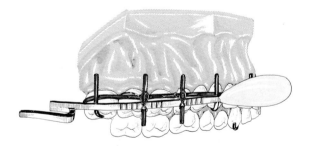

Fig. 12.90 Adjustable clamp with scale and plastic handle to hold the divided ascending ramus in its original position in central occlusion. Before beginning the osteotomy, the mandible is fixed in central occlusion. The clamp is placed in position on the denuded oblique line and the appropriate mark on the scale is determined. The clamp is then removed or retracted. After division of the ramus of the mandible, the clamp is reintroduced in the previously determined position.

prefer the latter since here in particular, Trauner's operation is too complicated both in planning and in execution.

It should be noted that, in all these displacement osteotomies, supplementary correction of the chin and the body of the mandible is often necessary in order to obtain satisfactory esthetic results, whether this is achieved by removal or levelling of prominent parts or by filling out flattened and/or sunken contours.

Important Modifications and Surgical Alternatives

Dal Pont's extension of the incision is undoubtedly an advance. This extension allows a considerably larger range for displacement of the fragments. Based on our experience, many of the advocated methods for the surgical treatment of prognathism have been made obsolete by this procedure.

Certainly, it is easier to split the ascending ramus above the angle of the mandible. Thus, Obwegeser's incision also suffices when the jaw must be mainly displaced posteriorly in a straight line. We prefer, however, Dal Pont's incision also in such cases because it permits stable fixation of the fragments.

Schuchardt's (1960) oblique osteotomy is easier to carry out, but the resulting contact surfaces of the fragments are smaller than after a sagittal split.

Transverse division of the mandible produces the smallest contact surfaces. For this reason the method is only of historical significance.

Caldwell and Letterman (1954) combined the transverse incision with a sagittal incision. In this procedure both fragments were correspondingly decorticated. Although the contact surfaces are increased, a scar on the neck and a deformed jaw angle on both sides must be tolerated. On the basis of histological studies of bone healing after oblique osteotomy on the ascending ramus, Boyne (1966) confirmed that decortication is unnecessary.

We do not divide the neck of the mandible either inside or outside the capsule. The difficulties which can develop after such an operation (relapse, deterioration as compared with the condition before

treatment in the form of an open bite, and compensation problems in regard to dentures in the edentulous mandible) speak against the use of such an operation, even if in edentulous patients the situation could be compensated by the use of dentures.

Landmarks and Danger Points

Landmarks

● For the mucosal incision: The oblique line.

● For access to the pterygomandibular space above the mandibular foramen: The base of the coronoid process; the notch and the neck of the mandible.

● For the superior bony incision: The notch, the posterior edge and the external surface of the ramus of the mandible, 1 cm below the notch. The external surface is kept in view in order to assess the depth of the incision. The inner layer of the cortex is concave internally.

● For the lower bony incision: The position of the second molar, the oblique line and the convex curve of the cortex.

● For the sagittal splitting: A line, 0.5 cm medial to the oblique line (see Fig. 12.81).

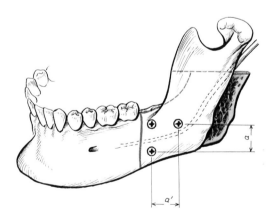

Fig. 12.91   Scheme for siting the screws in a prognathism operation taking into consideration the course of the nerve and the position of the second molar. The position of the two anterior screws is shown: One on the oblique line ("oblique screw") and one in the lower border of the mandible ("basal screw"). In both cases this is a clearly defined anatomical region. The third screw lies at an equal distance (a') behind the oblique screw.

● For the application of traction screws: Two screws are parallel to the edge of the incision of the proximal fragments; one passes through the oblique line ("oblique screw"); the other, through the lower border of the mandible 6 to 8 mm from its inferior edge ("basal screw"). The third lies an *equal distance* behind the oblique screw, parallel to the inferior edge of the mandible (Fig. 12.91).

Danger Points

● *Hemorrhage* can occur from the posterior facial vein, the inferior alveolar artery and the maxillary artery if the neurovascular bundle has not been carefully elevated along the base of the coronoid process to the posterior edge of the mandible. Sufficient room must also be created to allow insertion of the prognathism retractor. The posterior edge of the ascending ramus must be protected and kept under vision to prevent damaging the vessels with the drill.

● *Damage to the inferior alveolar nerve*:

1. During exposure of the superior osteotomy site,

2. During section of the ramus if the latter is not split far enough laterally,

3. During the lower bony incision if the curve of the cortex is not considered.

● *Iatrogenic fracture of the proximal fragment*:

1. If the superior incision is too deep,

2. If the sagittal split is too near or even on the oblique line,

3. If the posterior edge is not included when the incision is being made.

4. If chisels are used instead of fine, sharp osteotomes.

● *Complications after extubation*:

1. If the throat pack is not removed before intermaxillary fixation of the jaw,

2. If wire cutters are not sent with the patient to the recovery room so that the intermaxillary wires can be cut in case of emergency (e.g., vomiting).

Rules

● Exact planning on the simulation model.

● Prior removal of wisdom teeth.

● Controlled splitting. The groove must be positioned in such a way that the split is made exactly at the lateral border between the cortex and the cancellous bone. Extra-sharp osteotomes should be used! Attention should be paid to the initial direction of the osteotome during postangular splitting; this should not be in a sagittal direction but at a 20° to 30° angle to the external surface of the ascending ramus (see Fig. 12.81).

● Guaranteed positioning of the occlusion.

● Reliable fixation and maximal adaption of the fragments by interfragmentary compression with traction screws.

● Irrigation of the wound at regular intervals during the operation, preferably with a pulsating jet of water (Surgical Jet Spray) with Ringer's or polybactrin solution.

● Vacuum drain which is removed on the third day.

● Sufficiently wide wound edges on the alveolus to permit secure wound closure.

● 40 mg methyl prednisolone is given intravenously toward the end of the operation; an additional 40 mg is given 4 hours after the operation.

Postoperative Care

In-Patient Care

● If an atraumatic operative technique and regular wound irrigation have been used, antibiotic cover is not necessary. Appropriate antibiotic treatment is given when signs of infection become apparent.

● A nasogastric tube is used for feeding. If the tube is not tolerated, a purée rich in proteins and vitamins is given.

● The oral cavity is cleaned thoroughly twice a day with cetrimide spray; the teeth are brushed 3 times a day.

- The bottle on the suction drain is changed 3 times a day.

- The sutures are removed and the patient is released 8 days after the operation.

Out-Patient Care

- If ideal occlusion and a good frontal overbite are achieved via internal fixation with 3 lag screws on each side, the patient is checked once a week.

- If there is a tight overbite, monoblock treatment (i.e., correction of incisor relations with an acrylic plate) is begun during the second week after the operation.

- If only 2 traction screws have been applied on each side the intermaxillary fixation is removed after 3 weeks.

- If the fragments have been fixed with wire, the intermaxillary fixation is removed after 6 weeks (not after 3 weeks!). Intermaxillary fixation with rubber bands is employed for an additional 2 weeks. If there is a tight frontal overbite, the fixation is removed after 6 weeks, at the earliest, and immediate monoblock treatment is begun.

Functional Sequelae

Normal occlusion is achieved in almost 100% of the cases with Dal Pont's osteotomy and secure fixation via 3 traction screws on each side.

Trauner reports a two-thirds failure rate for 38 patients operated on by Obwegeser's and Dal Pont's method. The sequelae included recurrence, open bite, pseudarthrosis and permanent anesthesia of the lower lip. These results can, however, be traced back to certain unfavorable circumstances.

The disadvantage of the sagittal splitting is the danger of damaging the nerve in the postangular part of the mandible, particularly if the technique described above is not followed precisely. For the most part, paresthesia resolves within 6 months if the nerve has not been transected.

Sagittal Splitting as Lengthening Osteotomy

Principles of the Operation (see p. 190)

Indications

Sagittal splitting as a lengthening osteotomy is indicated for:

- Pseudounderdevelopment of the lower third of the face; main feature: *distal bite*.

- Underdevelopment of the lower third of the face; main feature: *retrognathia*.

- Unilateral underdevelopment of the lower third of the face; main feature: *unilateral retrognathia* (asymmetry of the face; underdeveloped, crooked chin).

In *pseudounderdevelopment of the lower third of the face, mandibular retrognathia is present*. Posterior displacement of the normally developed mandible by a distance equal to the breadth of 1 or 2 premolars produces the appearance of an underdevelopment of the lower third of the face (see Fig. 12.43).

The chief features are:

- Receding chin,

- Pronounced labiomental skin fold,

- Retracted lower lip which frequently lies behind the upper front teeth,

- Deep overbite.

In *underdevelopment of the lower part of the face, retrognathia* is present (synonyms: mandibular micrognathia, opisthognathia). The term retrognathia, as the opposite to prognathia, is more suitable for the surgeon both as a concept and for purposes of classification than the above-mentioned synonyms.

In the basic type of retrognathia, the appearance of underdevelopment of the lower third of the face almost always corresponds with the true situation since, in most cases, hypoplasia of the mandible (including underdevelopment of the chin) can be established on one or both sides. As a result lengthening osteotomy on the ascending ramus is a promising procedure.

The main features are:

● Absence of the prominence of the chin,

● Shortened ascending and/or horizontal rami,

● Posterior bite and usually a deep overbite.

In contrast there are cases of retrognathia in which the receding chin is not due to hypoplasia but rather is the result of the overly superior position of the temporomandibular joint. As a result the mandible and the teeth are rotated and displaced posteriorly. A corrective operation must then be performed on the chin itself.

The "bird face" is an extreme and rare form of retrognathia. It is caused by arrested development resulting from bilateral osteomyelitis of the mandible, with sequestrum formation during early childhood, or as a result of ankylosis. A displacement osteotomy alone is not adequate in these cases.

Unilateral underdevelopment of the mandible (unilateral retrognathia) is usually the result of arrested growth caused by infection or trauma.

The main features are:

● Displacement of the midline toward the diseased side,

● Flattened, mildly scoliotic mandible on the healthy side,

● Usually restricted opening of the mouth (ankylosis).

In osseous ankylosis a displacement osteotomy is not feasible because of the good occlusion. In practice all that is required is an ankylosis operation (see p. 259) and, if necessary, augmentation of the chin. For all patients with satisfactory occlusion, a displacement operation on the chin is the only operation possible.

Preoperative Diagnosis (see p. 191)

The presence of a distal bite is apparent from the occlusion (see p. 171).

Teleradiographic analysis shows the typical features of an underdeveloped lower part of the face (retrognathia) (Fig. 12.92).

Routine radiographs are described on page 191.

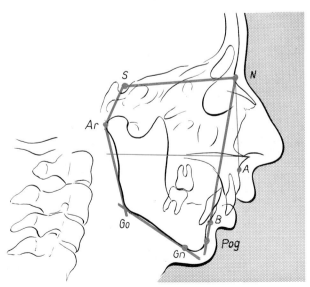

Fig. 12.92 Retrognathia, mandibular micrognathia). Go-Gn, S-N-B and S-N-Pog are small; N-S-Ar and S-Ar-Go are large.

Preparation for Surgery

Out-Patient Preparation

Simulation. Detailed simulation of a displacement osteotomy should be considered for bilateral and unilateral retrognathia.

In *distal bite* simple anterior displacement of the peripheral fragment suffices; a simple plaster-of-Paris model is adequate.

In *retrognathia*, however, the skeletal correction consists of displacement in two planes: anteriorly along the horizontal axis and inferiorly along the ascending axis (Fig. 12.93). The skeletal correction does not restore normal relationship between the upper and lower teeth since a deep bite is usually also present in these patients. Due to the extreme posterior position of the lower arch, the alveolus and the teeth compensate by growing obliquely in an anterosuperior direction. The result is that the lower teeth bite on the palatal mucosa immediately behind the upper front teeth. In such cases the skeletal correction is supplemented by dentoalveolar correction. Since this is a complex operation, an exact simulation should be carried out on the model.

The following should be determined:

- Required lengthening of the horizontal and ascending rami,
- Shape of the angle of the jaw,
- Segmental shortening of protrusion of the front teeth,
- Shape of the occlusal overlay,
- Technique of fixation: splinting and internal fixation,
- Type of occlusal adjustment,
- Correction of the chin.

The related technique for the simulation is illustrated in Figure 12.94.

In-Patient Preparation (see p. 192)

Special Instruments (see p. 193)

Anesthesia (see p. 192)

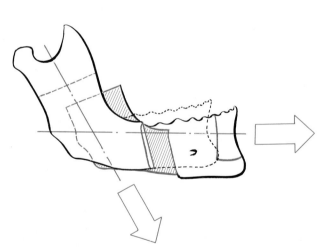

Fig. 12.93 Lengthening osteotomy by sagittal splitting of the rami of the mandible. The horizontal ramus (ventral arrow) and the ascending ramus (caudal arrow) are lengthened.

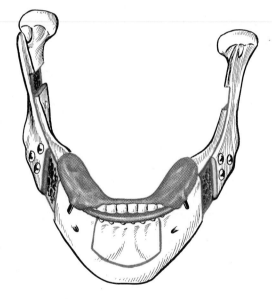

Fig. 12.94 The model after simulation of an operation for retrognathia: Lengthening osteotomy by a sagittal split of the mandible, stable fixation with 3 lag screws on each side.

Transposition osteotomy of the center of the mandible, rigid fixation of the anterior fragment with a wire-Palavit splint, combined with bite blocks to compensate for posterior open bite as a result of the displacement osteotomy.

Operative Technique

The technique, in principle, is the same as that described on page 195.

Remarks on the Individual Corrective Operations

A *distal overbite* is *corrected* in exactly the opposite way to a simple prognathism. The mandible is displaced anteriorly after sagittal splitting, the occlusion is fixed provisionally by intermaxillary fixation and the fragments are then fixed under pressure with 3 traction screws.

Correction of retrognathia is complex. The initial situation is shown in Fig. 12.95: a) the profile in retrognathism; b) the *skeletal anomaly*: a shortened mandible, posterior bite and absence of the prominence of the chin; *dentoalveolar anomaly*: deep overbite with relative protrusion of the front teeth, lower teeth engage against the palatal mucosa.

In addition to ramisection, correction osteotomies of the anterior part of the alveolus and the prominence of the chin as well as modification of the occlusion by a bite splint are almost always necessary. In many patients simulation on the model allows the entire correction to be carried out in one operation (see Fig. 12.94). Only when a more extensive correction of the chin is required, it is advisable to carry this out at a second operation.

Sequence of osteotomies:

● Chin correction,

● Frontal transposition osteotomy,

● Sagittal osteotomy of the rami of the mandible.

The entire chin is exposed using the technique described on page 238. The chin is corrected by simple removal of the required amount of bone.

Protrusion of the front teeth is dealt with by an osteotomy of the anterior alveolus. Figure 12.96 shows a frontal displacement osteotomy as part of an operation for retrognathia intended to achieve a normal frontal overbite. The lingually pedicled fragment is lowered by removing bone and is tilted, depending on the position and shape of the upper front teeth (the operative technique is described on page 238).

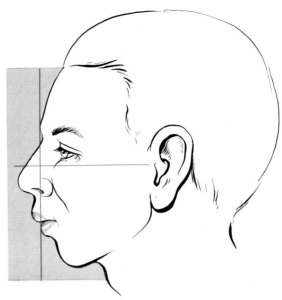

Fig. 12.95 a

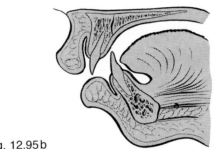

Fig. 12.95 b

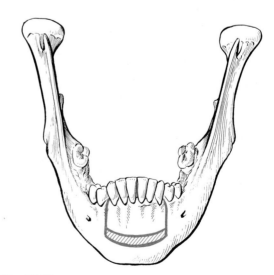

Fig. 12.96

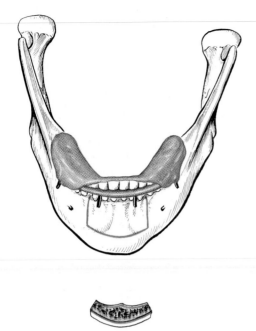

Fig. 12.97

Exact adjustment and fixation of the fragments is guaranteed by an occlusal overlay. It is used as a splint and for occlusal adjustment. Figure 12.97 shows adjustment of the fragments and fixation in a frontal displacement osteotomy using the occlusal splint (lingual splint and an alveolar block prepared preoperatively on the simulation model) and the wire-Palavit splint. Intermaxillary fixation is not necessary. The mucosal wound is closed after the fragments have been exactly positioned.

Sagittal splitting with anteroinferior adjustment of the fragments is then carried out.

This movement in two planes produces normal overbite but nonocclusion in the molar area. The nonocclusion (lateral open bite) is compensated by an acrylic occlusal overlay utilizing the principle of self-regulation of the bite (Fig. 12.98a). The overlay is ground down in stages during the postoperative period until the molars come into contact with each other. Figure 12.98b shows the same patient as in Figure 12.98a after successive reductions of the overlay over a period of 9 months. The first premolar now occludes with its antagonist; the second is lying visibly higher. Figure 12.98c shows the position after 18 months of treatment with an overlay; normal occlusion is now present.

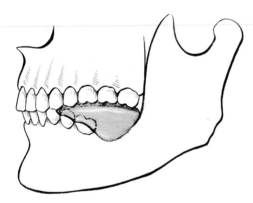

Fig. 12.98a

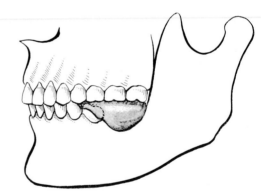

Fig. 12.98b

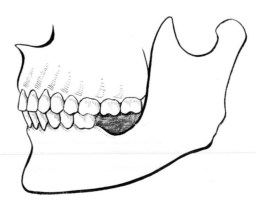

Fig. 12.98c

Fixation is achieved with 3 traction screws as shown in Figure 12.99. The location of these screws in an operation for retrognathia is shown; the course of the nerve must be taken into consideration. One of the anterior screws passes through the oblique line ("oblique screw") and one through the lower border of the mandible ("basal screw"). The third screw lies at an equal distance (a') behind the basal screw.

Figure 12.100 shows an overall picture of a corrective operation for a unilateral skeletal and dentoalveolar anomaly in a retrognathia. The steps may be summarized as follows:

1. Frontal displacement osteotomy,
2. Rigid fixation and adjustment of the occlusion with a wire-Palavit splint and an occlusal overlay,
3. Sagittal splitting and anterior displacement of the peripheral fragments according to a preoperatively determined occlusal overlay,
4. Exact internal fixation of the fragments with temporary intermaxillary fixation,
5. After application of the traction screws: removal of the intermaxillary fixation and closure of the mucosal wound with the mouth open.

If the correction must be carried out in several operations, dentoalveolar correction precedes sagittal splitting. Operation on the ascending ramus takes place 6 weeks later, at the earliest.

Correction of a *unilateral retrognathia* almost always requires an operation on both sides and only rarely on one side. The operation is, of course, indicated only in disordered occlusion. In patients with functionally normal occlusion in which the condition results from a developmental failure in childhood, only a displacement operation to improve the profile of the chin should be considered. In such patients a fibrous or osseous ankylosis is also present. Mastication must then be restored first.

The possibility of achieving the required displacement by sagittal splitting in patients with a markedly shortened half of the mandible on the affected side is often underestimated. For these patients the displacement during unilateral lengthening of the peripheral fragment takes place not only in an axial direction, but also around a vertical axis which passes through the center of the mandible. The effective displacement between the osteotomy surfaces is, therefore, relatively small. In other words, bilateral sagittal splitting is almost always the correct procedure for this type of anomaly.

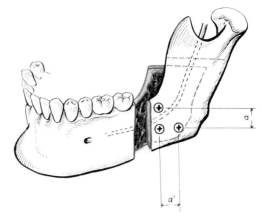

Fig. 12.99

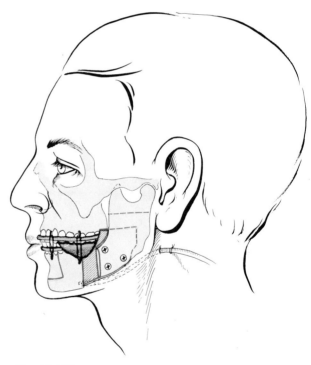

Fig. 12.100

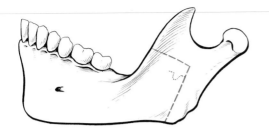

Fig. 12.101   Wassmund's incision for correction of retrognathia (reversed L-shaped osteotomy).

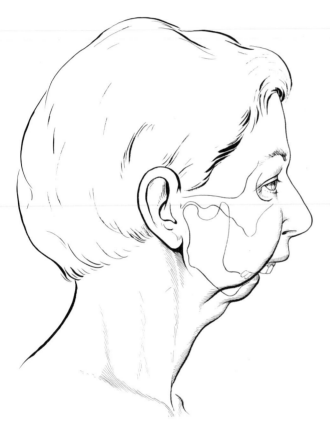

Fig. 12.102   Bird-face resulting from osteomyelitis of the mandible involving the head of the mandible during childhood: Extreme hypoplasia of the mandible and dysgnathia; deformed profile.

Modifications and Surgical Alternatives

In our experience sagittal splitting as a displacement osteotomy is the method of choice for distal bite and retrognathia.

Trauner's operation (1954) for anterior displacement of the mandible in distal bite via retrocondylar implantation of cartilage has almost no practical application.

Longitudinal division of the ascending ramus (Wassmund 1952) is not a satisfactory alternative. Wassmund's incision (Fig. 12.101) with interpositioning of a bony autograft, however, achieves not only true lengthening of the mandible but also favorable conditions for healing. This procedure has been recommended by many authors with various modifications (Pichler 1919, Trauner 1954, Immenkamp 1957, Robinson 1957, Schuchardt 1958, Thoma 1961).

This method cannot be considered as an alternative method to sagittal splitting, but it can be particularly recommended for correction of the *"bird face"* in which an extreme degree of retrognathia is present. Here the rudimentary rami cannot be split sagittally in the hope of achieving successful displacement. A satisfactory standard operation is preferable for such extreme cases. In our opinion the reversed L-shaped osteotomy with interpositioning of a bony autograft is a useful method (Schuchardt and Immenkamp).

Depending on the initial anatomical and functional situation for a patient with a "bird face" (Fig. 12.102), two operations are needed:

● A displacement (lengthening) operation on the ascending ramus as described above (Schuchardt and Immenkamp);

● Augmentation of the chin (see p. 243).

The two operations are carried out 6 months apart.

Interosseous fixation. All the authors who ad-
vocate the above-mentioned method use a
wire suture at the angle of the jaw to coapt the
contact surfaces between the graft and the
fragments in order to provide fixation. This unstable fixation causes traction on this side
which disturbs the healing of the graft after
early intermaxillary fixation has been removed. Not only a pseudarthrosis is the result
but also an open bite.

To prevent this complication, a wire ligature,
preferably a strong circular suture, should be
introduced on the side of the tractional stress
(Fig. 12.106). Before finally introducing the
graft, a hole is bored in the upper part of the
distal fragment and a 0.7 mm wire is inserted
through it and through the proximal fragment.
The graft is inserted and the circular suture is
drawn tight. This ensures a firm bed for the fixation of the plate on the lower aspect of the
angle of the jaw. To ensure an optimal contact
between plate and mandible, part of the cortex
of the graft is removed before application of
the plate. Figure 12.107 shows stable fixation
of the graft between the fragments. The circular suture and the compression plate together
form a load-carrying system.

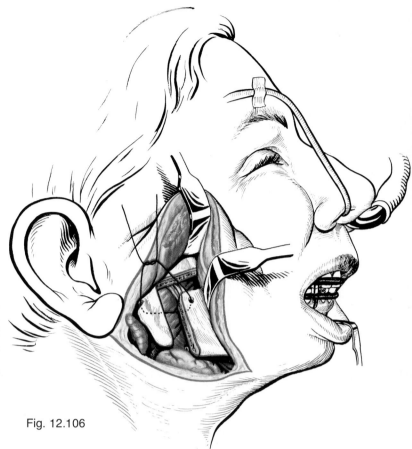

Fig. 12.106

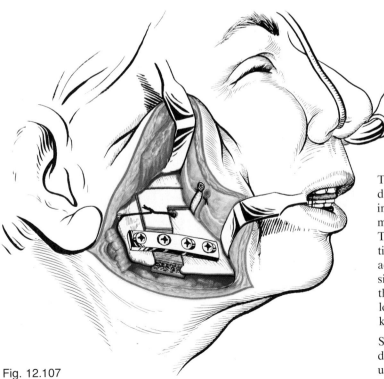

Fig. 12.107

The fixation system formed in the manner
described above permits rapid ingrowth
into the graft. The mandible can then be
mobilized early (after the fourth week).
This is particularly important for rehabilitation since the "bird face" is almost always
accompanied by a fibrous ankylosis. This
situation requires early functional orthodontic maneuvers since fixation for too
long an interval tends to produce total ankylosis.

Suturing and suction drainage are used as
described on page 146 and illustrated in Figure 12.108.

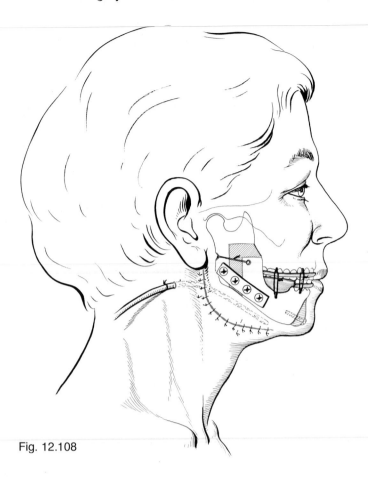

Fig. 12.108

Figure 12.108 shows a composite view of this corrective operation. The sequence of steps is as follows:

1. Reversed L-shaped osteotomy,
2. Anterior displacement and intermaxillary fixation of the peripheral fragment in optimal occlusion,
3. Preparation of the circular suture on the tension side,
4. Interposition of the graft,
5. Fixation with a 0.7 mm circular wire suture and a compression plate,
6. Chin augmentation with a bone graft, usually carried out as a second operation,
7. Removal of the intermaxillary fixation after 3 weeks, at the latest.

A further alternative operation is stepped osteotomy on the ramus of the mandible. A step is cut between the angle of the jaw and the canine tooth. This allows displacement of the peripheral fragments at a distance equal to the width of a tooth. Von Eiselsberg (1906), Dingman (1948), Pichler (1919) and Kazanjian (1932) preserve the nerve by removing the bone along the entire length of the canal (Fig. 12.109 a).

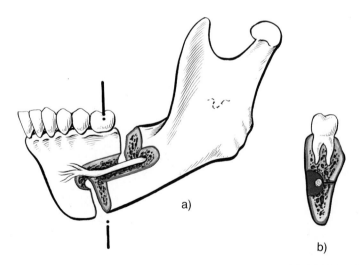

Fig. 12.109 a   Stepped displacement osteotomy (Pichler/Kazanjian) with exposure of the nerve canal.

Fig. 12.109 b   Frontal section through the divided mandible at the point marked (that is the first molar). The result of boring out the nerve canal is minimal cortical contact between the fragments.

This method cannot be recommended for several reasons. The expenditure of time and effort is too great in comparison with the end results. Lengthening of the jaw by a distance equal to that of a molar tooth demands that the vestibular side be almost totally denuded and drilled out. This method is unsuitable because the mandibular canal always runs on the lingual side. Due to the inevitable weakening of the ramus, which is usually hypoplastic, it is impossible to actually obtain good contact of the fragments since all that remains after drilling of the bone down to the canal is a marginal zone at most 1 mm thick on the lingual side (Fig. 12.109b). It is obvious that this allows neither exact approximation nor secure fixation of the fragments to each other.

Landmarks and Danger Points
(see p. 204)

Rules, Hints and Typical Errors
(see p. 205)

Postoperative Care

In-patient care: see page 205

Out-patient care: The patient is examined weekly if ideal occlusion has been achieved by fixation with 3 traction screws on each side. The plastic overlay splint (see p. 210) is ground down gradually during the follow-up period until the molars come into contact with each other.

Functional Sequelae (see p. 206)

Resection Osteotomy and Displacement Osteotomy of the Horizontal Ramus

Lateral Resection Osteotomy

Principles of the Operation

Shortening of the horizontal ramus by resecting a lateral transverse segment (Hullimen 1849, [cited by Wassmund 1935], Angle 1897, Pichler 1919) with preservation of the inferior alveolar nerve (Dingman 1944).

Indications

- True prognathism with an extremely long mandibular body and a moderately flat or normal angle of the jaw,
- True prognathism and open bite extending as far as the molar teeth,
- True prognathism with deep overbite.

An extreme reversed overbite of as much as 15 mm is characteristic of these patients. One of the obvious causes of overdevelopment of the mandible is an extremely enlarged tongue. An open bite develops simultaneously due to the increased pressure of the tongue. Only the posterior molars occlude when the patient bites.

Deep overbite is the opposite of open bite. The lower front teeth cover the upper ones as a result of the reversed overbite.

The question of diminution of the tongue must always be considered before treatment for these anomalies is begun. Many authors recommend it as a routine practice if the disproportion is limited to the body of the mandible. Since a seemingly normal tongue is occasionally found together with an enlarged mandibular arch, reduction should be undertaken only when the tip of the tongue (maximal protrusion) reaches the labiomental groove or when the edges of the tongue extend over the occlusal surfaces of the teeth on speaking or swallowing.

Principles of the Technique of Reduction of the Tongue

The main principle for this technically uncomplicated operation is the removal of a wedge from the tip of the tongue. To prevent scar contracture of the tip of the tongue, a flap of mucosa and muscle is formed at the tip and stitched to the corresponding side of the other half of the tongue.

The muscle is removed in full thickness of the tip of the tongue. The muscle mass in the center of the tongue is reduced; care should be taken to preserve the large vessels in the deeper part. Hemostasis is achieved and the wound is closed in layers. The mucosa is closed with 4×0 atraumatic Supramid sutures.

Diagnostic Preoperative Measures

The basic anomaly is overdevelopment of the lower third of the face. **Teleradiographs** show true prognathism (see Fig. 12.37).

Routine Radiographs

These include:

- Mandibular views centered on the chin: good views of the premolar and canine regions, the mental foramen, the interdental septa and the relationship of the mandibular canal to the roots of the teeth and to the border of the mandible.

- Separate views of each half of the mandible to demonstrate the ascending ramus, the molar region and the mandibular canal.

- Intraoral views of the mandible in a vertical plane: assessment of the outer and inner cortex.

- Dental films $\overline{6543} \mid \overline{3456}$ to assess the apical region, the interdental septa and the mental foramen.

Plaster-of-Paris model and **profile photographs** are made as described on page 172.

Preparation for Surgery

Out-Patient Preparation

Extraction of displaced and nonerupted wisdom teeth is carried out and dental treatment if necessary.

Simulation

Simulation is carried out on a model of the body of the mandible to accurately establish:

- The shape and extent of the resection,

- The detailed technique of fixation.

Axial shortening alone seldom suffices for extreme cases of overdevelopment of the horizontal ramus. Depending on the severity of the occlusal abnormality (open or deep occlusion), the anterior fragment must, at the same time, be slightly elevated or lowered. The cut surfaces on the resected piece of bone must be shaped accordingly. In an open bite, the incision is trapezoid in shape (wider above and narrower below); in deep overbite the trapezoid is reversed. This rule of thumb should be applied for each individual patient. It is particularly important that apposition of the fragment surfaces correlate with the desired adjustment of occlusion.

The desired shortening in the longitudinal direction is, therefore, simulated on the model by removing a corresponding segment with surfaces which converge slightly inward. Bending of the axis may possibly be indicated superiorly for overbite or inferiorly for a deep open bite. This is achieved by bevelling the ends of the fragments in one direction or the other. The external contour of the resulting defects on the model are retained by a lead template which defines the limits of the resection at the operation.

The program of simulation must include the following points:

- Resection osteotomy on the model,

- Preparation of the technical adjuncts:

1. Lead template for the incision and for shaping the end of the fragments,

2. Occlusal overlay for adjustment of the occlusion,

3. Splint in 3 parts and possibly previously bent dynamic compression plate for the fixation.

Operation on the model. Shortening the mandible is determined by the extent of the reversed overbite as measured in millimeters with calipers. As a rule, the distance is the width of one molar or premolar. If the required width exceeds that of one tooth on each side the transverse osteotomy on the angle of the jaw or a sagittal splitting of the ascending ramus should be simulated on the model. Paying careful attention to the neighboring teeth, the segments are cut out and the mandible falls into 3 separate pieces. These pieces retain their original position in the simulator.

The next step is adjustment of both rami in occlusion with the upper molars, as well as provisional fixation. The arch of the chin is then set backward. The extent of step formation or incongruity of the fragment ends appears when the occlusion is adjusted. The corresponding surfaces of the fragments are apposed, protruding ridges and cusps are removed and the grinding surfaces are marked with a colored pencil.

The final result should be ideal occlusion with optimal adaptation of the fragments.

Lead template (Fig. 12.110). Before final fixation of the fragments, the 3 pieces of the jaw are replaced in their original position; according to existing defects the lead templates are shaped.

Occlusal splint. An occlusal overlay constructed on the operative model is used to facilitate adjustment of the fragments. The splint should grasp the linguoocclusal part of the dental arch (including the alveolus to the circumlingual sulcus, if possible). In this way the adjusted fragments are held in the correct position and movement during adjustment of other fragments is prevented.

Intraoperative use of the splint is described on page 223.

Splinting. For both the resident physician and the patient, it is more practical to carry out splinting shortly before the hospital admission. In this way the splint can be checked. Thorough scaling should be carried out before the splinting.

The tripartite splint is prepared on the simulation model. An auxiliary splint is always carefully fastened to the maxilla.

In-Patient Preparation

On the day before the operation:

● Grinding down the teeth on the basis of the simulation model,

● Disinfection of the oral cavity and the splints

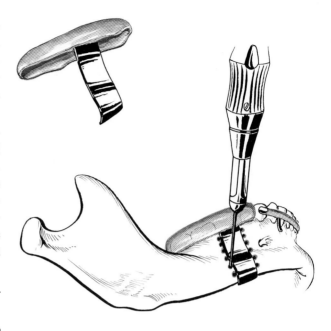

Fig. 12.110   Lead template with occlusal anchoring.

with 0.5% cetrimide spray at the end of this sitting.

● Routine premedication.

On the day of operation (in the anesthesia room):

● Position: For intraoral access to the mouth, the head of the patient is deflected slightly and is turned to the opposite side during extraoral exposure of the lower border of the mandible so that the submandibular triangle can be exposed in the greatest extent.

● The oral cavity is cleaned for 3 minutes with cetrimide spray with simultaneous suction. The skin of the neck and face are cleaned 3 times with 80% alcohol and clear 2% cetrimide. The lips and the angle of the mouth are smeared with Vaseline. The eyes are held shut with nonirritant adhesive tape.

Special Instruments

See Figures 12.63–12.65, 12.72 and 12.73.

Anesthesia

Resection osteotomies are painful and time-consuming operations which must be carried out under endotracheal anesthesia. Nasal intubation must be used to allow adjustment of the occlusion. A nasogastric tube should be introduced for at least 3 days. The anesthetic tube should be sealed with paraffin impregnated gauze; inflation of the cuff alone is inadequate.

Operative Technique

We prefer the one-stage intraoral – extraoral procedure because, with this procedure, good access, a rapid and atraumatic operation as well as stable fixation are made possible.

Intraoral Incision

The operation begins in the oral cavity. The scalpel (No. 15 blade) is introduced lateral to the last molar and is carried firmly down to the bone and then forward in the paragingival sulcus almost to the midline. With the tongue retracted and the floor of the mouth under tension, a similar incision is made on the lingual side. The periosteum is elevated widely and cleanly on both sides as far as the edge of the mandible; the mental foramen is exposed on one side and the insertion of the mylohyoid muscle is detached on the other side.

Intraoral Resection

The planned extraction is now carried out. The prognathism retractors are introduced (broad one on the vestibular side and narrow one on the lingual side) so that they both engage the lower edge of the mandible. The alveolus is removed completely using Luer's forceps. The lead template fitted with an occlusal overlay is now introduced (Fig. 12.110). A similar operation is carried out on the opposite side. Before continuing the operation externally, the wound is covered with saline compresses, the mouth and cheeks are draped with a towel and the head is turned toward the opposite side.

Extraoral Incision (Fig. 12.111)

The incision lies exactly in a skin crease of the neck so that the skin and then the platysma and the fascia over the submandibular gland can be divided with one stroke of the knife (No. 15 blade). Remaining in this plane, the flap of skin and platysma are elevated obliquely in a posterior direction up to the border of the mandible. This procedure leaves the branches of the facial nerve undisturbed. The facial vessels, as a rule, must be ligated. The lead template is encountered at the edge of the mandible. The periosteum has already been detached in this area.

Extraoral Resection

Small holes are bored in the outer cortex, along the edge of the template. The template and the soft tissues of the cheek are then elevated with a Langenbeck hook. As the final step of this phase, the mandibular canal is marked with fine burr holes, beginning at the mental foramen (Fig. 12.112).

The burr holes are united on the left and right sides with a Lindemann drill. Puncture holes are made with a spear burr on the lower edge in order to weaken the inferior margin. This facilitates removal of the lateral cortex with an osteotome (Fig. 12.113). Usually the nerve canal can be seen shining through in the exposed cancellous bone. The canal is carefully opened with Luer's forceps and the bone is removed (Fig. 12.114).

The neurovascular bundle is now mobilized with a fine Joseph's spatula and the lingual side cortex is "nibbled"

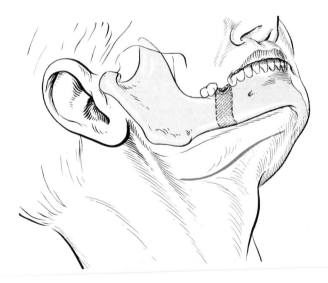

Fig. 12.111

away down to the canal with Luer's forceps. The neurovascular bundle is then freed from its remaining bony surroundings. It is protected on the lingual side by an extra-wide elevator (Fig. 12.115).

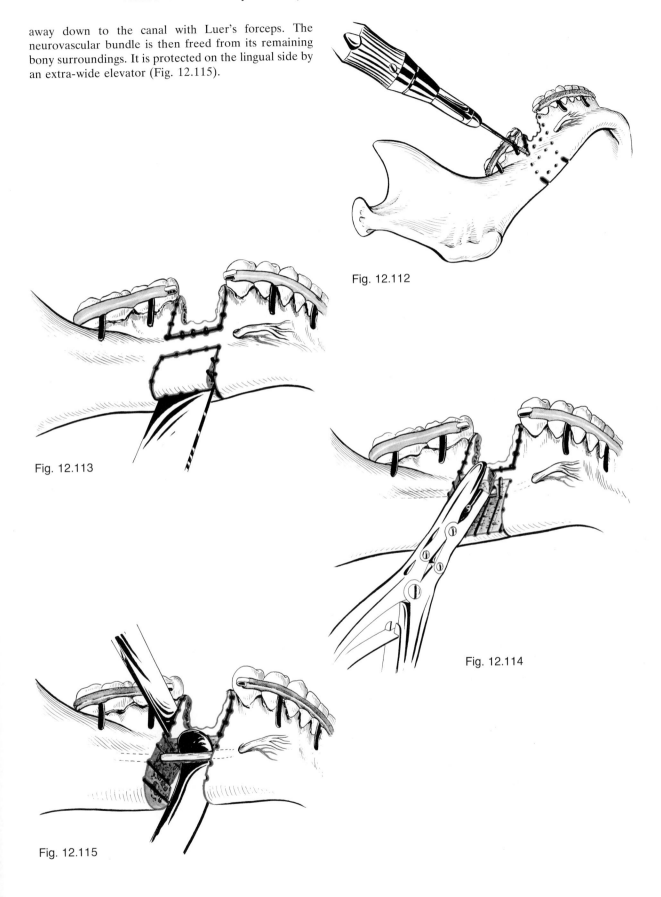

Fig. 12.112

Fig. 12.113

Fig. 12.114

Fig. 12.115

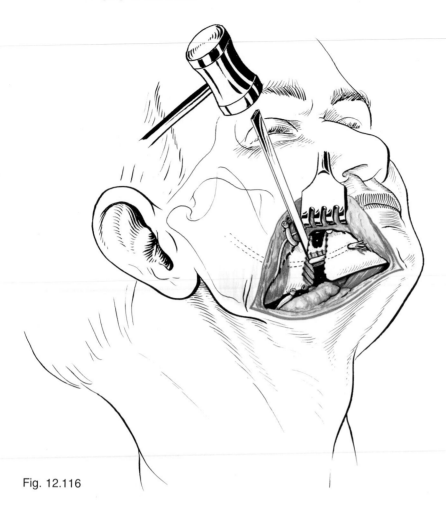

Fig. 12.116

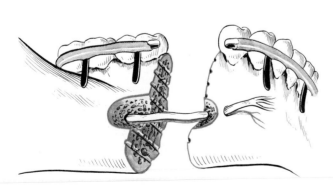

Fig. 12.117

Above the elevator, the outer cortex can be removed smoothly with a chisel (Fig. 12.116). The remaining cancellous bone is removed with the burr.

Before removing the lingual bridge of bone, a hollow is nibbled laterally in the ends of each fragment in order to avoid damaging the nerve when the fragments are apposed (Fig. 12.117).

The interposed elevator remains in place until the rest of the lingual cortex is removed, the edges of the bone are smoothed and the defect is washed out and packed. The wound is covered with a cetrimide pack.

Adjustment and Intraoral Fixation of the Fragments

After the osteotomy has been carried out on the opposite side and the wound has been carefully covered, the head is returned to its original position and the oral cavity is clearly displayed with 2 Langenbeck retractors.

The correct occlusion as determined on the model is the vital factor in adjusting the fragments. The position of the 3 fragments is secured by the occlusal overlay and the tripartite splint. The splint is first attached loosely with a 0.6 mm wire suture, then the occlusal overlay is introduced.

Due to the tendency toward torsion on the part of the fragments, a firm base is created with the occlusal overlay. The middle fragment is anchored to this base with two 0.6 mm ligatures around the splint (Fig. 12.118, above). This prevents the fragment from slipping during adjustment of the remaining fragments. The lateral fragments are each fixed with one ligature.

Perfect positioning of the occlusal overlay shows that the oral fragments are in the correct position (Fig. 12.118, below). The tripartite splint is now wired securely by drawing the wires tight and reinforcing them with acrylate. The overlay is then removed, the occlusion is checked and intermaxillary fixation is applied using 0.5 mm wire sutures drawn tight between the splints on the upper and lower jaw. Before final fixation is carried out, the throat pack must be removed and the mucosal incision on the lingual side must be closed.

The vestibule of the mouth is now thoroughly cleaned with Surgical Jet Lavage or with a cetrimide spray and is closed with continuous 4 × 0 Supramid sutures.

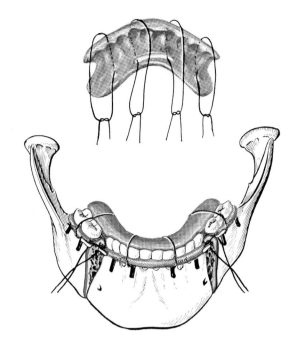

Fig. 12.118

Internal Fixation

After occlusion has been secured, absolute stabilization of the fragments is carried out through the extraoral access.

The last correction of the position of the fragments is carried out on the basal side. The adjustment planned on the model can now be easily achieved since the intermaxillary fixation prevents the fragments from deviating on the oral side. Interfragmentary compression is applicable using repositioning compression forceps (see Fig. 12.63). Finally, the dynamic compression plate is applied (Fig. 12.119).

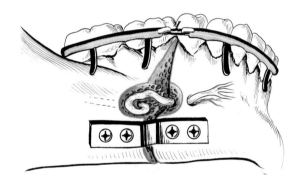

Fig. 12.119

Wound Closure

The platsyma is closed with continuous 4 × 0 Dexon (polyglycolic acid) sutures. This prevents postoperative deformity of the angle of the mouth. Four or five mattress sutures are introduced through all layers of the skin. The wound is closed with 5 × 0 Supramid sutures without a subcutaneous suture; a suction drain is introduced on both sides.

Important Modifications and Surgical Alternatives

Originally, Dingman (1944) carried out the ostectomy in 2 sittings at 3 to 4 week intervals. At the first operation, an intraoral resection of the alveolus of the extracted teeth was carried out; at the second stage, an extraoral resection of the remaining segment of bone was carried out with preservation of the inferior alveolar nerve.

Since the widespread use of prophylactic antibiotics, the operation has been carried out by many authors in one sitting, either by the intraoral and extraoral route (Dingman 1948, Kapovits and Pfeifer 1961), exclusively by the intraoral route (Aller 1917, Converse and Schapiro 1952, Ernst 1927, Thoma 1945) or exclusively by the extraoral route (Gabka 1961, Köle 1961). Apart from damage to the nerve, "infection, necrosis of the jaw, pseudarthrosis and postoperative disturbances of occlusion" (Köle) constitute the problems occurring with a lateral resection osteotomy. The complication rate has been reduced by broader use of the two-stage operation (Dingman) because the second operation is carried out under aseptic conditions via an external approach. In our opinion an increased danger of pseudarthrosis and late infection remains. This is due to the often unstable fixation which can be prevented neither by prophylactic antibiotics nor by staging the operation.

Absolute fixation of the fragments is imperative for preventing complications because, in this way, bone healing is not so much a matter of chance. Stability is crucial in this case since the contact surface of the fragments has been reduced as a result of the bilateral shortening of the mandibular arch and since primarily cortical bone is present. This can result in necrosis of the ends of the fragments and formation of a decalcified zone (Böhler 1957, Eggers et al. 1951). Stepping the ends of the fragments (Pichler 1919, Converse and Schapiro 1952) was supposed to help solve this problem. The modification is based on the idea of increasing interfragmentary contact and preventing elevation of the distal fragment in the absence of support of the molar teeth.

In fact the stepped ostectomy does not provide a satisfactory solution. The gain in contact surface achieved by the additional bony notch is insignificant since the ends of the fragments remain largely out of contact due to the shortening of the mandibular arch. Elevation of the distal fragment is more easily and securely prevented by intermaxillary fixation and support with dental overlays than by notching the ends of the fragments.

An additional attempt to achieve interfragmentary retention without using fixation is the "inlay ostectomy" (Thoma 1958). It is used for the edentulous mandible or where molars are missing. A mortice joint is made of the ends of the fragments; the distal end forms the tenon and the proximal end forms the slot. This is a more complicated operation than the step ostectomy; interfragmentary notching should not be used in lieu of fixation.

Trauner's (1973) "right-angled ostectomy plus osteotomy of the angle of the jaw" is a real alternative method (Fig. 12.120a, b). It has the following advantages: Exposure of the osteotomy site at the angle of the jaw is both technically and cosmetically more favorable. Resection combined with an osteotomy is easier and quicker. The angle of the jaw can be molded under direct vision. Functioning teeth are not extracted. The adjustment with the appropriate correlation between optimal occlusion and adaption of the fragments is less complicated. Superfluous bone on the ends of the stumps of the horizontal ramus can be removed and used for filling interfragmentary defects. Finally, splinting and intraosseous fixation is considerably easier to carry out.

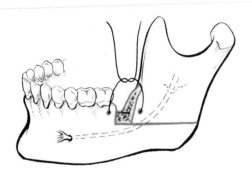

Fig. 12.120a

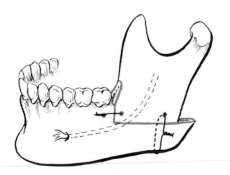

Fig. 12.120b

Technique. In many respects we perform this operation differently from Trauner. When Trauner postulates "carrying out the ostectomy in the region behind the last molar tooth", the methodology of the procedure is called into question, since the ostectomy is then not carried out on the angle of the jaw but on the ascending ramus. As a result, many of the advantages described above are sacrificed.

We carry out a segmental ostectomy (Fig. 12.121a); the wisdom teeth are removed 3 months before the operation. The bone is exposed both intraorally and extraorally. The fact that the masseter muscle can be elevated from within the mouth subperiostally and atraumatically to the posterior and inferior edge of the mandible is a distinct technical advantage. The template for the excision can be introduced under vision and can be fixed to the neighboring teeth. It is not clear from Trauner's description how this can be achieved through a 3 cm extraoral incision. Moreover, his geometrical planning of the excision on the teleroentgenograph without the use of a template is of little value.

In our experience a preangular resection osteotomy carried out via the oral cavity is quicker because the soft tissues, including the lingual nerve, can be better retracted on both sides from the resection site. The origin of the pterygoids need not be freed. This is an important consideration for revascularization of the periphery of the fragments since these have been completely denuded on the lateral side.

The extraoral access is exposed generously. The transangular osteotomy (with preservation of the inferior alveolar nerve) is facilitated by using Liston's scissors after grooving the outer cortex along the previously marked osteotomy line. The mobile ascending ramus is retracted outward with an angled retractor so that the canal in the region of the osteotomy site can be enlarged under vision in order to protect the nerve. The lingual cortex may also be removed.

The next important step is firm fixation of the occlusion with intermaxillary wiring. Grinding down the occlusion toward the end of the operation, as Trauner recommends, is inexact and complicated and it prolongs the operating and anesthetic time.

A two-hole tension-band and a four-hole stabilization plate are used for the internal fixation (Fig. 12.121b). Tension is provided by this arrangement of the plates which guarantees sufficient stability in spite of the weakness of the ascending ramus and the low number of holes in the plate. This technique allows immediate opening of the mouth. The anterior screw of the traction plate engages only the outer cortex.

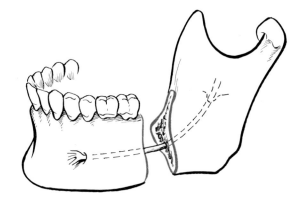

Fig. 12.121 a

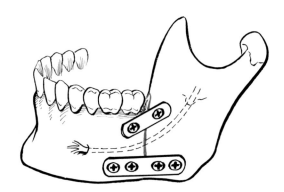

Fig. 12.121 b

Landmarks and Danger Points

Landmarks

● For the intraoral incision: Gingival margin.

● For access to the resection site: The edge of the incision in the periosteum, the mental foramen and the mental nerve, the lower border of the mandible, the mylohyoid line and the insertion of the muscles.

● For the intraoral resection: The walls and fundus of the alveolar socket, the mental foramen and the mental nerve, the neighboring teeth for the correct positioning of the lead template.

● For the extraoral incision: A lateral skin crease and the hyoid bone.

● For extraoral access to the resection site: Formation of a flap of skin and platysma; the capsule of submandibular gland for the plane of cleavage for sharp dissection.

● For the extraoral resection:

a) The thickness of the bone on the vestibular side down to the mandibular canal is:
At the level of the mental foramen: 1.5 mm
At the premolar: 5–6 mm
At the first molar: 8–9 mm;

b) The height of the lower border of the mandible up to the mandibular canal measured from the lower border is:
At the site of the mental foramen: 13–16 mm
At the premolar: about 10 mm
At the first molar: 10 mm.

Danger Points

● Damage to the mandibular nerve in its course within and beyond the canal.

● Detachment of the mylohyoid muscles; bleeding from one of the large veins of the floor of the mouth.

● Damage to the roots of neighboring teeth.

● Division of the marginal branch of the facial nerve if the skin incision lies superior to the natural skin crease, if the platysma and the fascia are elevated from posterior rather than in the reverse direction and if the correct depth of the incision relative to the capsule of submandibular gland is not maintained.

Rules, Hints and Typical Errors

Rules

● Simulation must be as exact and detailed as possible.

● Access must provide as good a view as possible.

● Incision of the bone must be as simple as possible.

● Fixation must be as stable as possible.

Hints

● For prevention of infection, edema and postoperative pain:
a) Thorough cleaning of the oral cavity on the day before operation.
b) Spraying for 3 minutes with cetrimide or a pulsating jet of sodium chloride solution when preparing the oral cavity for the operation.
c) A pulsating jet of Ringer's solution should be used frequently during the operation, particularly on the bone incision.
d) Suction should be used instead of pledgets!
e) Bone retractors should be used gently.
f) A sterile mixture of Ringer's solution and air should be used during the osteotomy for cooling.
g) Suction drainage.
h) 40 mg of prednisolone should be administered intravenously toward the end of the operation and 40 mg 4 to 5 hours later.

● The skin is always divided in a skin crease when making the submandibular incision; anteriorly, the incision should not be curved in order not to cross a tension line of the skin. If necessary, it should be extended in the line of a skin crease.

● The periosteum should be elevated only from within the mouth when carrying out intraoral-extraoral exposure of the bone.

● During the resection a planned dental extraction can be combined with the ostectomy (with the exception of an alveolar ostectomy). The template should be used as a resection model. The major part of the resection is carried out with an osteotome and Luer's forceps.

● For adjustment of the occlusion:
Grinding down the teeth before the operation; use of the occlusal overlay; provisional fixation of the fragments by joining the divided splint with a wire ligature; preoperative splinting.

● For the fixation:
Intermaxillary fixation with strong wire sutures (which requires application of a rigidly fixed splint). A stable screwed plate rather than an unstable wire suture.

● For the suturing:
Continuous atraumatic sutures, where advantages are tension-free adaptation of the wound edges, wound edges not disturbed by circulatory deficiency and economical use of time and materials. Mattress sutures are used instead of subcutaneous sutures.

Typical Errors

During the operation:

● Too small incisions, both intraorally and extraorally.

● An inadequate view of the operative site results in unnecessary trauma.

● Crushing the soft tissues causes edema, hematoma and pain.

● Tearing the periosteum results in delayed revascularization.

● Excessive elevation of the periosteum causes excess devitalization of the fragment ends.

● Excessive speed and insufficient irrigation or cooling of the drill causes necrotic foci.

During the fixation:

● Adjustment and fixation of the fragments may never be carried out in the same manner as for a double fracture of the mandible.

● Delayed bone healing and pseudarthrosis do not result from macroglossia or increased tongue pressure; in fact, unstable fixation is the basic cause of these complications. The risk of complications due to macroglossia may be during removal of the fixation. It is more likely to occur when the occlusion has been badly adjusted or when overbite is absent.

Postoperative Care

In-Patient Care

If the operation extends over more than 2 hours, antibiotic cover should be given according to the following schedule: penicillin (20–40 million I.U.) per day and streptomycin 1 g administered intravenously by continuous infusion (usually for 5 days). 40 mg prednisolone are given intravenously

during the operation and 40 mg intravenously 4 to 5 hours after the operation.

The patient should be tube fed for the first 3 days. A diet rich in proteins and vitamins is given beginning on the fourth day.

Wound care: The oral cavity is cleaned thoroughly twice daily with cetrimide. The teeth are also cleaned 3 times a day.

The external wound remains uncovered and is cleaned once a day with cetrimide.

Wound drainage: The suction drainage is changed 3 times a day and the drain is removed on the third day.

Removal of the sutures: The extraoral sutures are removed on the fifth day after operation, the intraoral sutures on the eighth day.

The patient is discharged from hospital on the eighth day.

Out-Patient Care

If stable fixation has been used, early mobilization is begun during the third week; a puréed diet is given.

If unstable intraosseous fixation with wire has been used, mobilization is begun during the sixth week, at the earliest.

Check up: The patient is checked twice a week.

Functional treatment: Monoblock treatment is begun immediately after removal of the intermaxillary fixation if there is an accurate frontal overbite. Average duration is 6 months.

Functional Sequelae

Sensory disturbances in the area supplied by the mental nerve seldom occur with the technique described above. We do not agree with Köle's statement that "most authors consider division of the nerve to be of no practical significance". The obvious excess of tissue on the cheek, which occurs as a direct result of shortening of the ramus of the mandible, is more an esthetic than a functional disadvantage. The "baroque angel's face" occurs only in extreme cases. The soft tissue contours harmonize spontaneously after 1 year, at the latest.

The lack in the literature of a statistical analysis of the success of this operation is conspicuous even though relapses are seldom observed. Certainly, this is due to the low number of cases and, as such, is proof that a displacement osteotomy on the ascending ramus is usually preferred to a resection osteotomy on the horizontal ramus. On the other hand, the low tendency toward recurrence can be explained by the fact that the real shortening of the body of the mandible occurs outside the direct functional area of the masticatory muscles.

The incision in a skin crease fades after 1 year and is barely visible after an additional year. Occasionally, a hyperplastic scar may develop; it should be corrected 1 year later, at the earliest.

Anterior Resection Osteotomy

Principles of the Operation

Shortening and narrowing of the mandibular arch by resecting a segment of the center of the chin.

Indications

Extreme prognathism with bilateral crossbite due to overdevelopment of the mandible and simultaneous underdevelopment of the upper jaw (Figs. 12.122, 12.123).

In prognathism with bilateral crossbite, the individual cusps of the last molars just make contact on occlusion (Fig. 12.124).

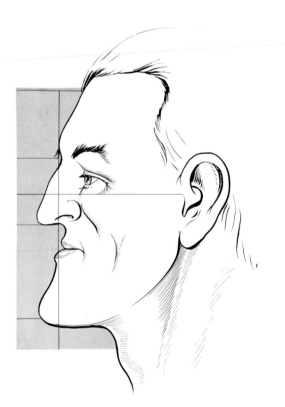

Fig. 12.122   Profile of an overdeveloped lower third of the face (widely projecting mandibular arch) and underdevelopment of the middle third of the face.

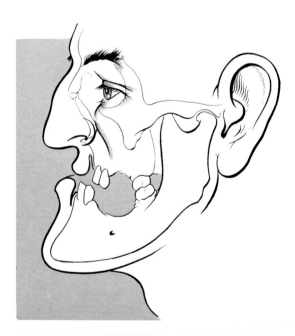

Fig. 12.123   Gnathic anomaly: Base of the maxilla is underdeveloped while the lower border of the mandible and the ascending ramus are overdeveloped.

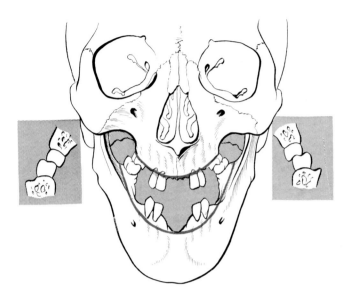

Fig. 12.124   Bilateral crossbite.

Diagnostic Preoperative Measures

● Analysis of the teleroentgenograms: The typical picture of prognathism with bilateral crossbite is hypoplasia of the upper jaw and hyperplasia of the lower jaw (Fig. 12.125).

● Plaster of Paris model and profile photographs.

● Routine radiographs:

1. Contact occipitomental views of the mandible: Demonstration of the mandible, particularly the chin region against a blurred vertebral column.

2. Dentosubmental views of the mandible: Assessment of the anterior edge of the chin up to the alveolus without superimposition of the vertebral column, the apices of the teeth and the interdental septa from canine tooth to canine tooth.

3. Dental films: $\overline{54321 \mid 12345}$.

4. Possibly, orthopantomograms of the mandible.

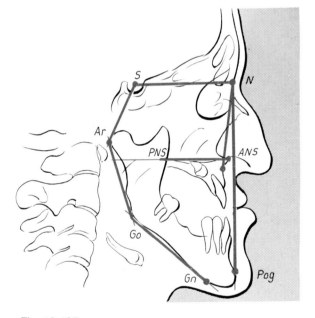

Fig. 12.125

ANS-PNS and SNA
N-S-Ar, S-Ar-Go } small

Go-Gn
Ar-Go-Gn } large
S-N-Pog

Preparation for Surgery

Out-Patient Preparation

Simulation. In prognathism with bilateral crossbite, the intermaxillary proportions are so distorted by the hyperplasia of the mandible and hypoplasia of the upper jaw that conventional osteotomies alone are inadequate. Simulation shows that occlusion cannot be achieved solely with a lateral resection osteotomy nor with a sole sagittal split of the ascending ramus. In such a case, the center of the chin should be resected and a sagittal osteotomy should be carried out on the ascending ramus. At the same time, a strongly protruding chin is shortened (Fig. 12.126).

The advantages of simulating the operation on the model are clearly demonstrated in this case. The extent of narrowing and posterior displacement of the mandible required, including modification of the angle of the mandible, can be determined exactly on the simulator (see Fig. 12.47). Usually premature loss of teeth or periodontal disease, particularly of the incisors, is present. In such cases, re-

section of a transverse segment from the center of the chin should be considered.

The result of operative simulation on the model is the separation of the mandible into 4 pieces (Fig. 12.127). This, however, brings up the problem of fixation. Stabilization of the fragments in the midline is particularly important because the danger of pseudarthrosis is greatest here. If dentition is adequate, strong wire and a rigid splint suffice. Intermaxillary fixation should be continued at least for 6 weeks. Most patients present an edentulous jaw; here fixation is difficult, but essential.

The method of internal fixation using screws and plates is the most suitable and certain. It is suitable because intermaxillary fixation time can be shortened to 2 or 3 weeks with this method. It is certain because both halves of the mandible can be united under pressure in the midline. The sagittally split ascending ramus must be fixed not only with wire but also with traction screws (Fig. 12.127).

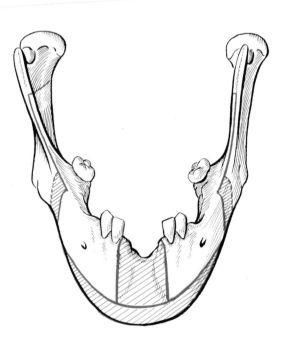

Fig. 12.126   Incision for narrowing and shortening the mandible in bilateral crossbite. Anterior: Resection osteotomy. Posterior: Displacement osteotomy.

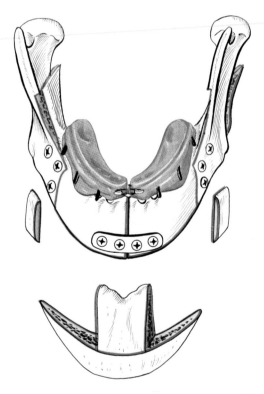

Fig. 12.127   Simulation of the resection and fixation (patient in Fig. 12.126). Anterior: A bipartite traction archbar with bite blocks and screw plate. Posterior: 3 lag screws on each side.

Provision of a denture for the edentulous patient should be included in the planning of the operation. The intended overbite and the height of the bite are established on the basis of the articulated, simulated operative model. Dental overlays are used which serve both as an occlusal key for the intraoperative adjustment of the fragments and for the 3-week intermaxillary fixation. At the end of this period, the overlays are reshaped for the orthodontic treatment (see Fig. 12.47).

Splinting. If the patient has teeth, a splint which is divided in the middle is used; as usual, on the upper jaw an auxiliary splint is applied. In the edentulous patient the prosthetic splint is fastened, under anesthesia, immediately before the beginning of the operation (see below).

In-Patient Preparation

On the day before the operation:

- Grinding down the teeth as described on page 219.

- Cleaning the oral cavity as described on page 223.

- Premedication according to the schedule already described.

On the day of the operation (in the anesthesia room):

- Splinting of the edentulous jaw: After the patient has been intubated, the divided splint is fixed to the mandible with circumferential wiring (2 loops for each half of the jaw) and to the upper jaw with 2 or 3 peralveolar wires, laterally and anteriorly (possibly combined with zygomaticomaxillary suspension). The standard awl is used for the circummandibular loops; a bore is used for the peralveolar fixation to pierce the base of the alveolus in the region of the canine teeth and in the region of the incisors if necessary. 0.6 mm wire is used.

- The position of the patient and all other measures are described on page 219.

Special Instruments (see p. 220)

Anesthesia (see page 220)

Operative Technique

The operation may be carried out either via the intraoral or the extraoral route. We usually select the extraoral route because intraosseous fixation can be carried out more easily by this route and there is less danger of infection.

The central incisors must be extracted 3 months before the operation. If the front teeth are healthy and there is no periodontal disease, we select an alternative incision (see alternatives p. 233).

Submental Incision

A curved incision is made immediately posterior to the border of the mandible (Fig. 12.128). The submental region is exposed while the wound edges are elevated with sharp hooks. The adherent periosteum which intermingles with the insertion of the digastric muscle must be repeatedly incised in the same location and completely freed from the bone if possible. To achieve this, it is best to start in the midline and proceed up to the alveolus. The mucoperiosteum is undermined as far as the edge of the alveolus with a curved elevator. Laterally, the lower border of the mandible is exposed as far as the mental foramen. The inner surface of the lower border of the mandible remains intact.

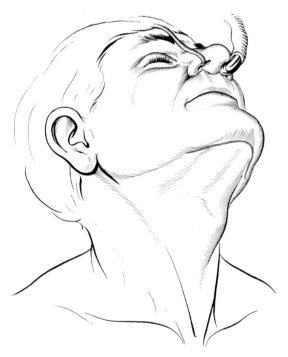

Fig. 12.128

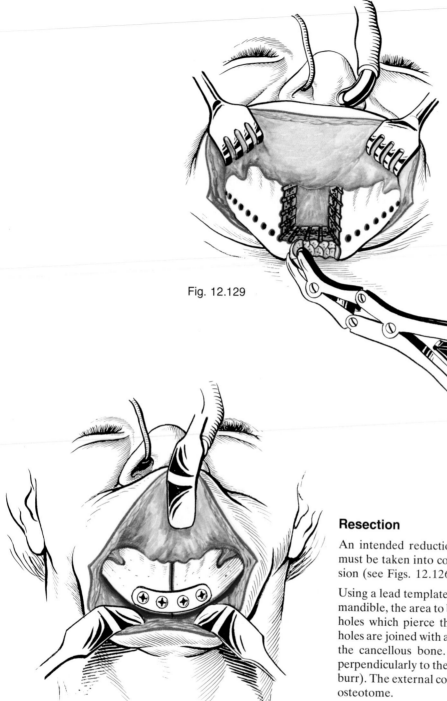

Fig. 12.129

Fig. 12.130

Resection

An intended reduction of the prominence of the chin must be taken into consideration when making the incision (see Figs. 12.126, 12.127).

Using a lead template applied to the lower border of the mandible, the area to be resected is marked out with burr holes which pierce the cortex on both sides. The burr holes are joined with a fissure burr which reaches as far as the cancellous bone. Additional holes are then made perpendicularly to the lower edge of the mandible (flame burr). The external cortex can then be levered off with an osteotome.

The resection should not be carried out in one piece. The following method is less damaging and quicker: As soon as the cancellous layer of bone has been exposed, the burr holes of the inner cortex are joined; the periosteum is preserved. Only the base of the mandible is exposed in order to prevent tearing of the aponeurosis which is attached to the mental spine and the symphysis. The bone is removed in stages with a rongeur. In this way the aponeurosis remains intact (Fig. 12.129).

Adjustment and Intraoral Fixation of the Fragments

The stumps are beveled internally to provide wide contact surfaces. Adaptation of the fragments can be disturbed by the excess mucosa. Since both parts of the splint must be joined together without an intervening gap in any case, the mucosa is excised from the alveolar sockets. Both splints are joined in the center with a 0.6 mm wire suture (see Fig. 12.127).

Intraosseous Fixation (see Fig. 12.130)

Wound Closure

Suction drains are inserted, 3 to 4 mattress sutures are inserted and the skin is closed with continuous Supramid 5 × 0 sutures.

The second part of the operation now follows, that is the posterior displacement of the body of the mandible by sagittal splitting of the ascending ramus. The technique is described on page 195. The situation at the end of the operation is illustrated in Figure 12.131.

Important Modifications and Surgical Alternatives

If the front teeth are intact, the central incisors are not sacrificed. The basal resection is then combined with an alveolar resection as follows: The dental arch is shortened by the width of one premolar segment on each side, and the frontal segment of the alveolus is detached from the body of the mandible. In addition the lower border of the mandible is shortened by removing a central piece of bone the width of 2 premolar segments combined (Fig. 12.132).

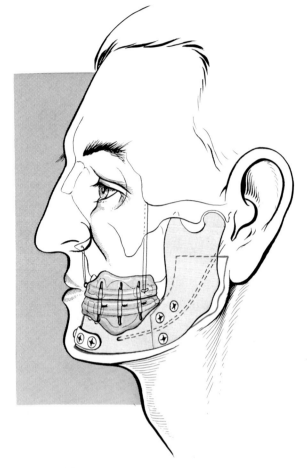

Fig. 12.131

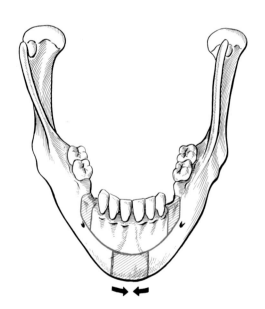

Fig. 12.132   Excision for narrowing and shortening of the mandible in bilateral crossbite: Stepped resection osteotomy.

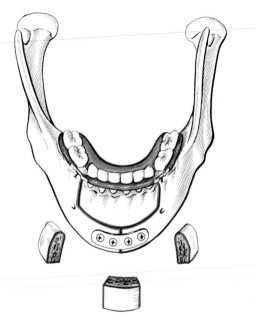

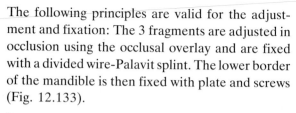

The following principles are valid for the adjustment and fixation: The 3 fragments are adjusted in occlusion using the occlusal overlay and are fixed with a divided wire-Palavit splint. The lower border of the mandible is then fixed with plate and screws (Fig. 12.133).

In contrast to median resection, this stepped resection is carried out only from the intraoral side.

The same principle of stepped osteotomy is used to expand the mandibular arch (Fig. 12.134). In this case a bony defect is produced which is then filled with a bony allograft consisting of cortical and cancellous bone on the basal side and cancellous bone on the alveolar side (Fig. 12.135). The operation is carried out via the intraoral approach.

Fig. 12.133 Resection and fixation (case in Fig. 12.132): Occlusal overlay for securing the position of the fragments, a tripartite archbar and a dynamic compression plate are shown.

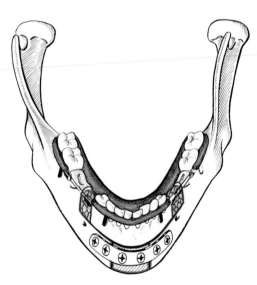

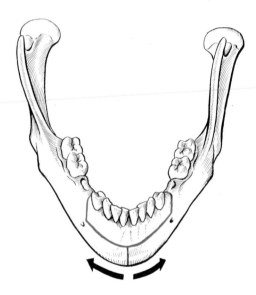

Fig. 12.134 Incision for widening the mandible in bilateral overbite with a narrow jaw.

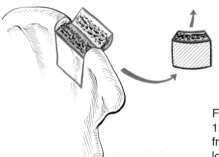

Fig. 12.135 Osteotomy and fixation (case in Fig. 12.134): Occlusal overlay for securing the position of the fragments, tripartite archbar, interfragmentary cancellous graft and a dynamic compression plate with graft of cortical and cancellous bone.

Vestibular flaps are used to close the mucosal defect (Fig. 12.136). Generous exposure of the mandibular arch is needed for the osteotomy (Fig. 12.137). After transposition of the vestibular flaps continuous sutures are applied (Fig. 12.138).

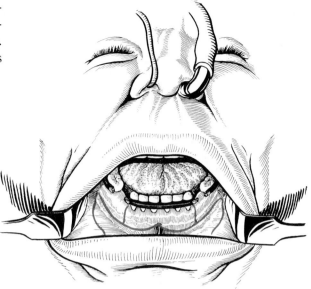

Fig. 12.136

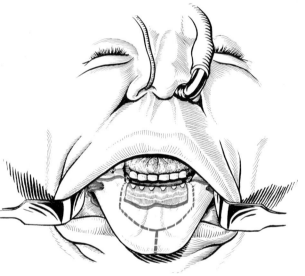

Fig. 12.137

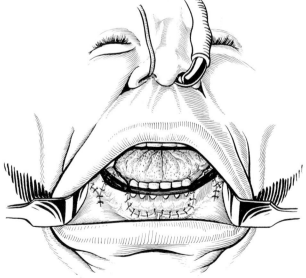

Fig. 12.138

Landmarks and Danger Points

Landmarks

- For the submental incision: The lower border of the mandible.
- For extraoral access to the site of resection: The aponeurosis of the mentalis muscle, the depressor labii inferioris muscle, the depressor anguli oris muscle and the mental foramen.
- For the resection: The alveolar ridges over the tooth roots, the mental protuberance, the mental spine, the digastric fossa and the sublingual fovea.

Danger Points

- Damage to the roots of neighboring teeth.
- Damage to the mental nerve.

Rules, Hints and Typical Errors

Rules. See page 226.

Hints. Resection should not be carried out in one piece but rather by removing the bone in layers. (The symphyseal aponeurosis should be preserved).

Postoperative Care (see p. 227)

Functional Sequelae

In spite of internal or external rotation of both halves of the mandible, disturbances of the temporomandibular joint are hardly ever observed. This may be due to the shape of this joint which functions as a ball-and-socket joint. Furthermore, the inward or outward rotation of the head of the mandible when the halves of the mandible are reunited is negligible because of the length of the ramus of the mandible. The simultaneous posterior displacement of the body of the mandible also generally produces no late effects. The scar beneath the chin is barely noticeable and is seldom esthetically disturbing.

Frontal Displacement Osteotomy

Principle of the Operation

Displacement of the center of the mandible by a right angled osteotomy on the alveolus; the fragment remains pedicled lingually.

Indications

- Protrusion,
- Elevation of the front teeth above the occlusal plane,
- Infraposition of the front teeth below the occlusal plane.

Protrusion of the tooth-bearing front of the mandible is referred to as *alveolar protrusion*. In contrast to true prognathism, the lower border of the mandible is normally developed. The developmental anomaly is confined to the alveolus and the teeth. Protrusion of the front of the mandible is often accompanied by protrusion of the upper jaw (*bialveolar protrusion*).

Elevation of the front teeth of the mandible above the occlusal plane is a fairly common feature accompanying prognathism and alveolar protrusion of the upper jaw (see p. 265).

Infraposition of the front teeth of the mandible below the occlusal plane often occurs with the rachitic open bite (see p. 274).

Diagnostic Preoperative Procedures

- Analysis of the teleradiographs. An example of bialveolar protrusion is shown in Figure 12.139.
- **Plaster-of-Paris model** and **profile photographs.**
- **Routine radiographs.** The same projections are required here as for anterior resection osteotomy (see p. 229).

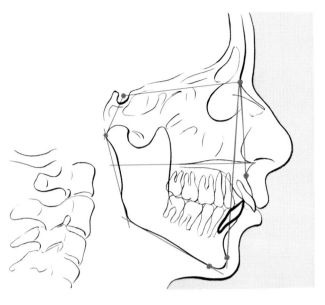

Fig. 12.139 Bialveolar protrusion with stepping of the incisor teeth and distal bite. Lower border of the mandible and the ascending ramus normally developed.

If the lateral teeth are missing, the overlay also serves as a prosthetic splint which is introduced during the operation. The anterior arch of the splint is stiffened with self-hardening acrylate so that the fragment is blocked on the vestibular and the lingual side. Intermaxillary fixation is not used with this type of fixation.

If the front teeth are elevated, only the affected segment is freed from the alveolus and shortened as necessary.

If, however, the front teeth are deep-seated, the fragment is raised and supported with a graft. The adjustment of the fragment by means of the occlusal overlay and fixation by means of a splint is achieved in a similar way as described above.

In-Patient Preparation (see p. 231)

Special Instruments (see pp. 193, 194)

Anesthesia

In some cases a frontal displacement osteotomy can be carried out under local anesthesia. A bilateral nerve block at the mandibular foramen is combined with infiltration anesthesia in the vestibule and the floor of the mouth. It must be assumed, however, that the operation will last longer than 30 minutes and that application of more analgesics will be necessary.

Extensive infiltration of the operative area with a vasoconstricting local anesthetic is not advisable for operations on the mandible since this limits the methods available to the anesthetist. It is generally accepted that fluothane ought not be used if epinephrine or norepinephrine is to be used. Experience has also shown that if the operation is carried out without local anesthesia, almost no postoperative pain or edema develops. We consider this a greater advantage than the blood-free operative field acquired via infiltration.

Preparation for Surgery

Out-Patient Preparation

Simulation. A simple plaster-of-Paris model suffices. Correction of reversed overbite is achieved by displacing the protruding front teeth posteriorly by a distance equal to 1 premolar. The appropriate premolar on each side of the plaster-of-Paris model is ground down; the segment holding the front teeth is sawed out at approximately a right angle. The 3 incisional surfaces must be shaped in such a manner that they form a smooth mandibular arch with normal frontal overbite. The occlusal overlay is prepared on the corrected model. At the same time, a splint is prepared. A tripartite splint is used for a mandible with a complete dentition.

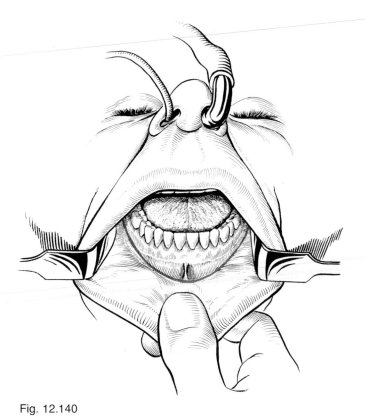

Fig. 12.140

Operative Technique

Intraoral Incision

While an assistant retracts the lower lip and stretches the vestibule, the mucosa is incised using a curved incision extending from $\overline{6}$ to $\overline{6}$. The apex of the curve lies on the labial mucosa (Fig. 12.140). This incision prevents wound dehiscence.

Sharp dissection is carried down to the bone (Fig. 12.141) and the periosteum is repeatedly incised in the same location. Atraumatic release of the adherent tendon of the mentalis muscle is best achieved with a sharp-edged, narrow elevator. Since the muscles of facial expression inserted laterally around the mouth must be elevated cleanly, it is advisable to begin the subperiosteal elevation at the level of the mental foramen and then, from below (from the mental tubercle), to free the adherent insertion of the mentalis muscle up to the alveolus of the incisors without tearing.

The soft tissues are mobilized over the edge of the mandible, particularly if reduction of the point of the chin has been planned (see Fig. 12.147). Clear exposure of the labial bone surface up to and including the mental foramen is necessary. Since the alveolar eminences are distinctly raised, the height of the root apices can be easily determined; the osteotomy is carried out 1 cm below in a transverse direction.

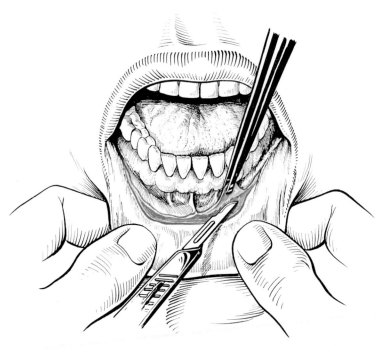

Fig. 12.141

Osteotomy

First, a premolar is extracted on each side and the alveolus is removed (Fig. 12.142). Burr holes are made along the incision (marked with gentian violet) and a small gutter is drilled along the cortical perforations. The segment is then mobilized with a narrow osteotome using quick, light hammer blows and slight elevatory movements. The fragment can then be elevated and tilted, pedicled on the muscles and mucosa of the lingual side. A narrow pear burr is used to shape the surfaces so that they correspond with the pattern on the model.

A normal overbite is achieved by posterior displacement, depression or elevation and turning of the fragment. A resulting anterior open cleft or a through-and-through dehiscence (Fig. 12.143) is filled with a bone graft taken from the inferior edge of the chin. In many cases of alveolar protrusion, the mental part of the lower third of the face appears overdeveloped; shortening of the chin is indicated.

Adjustment of the Fragment and Intraoral Fixation

After testing occlusion by adduction of the jaw, the fragment is adjusted exactly using the prepared occlusal overlay. The position of the fragment is thus ensured; the tripartite splint (see Fig. 12.142) is coupled together and fixed to the template with wire ligatures and Palavit. The fragment is thus firmly fixed in its new position. Intermaxillary fixation is unnecessary.

The overlay is removed 2 weeks later to prevent gingivitis on the lingual side caused by debris accumulation. Since a rigid wire-Palavit splint is present on the labial side, the overlay need not be used after this short period of time.

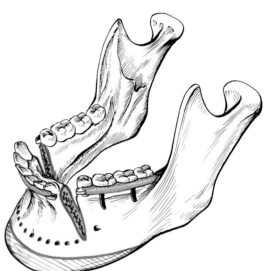

Fig. 12.142

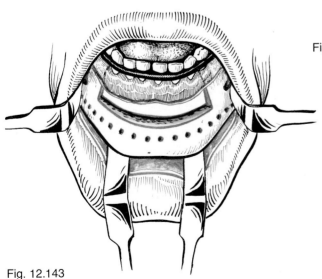

Fig. 12.143

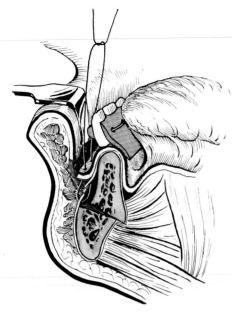

Fig. 12.144

Wound Closure

For practical reasons the wound is closed after fixation has been completed. Manipulation of the splint tears the mucosal suture. The wound, therefore, is covered with a saline compress during splinting. The wound and the oral cavity are then thoroughly cleaned with cetrimide spray or the Surgical Jet Lavage with continuous suction. The wound is closed in 2 layers: The periosteum and muscles are stitched to the bone with 4×0 Supramid mattress sutures (Fig. 12.144). This can easily be carried out laterally; but, in the central area, incisions in the periosteum may be necessary since the aponeurosis of the mentalis muscle cannot be elevated easily. The mucosa is closed with continuous 5×0 Supramid sutures.

Important Modifications and Surgical Alternatives

None.

Landmarks and Danger Points

Landmarks

- For the incision: The edge of the gingiva; the labial origin of the frenulum.

- For access to the site of the osteotomy: The aponeuroses of the following muscles: Mentalis muscle, depressor labii inferioris and depressor anguli oris muscles; mental foramen and lower border of the chin.

- For the ostectomy: The alveoli of the extracted premolar, the mental foramen, the alveolar eminence over the teeth roots.

Danger Points

- Damage to the neighboring teeth roots and root apices,

- Damage to the mental nerve.

Rules, Hints and Typical Errors

Rules (see p. 226)

Hints

- Labial extension of the incision in the edge of the gingival mucosa.

- An occlusal overlay has to be prepared in order to check and secure the position of the fragments.

- Closure of the wound only after splinting has been achieved.

- Thorough mechanical cleaning of the wound with a cetrimide spray or Surgical Jet Lavage with continuous suction before the sutures are introduced.

- Two-layer wound closure.

Typical Errors (see p. 226)

Postoperative Care

In-patient care. (see p. 227)

Out-patient care. Since intermaxillary fixation is not necessary, it is sufficient to see the patient twice a week initially and then once a week.

Functional Sequelae

Functional disorders have not been observed.

Corrections of the Chin

The chin is a distinct human feature which is as significant as the nose for determining the human profile. If we examine the bulky jaw of the Heidelberg man, no chin is evident.

In general an overly exaggerated contour is less disturbing esthetically than a receding chin.

Assessing the type of anomaly depends on a natural esthetic perception, but it is objectified by the position of the jaw relative to the orthograde profile line. The basic types of anomalies are: the *receding* chin, the *protruding* chin and the *asymmetric* chin.

Displacement osteotomy, *ostectomy* as well as *grafts* and *implants* come into consideration for corrective surgery. The operation may be carried out either alone or in combination with other orthopaedic procedures. Grafts and implants are not discussed in this chapter (see Vol. 1, Chapter 5).

Displacement osteotomy is used to:

● Build up the prominence of the chin,

● Straighten an asymmetric chin,

● Reduce the height of the chin,

● Heighten the chin when the lower third of the face is too short.

Ostectomy is used to:

● Reduce the length of the chin,

● Straighten an asymmetric chin.

Principles of the Operation

Displacement osteotomy. The lower border of the chin and, if necessary, the lateral part of the lower border of the mandible as far back as the angle of the jaw are divided by an osteotomy and fixed in the desired position.

Ostectomy. The mental protuberance is removed from the base of the mandible.

Grafts and implants. Implanting and fixation of endogenous or exogenous material which is either prepared during the operation using a plastic model or before the operation from a mask of the face (see Vol. 1, Chapter 5).

Indications

Displacement osteotomy is indicated:

● In a high lower third of the face if the height of the chin is the dominant factor; basically the contour may be positive (prognathic) or negative (retrognathic).

● In receding chin as an independent anomaly without malocclusion (micrognathia, see Fig. 12.145).

● In retrognathia, either bilateral or unilateral (see p. 207), if the results of the lengthening osteotomy on the ascending ramus are not esthetically satisfactory.

● If a strongly pronounced labiomental fold (e.g., as a result of a complete overbite) is esthetically disturbing.

Ostectomy is indicated as a modeling operation for the following conditions:

● An exaggerated pointed chin or an excessively protruding chin, without malocclusion;

● If the mental protuberance is too high (usually a component of a lower third of the face which is too high);

● Prognathism or pseudoprognathism if a shortening osteotomy does not provide satisfactory esthetic results (either a mental protuberance which is too high or a protuberance of the chin which is too pronounced anteriorly at the lower border of the mandible);

● Unilateral hyperplasia of the chin;

● Bilateral crossbite if anterior resection osteotomy alone does not provide satisfactory esthetic results (see p. 230).

Grafts and implants to provide a positive and symmetrical chin contour are indicated:

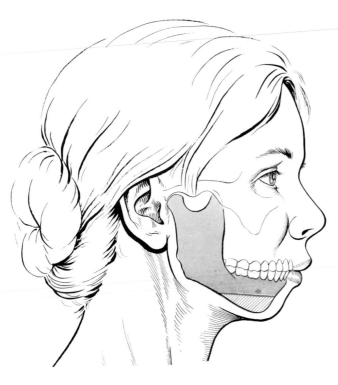

Fig. 12.145

- In extreme retrognathia. Lengthening the chin by a displacement osteotomy is limited, particularly in micrognathia, whose most extreme degree is bird face or Pierre-Robin syndrome, by the given strength of the bone of the lower border of the mandible;

- In scoliosis of the mandibular arch (e.g., hypoplasia of one half of the mandible);

- In asymmetry of various causes.

If correction of the chin and the jaw is planned as part of an orthopedic operation, this should be carried out in one sitting, if possible.

Preoperative Diagnosis

Radiographs

- Teleroentgenograms (underexposed and overexposed),

- Dental films from $\overline{6|}$ to $\overline{|6}$ to exclude the possibility of apical infection,

- Occlusal views to confirm the prominent lower border of the mandible in the horizontal plane.

Preparation for Surgery

The preparation is determined by the main surgical procedure planned (e.g., displacement osteotomy, resection osteotomy or graft). If the correction involves only the correction of the chin, the following measures are necessary:

On the day before operation: If necessary, a silicone or plastic implant is prepared on the basis of the facial mask. This implant is kept in antiseptic solution until the operation.

On the day of operation: The head is positioned straight; the mouth and the entire face and neck are cleaned as described above.

Special Instruments

- Oscillating saw (see Fig. 13.14b),

- Internal fixation set (see Fig. 12.63),

- Transbuccal intraosseous fixation instruments (see Fig. 12.72).

Anesthesia

Correction of the chin can be a very painful operation if the extent of deformity necessitates wide access as well as chiseling and burring for prolonged periods. Nasal intubation is justified in such cases.

On the other hand, minor displacements and removal of bone can be carried out under nerve blocking anesthesia combined with local infiltration.

A lidocaine-procaine solution (3 ml, 2% Xylocaine-Novocain) with norepinephrine is injected from outside on each side on the mental foramen. The submental region is infiltrated with 20 ml 1% plain lidocaine (Xylocaine) mainly in the immediate neighborhood of the mental spine. After this has been completed 4 ml 2% lidocaine (Xylocaine) with norepinephrine is injected in the sublingual fovea on the right and left sides as well as beneath the periosteum of the anterior part of the vestibule of the mouth.

Operative Technique

Displacement Osteotomy

Intraoral Incision and Exposure of the Site of Osteotomy (see p. 238)

Osteotomy. We prefer to use the saw for the excision. This not only saves time but also reduces the amount of bony substance lost, a situation which is useful when the chin is built up again (Fig. 12.146).

If the osteotomy extends posterior to the canine area, the drill and burr must, however, be used. When the base of the mandible is divided laterally, care should be taken to ensure that the burr holes extend to the lingual cortex. This prevents uncontrolled splintering of the bone when the osteotome is applied.

As soon as the bone graft is mobile, it is displaced anteriorly over the prominence of the chin. Heavy bleeding from the marrow cavity is controlled with wax.

In terms of method, *pedicled* grafts are differentiated from *free* grafts. For a *pedicled* graft the insertion of the digastric muscle is preserved in order to provide blood supply to the bone graft. In view of the danger of recurrence, *free* grafts are preferred in some cases. In this case the exposed insertion of the digastric muscles, together with the cortical bone, if possible, is resected and re-attached to the symphysis with a wire suture.

In pronounced asymmetry of the mandibular arch, the lower border of the mandible on the hypoplastic side is divided back to the angle of the jaw, and the lower border on the healthy side is divided as far as the mental foramen. In a few cases, displacement of the bone graft suffices until the typical depression between the 2 mental tubercles coincides with the midline.

After the insertions of the muscles have been divided, excess bone is removed from the lower border of the mandible, partly with the chisel and partly with the drill. In a marked deformity, a symmetrical mandibular arch is not always achieved. Additional bone or cartilage grafts may be needed to obtain an esthetically pleasing form.

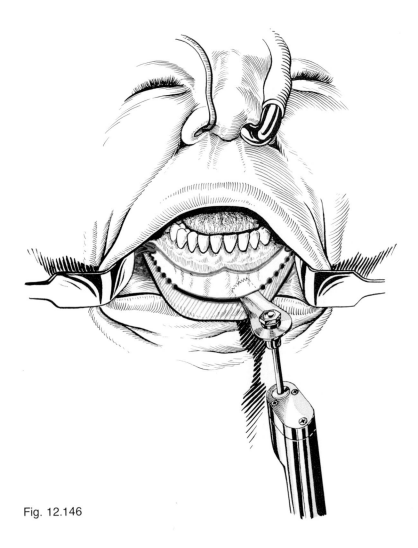

Fig. 12.146

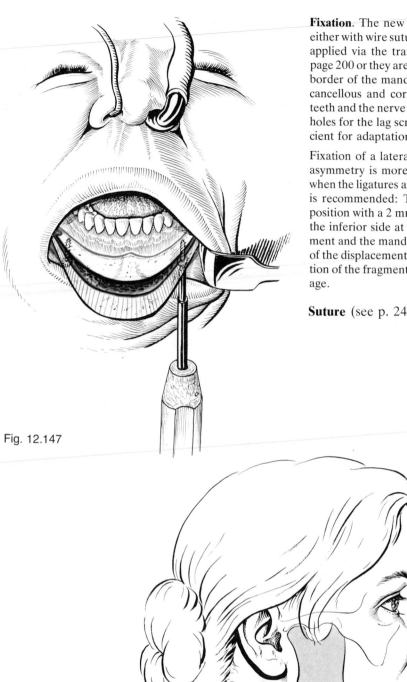

Fig. 12.147

Fixation. The new position of the fragments is secured either with wire sutures or with lag screws. The screws are applied via the transcutaneous technique described on page 200 or they are attached directly to the exposed lower border of the mandible (Fig. 12.147). A 3–4 mm thick cancellous and cortical layer between the roots of the teeth and the nerve canal is necessary in order to bore the holes for the lag screws. One screw on each side is sufficient for adaptation of the fragments (Fig. 12.148).

Fixation of a laterally displaced fragment to correct an asymmetry is more difficult because the fragment slips when the ligatures are tightened. The following procedure is recommended: The fragment is fixed in the correct position with a 2 mm AO cortical screw introduced from the inferior side at the point of intersection of the fragment and the mandibular arch. Depending on the extent of the displacement this point lies paramedian. The position of the fragment is secured through this fixed anchorage.

Suture (see p. 240)

Fig. 12.148

Important Modifications and Surgical Alternatives

One modification of the individual procedures is the choice between the intraoral access (Obwegeser 1966) and the extraoral approach (Hofer 1957). Corrective operations on the lower border of the chin can be carried out under adequate vision via an intraoral approach; there is no compelling reason to inflict the disadvantages of an external scar on the patient. Detachment of the insertion of the digastric muscle with its attached bony lamella is more difficult since the digastric fossa lies in a rather deep depression on the inner surface of the edge of the mandible. The position of the mental nerve also presents a problem if the curved resection must be extended backward to the angle of the jaw.

In marked micrognathia or asymmetry, Neuner (1967) uses 2 bone grafts and displaces these stepwise, anteriorly or laterally. In some cases this method may be very useful, but, in general, it is too complicated because the thinly divided bone segments are difficult to fix in the correct position.

Köle (1968) recommends the socalled chin ostectomy (Fig. 12.149a) for reducing the height of the chin and, at the same time, forming a positive chin prominence. This operation is a resection osteotomy in which the lower border of the mandible is first divided and a wedge-shaped segment 8–10 mm wide is resected. The anatomical curve of the lower border of the mandible is preserved by readapting the bony fragments (Fig. 12.149b). An excessively high chin and a sufficient mass of bone between the inferior edge of the mandible and the roots of the teeth are prerequisites for this operation regardless of whether prognathism or retrognathia is present.

There are cases (principally where the lower third of the face is too short, where the main feature is a complete overbite) in which the displacement osteotomy is restricted to localized removal of the mental protuberance.

Depending on whether the mental protuberance is displaced superiorly or inferiorly, an ugly labiomental fold can be compensated (Köle 1968). If, for example, complete overbite is the cause of the compression fold, compensation is achieved by

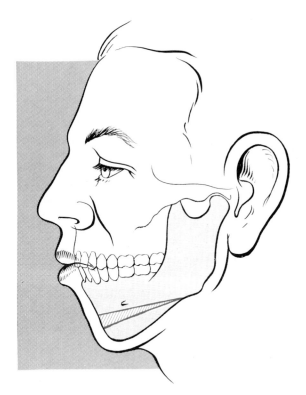

Fig. 12.149 a

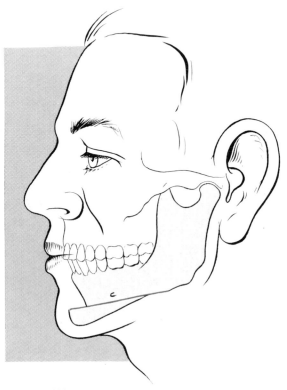

Fig. 12.149 b

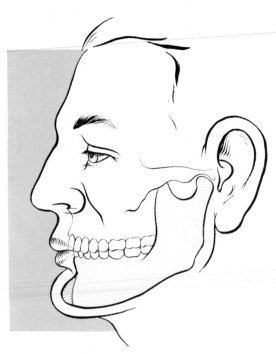

Fig. 12.150a

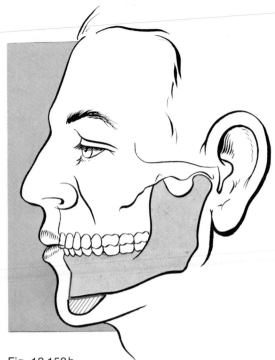

Fig. 12.150b

displacing the sawed-off mental protuberance onto the inferior surface of the edge of the chin (Fig. 12.150a, b).

Other cases with disproportionate protuberance of the chin and a deepened labiomental fold can be corrected by cranial displacement of the sawed-off mental protuberance (Fig. 12.151a, b).

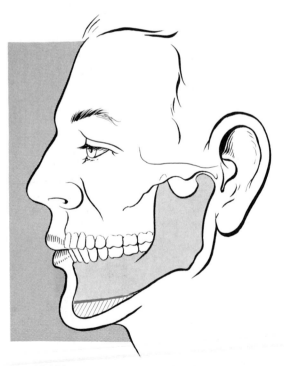

Fig. 12.151a

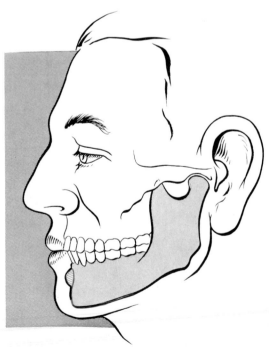

Fig. 12.151b

Ostectomy

Intraoral Incision and Exposure of the Site of the Ostectomy (see p. 238)

Reduction of the length and height of the chin is achieved either by simple modeling and removal of the edge of the mandible with a drill or by resection of the base of the chin.

Suture (see p. 240)

Landmarks and Danger Points

Only a few anatomical **landmarks** are important for corrective operations on the chin. They are:

- The anterior landmark: labial insertion of the frenulum;
- The mental foramen and the mental nerve;
- The mental protuberance which is narrow at its origin between the central incisors but expands as it approaches the lower border of the mandible on both sides at the mental tubercle which is the lateral limit of the muscles inserted into the chin;
- The alveolar eminences over the tooth roots;
- The lower border of the mandible;
- The digastric fossa.

Danger Points

- Division of the mental nerve;
- Hemorrhage from the facial vessels during exposure of the lateral part of the lower border of the mandible.

Rules, Hints and Typical Errors

- Wide access is necessary not only to preserve the soft tissues of the lip and cheek as well as the mental nerve but also to provide a good view during exposure of the lower border of the mandible for assessing the extent and site of the deformity correctly.
- If exposure of the lower border of the mandible as far as the angle of the jaw is necessary, grooving the mental foramen may be helpful for achieving more space between the elevated soft tissues and the bony surfaces.
- The fragments or the graft should, if possible, be fixed with lag screws, which are more easily introduced and more stable.
- Postoperative edema of the soft tissues of the lip and the edges of the wound should be prevented by an atraumatic technique since the tendency toward wound dehiscence and infection is particularly high in the mental region.

Typical Errors

- If would be wrong for extraoral access to leave the platysma on the divided bony segment. This results in the loss of functional relationship between the platysma and the muscles of expression around the mouth. Division of the terminal branches of the marginal mandibular branch of the facial nerve may produce weakness of the corner of the mouth.
- Not maintaining the divided digastric muscles results in a submandibular bulge which can be prevented by reinserting the belly of the muscle into the remaining edge of the mandible. To ensure that the suture does not tear out of the muscle tissue, the insertion together with the cortical plate is marked out with a fine burr and removed in 1 piece with the chisel and then reattached with a wire suture (see p. 243).
- Failure to make relief incisions when the soft tissues of the chin are placed under tension.

Postoperative Care (see p. 240)

The dressings are changed after 24 hours and, again 24 and 48 hours later. External bandages are removed on the eighth day.

Functional Sequelae

- Temporary paresthesia in the area supplied by the mental nerve;
- Occasional hypersensitization in the mental region.

Operations on the Temporomandibular Joint

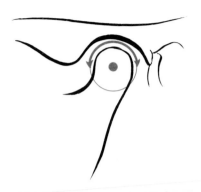

Fig. 12.152 a   Capitular rotation around an axis within the head of the mandible.

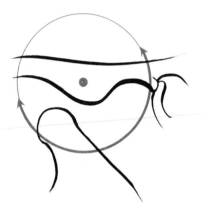

Fig. 12.152 b   Tubercular rotation around an axis within the articular tubercle.

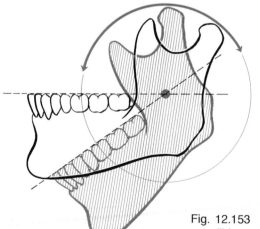

Fig. 12.153   Opening and closing movements of the mandible around an axis through the lingula.

The temporomandibular joint has a considerable freedom of movement. The only limitation to movement is that both joints must move at the same time. The interarticular disc divides the temporomandibular joint into 2 adjoining cavities in which two types of movement occur when the mandible is elevated or depressed:

1. Rotation of the head of the mandible around an axis located in the head (capitular rotation) (Fig. 12.152a).

2. Rotation of the head of the mandible around an axis located in the articular tubercle (tubercular rotation) (Fig. 12.152b).

If both movements of the head of the mandible are carried out at the same time, the mandible turns around an axis the center of which is located in the lingula (Fig. 12.153).

Since this axis is at the same level as the occlusal plane, the forces necessary for mastication are diverted away from the head of the mandible and directed on the axis of movement (Fig. 12.154). In this way the temporomandibular joint is subjected primarily to pushing and gliding movements which are dependent on the number, strength and direction of the involved muscles. The main task of the temporomandibular joint and its muscles is to guarantee stable fixation of the head of the mandible in every phase of movement. This is achieved by a complex reflex mechanism which originates in proprioceptive nerve endings within the muscles, joint capsule and periodontal ligaments (Sharpey's fibers). If disturbed muscular coordination is present or if the occlusal plane is altered by overbite, premature contact, etc., the rotation axis of the mandible is displaced. The functions of the individual muscles are, therefore, altered. This disturbs the subtle coordination of the mandibular muscles and eventually leads to muscular spasms, overstraining of the joint and related symptoms.

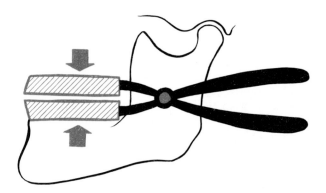

Fig. 12.154 Relieving the temporomandibular joint by transferring the masticatory force (arrow) to the axis of movement (joint of forceps).

Preoperative Diagnosis

Functional disturbances of the temporomandibular joint can have several causes:

- Malocclusion with the related disturbance of the proprioceptive reflex mechanism.

- Subluxation or luxation of the temporomandibular joint resulting from slackness of the joint capsule, the muscles and ligaments.

- Alterations in the region of the disc and the head of the mandible resulting from trauma and arthrosis.

- Ankylosis of the temporomandibular joint resulting from trauma and inflammation.

- Arthritic alterations in the temporomandibular joint as an accompanying symptom of generalized arthritis.

If these changes of the temporomandibular joint are suspected, the following diagnostic measures should be carried out:

History. A detailed history is just as important as the examination itself. Pain localized to the temporomandibular joint is generally caused by the head of the mandible or the interarticular disc pressing on the part of the capsule posterior to the disk. This part is innervated by the auriculotemporal nerve. This pain can be localized in the area supplied by the auriculotemporal nerve.

Dragging pains around the mandible itself are usually the expression of muscular spasms. Often the patient complains about "cracking" or "grinding" noises in the joint area. The teeth no longer occlude properly or the mandible seems to lock when the mouth is opened. For lack of a better term, the symptoms are referred to as the pain dysfunction syndrome.

Grinding the teeth, particularly during sleep (nocturnal bruxism), is typical of nervousness and states of psychomotor agitation which are expressed as a result of disturbances of the proprioceptive reflex mechanism. The condition is a vicious circle (see the following diagram).

Pain-Dysfunction Syndrome

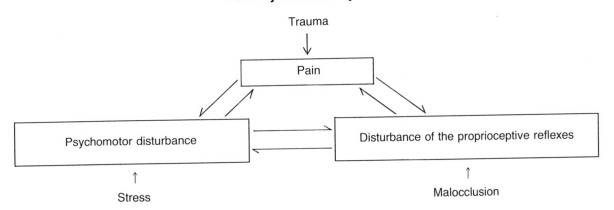

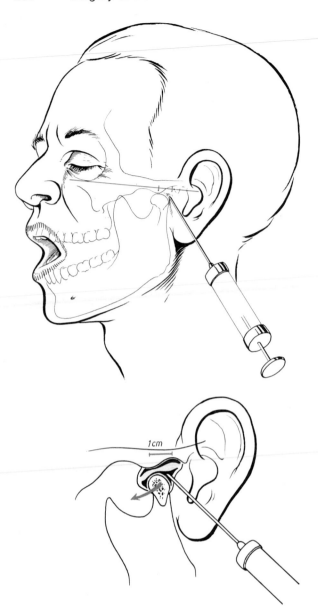

For mild cases conservative treatment with moist compresses, tranquilizers or sedatives as well as informing the patient of the cause and treatment of this condition is often successful.

For difficult cases local anesthesia, either with an ethyl chloride spray on the masseteric region or intraarticular injection of 2 % procaine (Novocain) or lidocaine (Xylocaine) are indicated (Fig. 12.155).

Inspection. The movement of the jaw is checked and the degree to which the mouth can be opened as well as any deviation from the midline are noted. The type of occlusion can be determined by a wax impression. Often a cross bite, premature contact, deviated bite or deep overbite is present which then puts an incorrect strain on the temporomandibular joint.

Palpation. Manual examination is carried out on both sides at the same time by palpating in front of the tragus and in the external auditory meatus. In this way the extent of movement of the head of the mandible when opening and closing the mouth can be tested. Intraoral and extraoral palpation of the jaw muscles completes this examination.

1 cm

Fig. 12.155 Intra-articular injection with the mouth open. A depression in the skin appears anterior to the tragus over the empty joint cavity. This is used as the site of injection.

Special radiographs of the temporomandibular joint. Before every operation the following special views of the temporomandibular joint are necessary:

● Suboccipitofrontal views of the joint with the mouth opened and closed (Clementschitsch-Altschul);

● Transbuccal views of the ascending ramus (Rösli);

● Transorbital views of the head of the mandible (Hofrath);

● Lateral views of the temporomandibular joint, with the mouth opened and closed (Schüller);

● Lateral contact views of the temporomandibular joint, with the mouth opened and closed (Parma);

● Lateral contact views of the temporomandibular joint (Steinhardt);

● Tomograms in the anteroposterior plane, and possibly in a laterolateral direction.

Arthrography. This investigation is fairly painful and usually provides no additional diagnostic information. It is carried out only in rare cases, e.g., for suspected lesions or perforation of the disc.

Electromyography. Increased electrical activity of the masticatory muscles, which appears as spasms of the individual muscles or muscle groups, can be confirmed by an EMG. This technique is used, for example, to clarify a myofascial pain syndrome which persists in spite of the use of a special onlay splint.

Manual Repositioning after Subluxation of the Temporomandibular Joint

Indications

Manual repositioning is indicated when dislocation does not resolve spontaneously. Luxation occurs when the mouth is opened too wide. The head of the mandible glides over the articular tubercle and into the infratemporal fossa; it remains there due to a spasm of the masseter and pterygoid muscles. The condition is caused by an alteration of the articulating joint surfaces (a flat type of joint) and a weakening of the capsular ligaments.

Principles of Treatment

The pain and associated muscle spasms are relieved by para-articular and intra-articular injection of a local anesthetic (see Fig. 12.155). With this treatment the mandible usually returns to its position spontaneously. If this is not the case, the mandible is manually repositioned.

Manual Repositioning

Two methods are in use:

1. Intraoral pressure is exerted inferiorly and posteriorly on both sides of the ascending ramus (not on the teeth!) with the index fingers. At the same time the mandible is pushed upward with the thumbs under the chin (Fig. 12.156). This is carried out from the front with the patient in the sitting position. The patient's head should be held in place by an assistant.

2. The physician stands behind the sitting patient and presses intraorally with both thumbs on the ascending ramus. At the same time, he pushes the chin upward and backward (Fig. 12.157). This method has the advantage that the head of the patient can be held between the hands and the body of the physician.

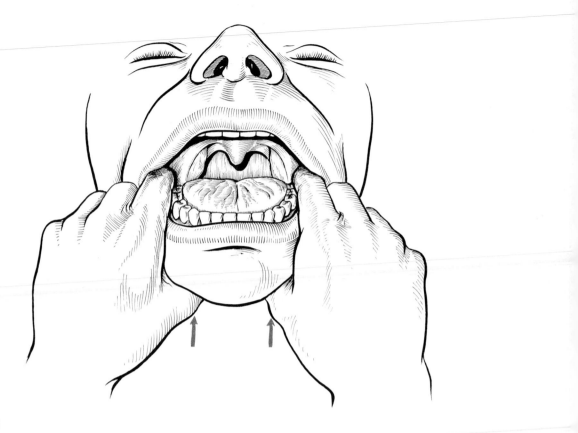

Fig. 12.156

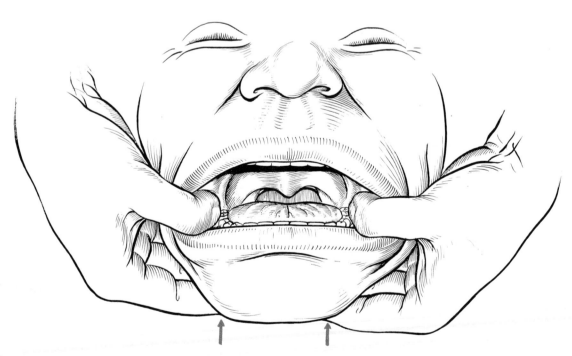

Fig. 12.157

Osteoplasty for Habitual Subluxation of the Temporomandibular Joint

Indications

This operation is indicated for repeated subluxation without spontaneous repositioning. The patient lives in constant fear of trismus due to uncontrolled opening of the mouth in yawning, laughing, etc.

Principle of the Operation

Increasing the height of the joint by implanting a bone graft via the temporal fossa.

Operative Technique

A preauricular incision curving anteriorly is made which ends in the hair bearing part of the temple (Fig. 12.158). The temporal artery and vein are ligated and the skin flap elevated. The temporal fascia and muscle are divided and detached from the squamous part of the temporal bone (see Fig. 12.159). This provides access to the infratemporal fossa.

The inner surface of the zygomatic arch is exposed (see Fig. 12.160). The size of the bony graft is determined by measuring the distance between the anterior edge of the inferiorly facing joint tubercle and the mandibular notch. One or two pieces of bone are removed from the iliac crest. The bone graft is shaped into the required size and thickness so that it can be wedged firmly between the zygomatic arch and the squamous part of the temporal bone at the anterior edge of the joint tubercle. A supplementary notch is made which engages the root of the zygoma and guarantees the correct position of the graft. The bone graft is then put in place with a hammer (see Fig. 12.161). Additional fixation is unnecessary.

The wound is closed in layers and a drain is inserted (see Fig. 12.162).

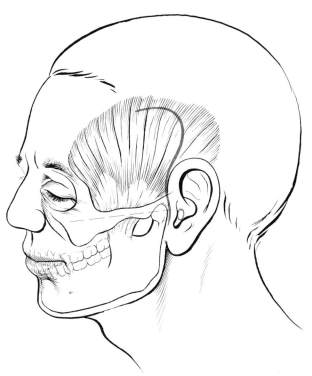

Fig. 12.158 Incision and landmarks for determining the length of the free end of the graft: distance between the anterior edge of the articular tuberosity and the sigmoid notch. Frankfurt horizontal plane parallels a line through the muscular tuberosity on the inferior edge of the zygoma.

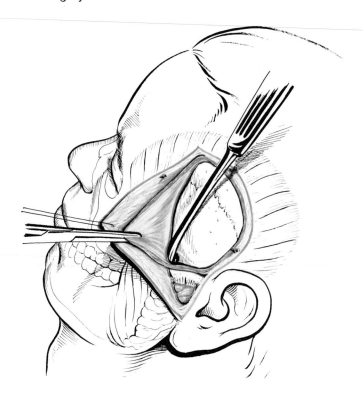

Fig. 12.159

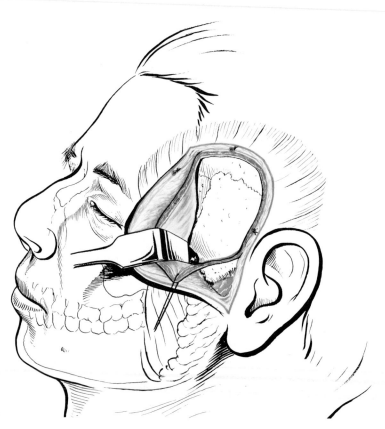

Fig. 12.160

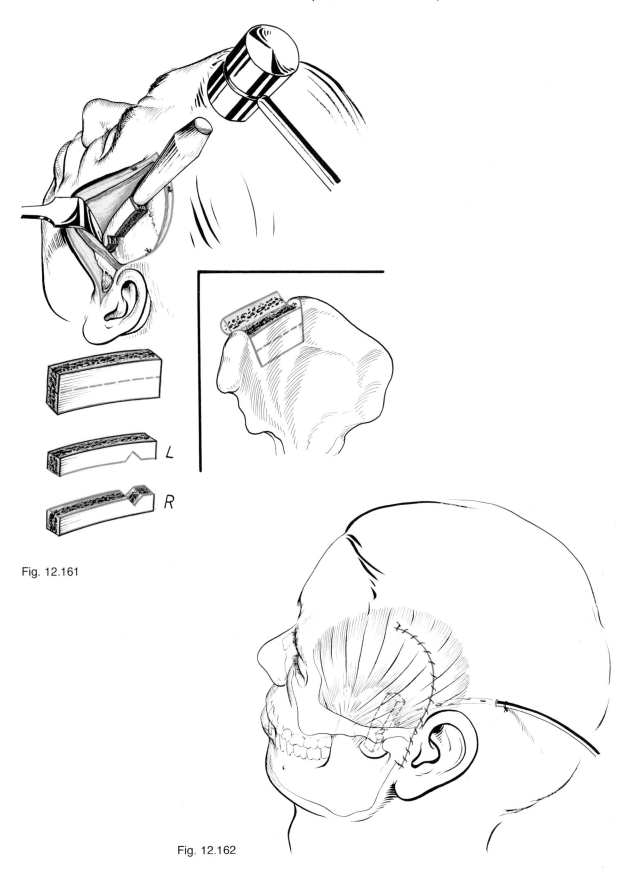

Fig. 12.161

Fig. 12.162

Landmarks and Danger Points

Landmarks

The length of the graft between the anterior surface of the articular tubercle and the mandibular notch can be determined before the operation on the basis of a line running along the inferior edge of the zygoma parallel to the Frankfurt horizontal plane.

Danger Points

None.

Rules, Hints and Typical Errors

● The graft of cancellous bone must be large enough to ensure that it can be wedged between the squamous part of the temporal bone and the zygomatic arch. The graft must lie perpendicular to the zygomatic arch with its point extending at most 1 cm beyond the articular eminence.

Only this position guarantees that the movement of the head of the mandible is limited and does not further glide forward when the jaw is opened wide.

● By taking the bone from the external surface of the iliac crest the graft acquires a natural, internally curved surface which corresponds to the convexity of the squamous part of the temporal bone.

Postoperative Care

Intermaxillary fixation for 2 to 3 weeks.

Functional Sequelae

Initially, opening of the mouth can be restricted which is desirable at this time. Resorption of the graft always occurs to some extent. The long-term results, however, are good.

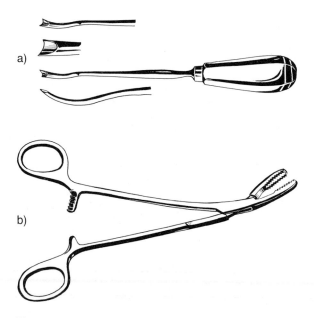

Fig. 12.163 a, b   The meniscotomes (a) and meniscus forceps (b).

Removal of the Disk

Indications

The operation is indicated only when all conservative measures such as physiotherapy, tranquilizers and pressure special onlay splints have failed.

The main indication is the myofascial pain syndrome associated with grinding and cracking. It is a symptom of degenerative disc disorders.

Principles of the Operation

Intracapsular extraction of the articular disc; the posterior extracapsular parts, (venous plexus and fatty tissue) are preserved.

Special Instruments (see Fig. 12.163 a, b)

Operative Technique

A preauricular incision with a curved extension into the temporal area is made (Fig. 12.164). The skin is elevated from the subcutaneous tissue and the flaps are turned backward. The temporal artery and vein as well as the auriculotemporal nerve are divided at the level of the insertion of the auricle. The temporomandibular ligament is exposed in the depths of the wound a fingerbreadth anterior to the auricular cartilage and superior to the parotid capsule. The ligament is split vertically. The incision is extended anteriorly in the shape of a hockey stick, through the temporal fascia parallel to the zygoma (Fig. 12.165). Opening the joint reveals the articular disc and the capillary clefts of the upper and lower joint cavities.

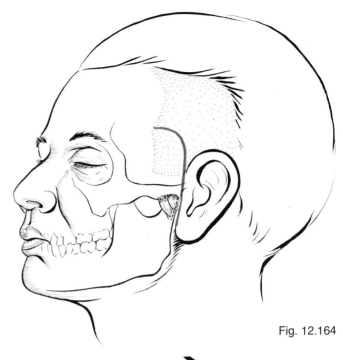

Fig. 12.164

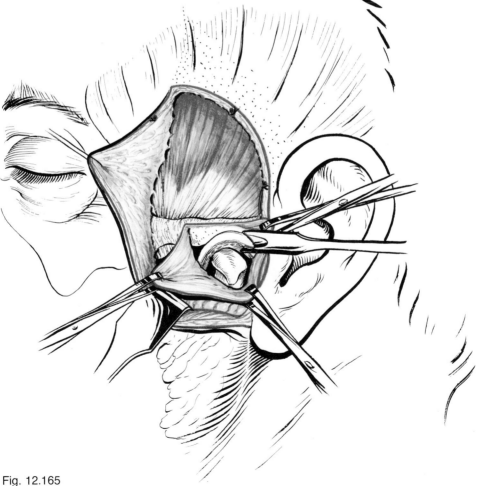

Fig. 12.165

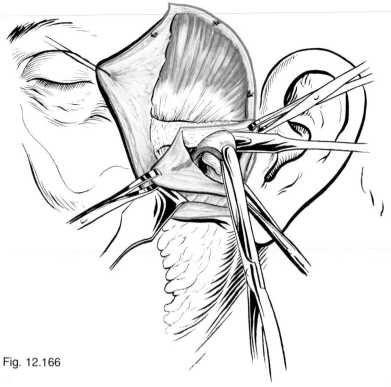

Fig. 12.166

The disc is put under tension with meniscus forceps and divided in the middle with a chisel. The anterior and posterior parts are subluxated and re-moved separately (Fig. 12.166). The loose connective tissue and the venous plexus in the extracapsular part of the articular fossa are preserved.

The capsule is closed and the wound is sutured in layers after a suction drain has been introduced (Fig. 12.167).

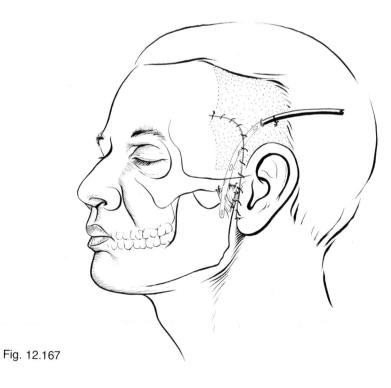

Fig. 12.167

Landmarks and Danger Points

The capsule of the joint can be determined by the intersection of the Frankfort horizontal plane and a point one fingerbreadth anterior to the tragus. The insertion of the lateral pterygoid muscle makes the anterior part of the disc difficult to remove. Tearing the capsule at this point can cause bleeding from the middle meningeal artery.

Rules, Hints and Typical Errors

Damage to the temporal and zygomatic branches of the facial nerve can be prevented by dissecting in depth 1 cm anterior to and along the tragal cartilage with fine, blunt scissors as far as the temporolateral ligament of the joint capsule. In most cases the temporal artery and vein must be ligated and divided.

Typical Errors

- The external auditory meatus may be perforated when dissection is carried out along the tragal cartilage.
- Omitting the formation of a flap (by a hockeystick incision) of the temporal fascia, the temporomandibular ligament and the joint capsule itself may lead to unsatisfactory closure of the joint and formation of an intra-articular scar tissue.
- Underestimation of the medial extent of the disc. Danger of incomplete extirpation.

Postoperative Care

Mobilization is begun early on the first day after surgery by systematic opening and chewing movements. A bland diet is given.

Functional Sequelae

Since the articular disc lies on the incongruent joint surfaces of the articular fossa and tubercle and the head of the mandible, there is a danger of premature wearing of the joint surfaces after the disc has been removed and of dysfunction with the related sequelae. Indications for this operation, therefore, must be very strict.

Operations for Ankylosis

Indications

Total (bony) or partial (fibrous) ankylosis of one or both joints. For partial ankylosis the operation is indicated only when intensive stretching exercises carried out over a period of several months have not been successful.

Principle of the Operation

Resection of the ankylosed head of the mandible and implantation of silicone to prevent reankylosis and to support the mandible during movement.

Special Instruments

- Gouge,
- Hammer,
- Rose and fissure burrs.

Anesthesia

Intubation anesthesia is always indicated for ankylosis operation which mostly must be carried out on both sides. If a tracheotomy is to be avoided the problems of blind intubation arising from the extreme degree of trismus must be taken into consideration. The first principle of blind intubation is to maintain spontaneous breathing and to avoid muscle relaxants. In total trismus the procedure with the least risk is chosen. The patient is intubated while still conscious either under neuroleptanalgesia or under sedation (diazepam [Valium] and meperidine hydrochloride [Demerol], intravenously). Passing the tube through the inferior part of the nasal cavity and pharynx is facilitated by using topical anesthesia and decongestants.

If intubation is to be carried out under general anesthesia, blind introduction of the tube is more likely to be successful when spontaneous breathing is intense. This is achieved either by inducing anesthesia with ether or by briefly raising the level of carbon dioxide in the inspired air (e.g., by temporarily disconnecting the absorber).

Techniques of Blind Intubation

First method. The tube is pushed blindly through the nose into the larynx with the head in the extended position. The anesthetist keeps his ear to the opening of the tube; respiratory sounds can be heard as soon as the tube is introduced into the nose but disappear if the tube is pushed into the esophagus, in which case the tube should be pulled back slightly. If the tube passes into the trachea, inspiratory sounds can be continuously heard and felt. The cough reflex is an additional positive sign.

Second method: A catheter is introduced into the trachea and the tube is threaded along it.

Third Method: If transnasal-translaryngeal intubation appears to be impossible, the tube is introduced with guidance from below through the cricothyroid ligament. A long Intracath is introduced percutaneously into the trachea below the thyroid cartilage and is pushed through the glottis into the pharynx. There it is grasped with forceps and brought out through either the mouth or the nose.

Fourth method: Flexible fiberoptics represent a new method to facilitate intubation.

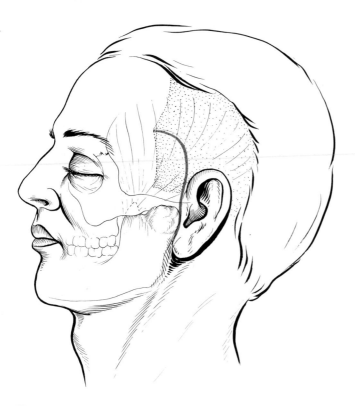

Fig. 12.168

Operative Technique

A preauricular incision is extended into the temporal region (Fig. 12.168). The skin flap is elevated and the superficial temporal artery and vein are ligated. The joint capsule or the ankylosed head of the mandible is exposed 1 cm anterior to the auricular cartilage by sharp dissection. The temporal fascia is divided parallel to the zygoma (Fig. 12.169). If the coronoid process is also involved, the incision is carefully extended inferiorly along the edge of the mandible so that the whole width of the ascending ramus can be grasped. The ostectomy is carried out with fissure or rose-head burrs and a gouge (Fig. 12.170).

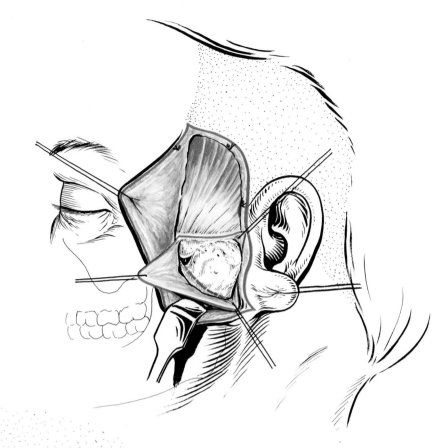

Fig. 12.169

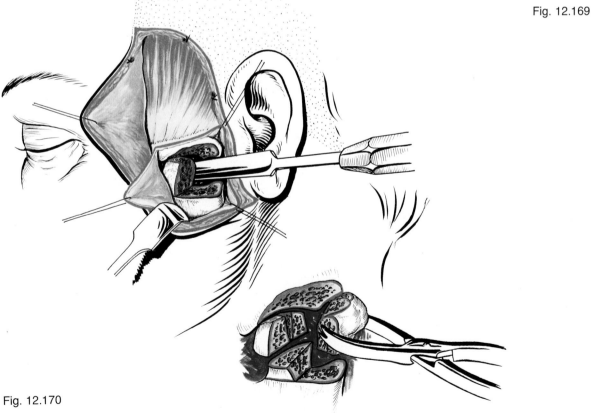

Fig. 12.170

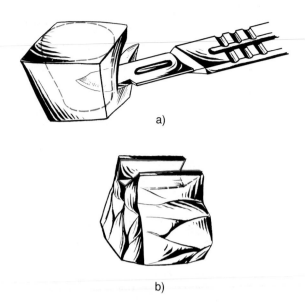

a)

b)

Fig. 12.171

Particular attention should be paid to restoring the articular fossa and exposing the articular surface itself. Remnants of the medial part of the head of the mandible can be easily overlooked, especially in ankylosis caused by a dislocation fracture. In such a case, the head of the mandible is dislocated and lies inferior to the tympanic plate deeper than the inexperienced operator suspects. Bony remnants left behind at this point can easily lead to recurrence.

A piece of Silastic in the shape of the condyle is introduced into the cavity as a support and to fill in the space (Figs. 12.171a, b; 12.172). It is important that the implantation be carried out with the mouth open. A mouth gag is used which, after the mouth has been opened as wide as possible, is replaced by an intermaxillary retaining block made of self-hardening plastic. The retaining block is secured with a stay suture (Fig. 12.173). The wound is closed with continuous sutures and a suction drain is introduced.

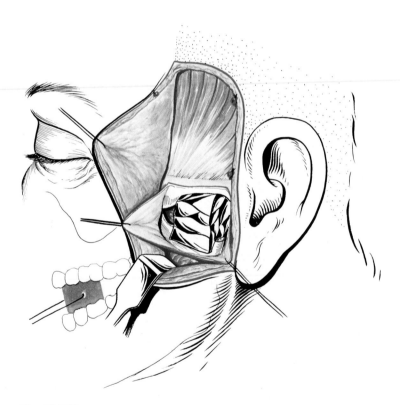

Fig. 12.172

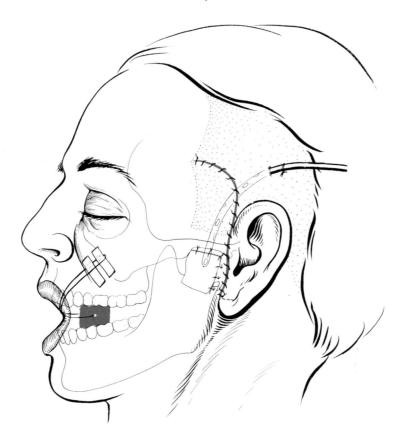

Fig. 12.173

Important Modifications and Surgical Alternatives

If the coronoid process is involved in the ankylotic process, the ascending ramus should be divided completely at the level of the sigmoid notch.

The easiest method for dealing with trismus produced by ankylosis consists of transverse division of the ascending ramus in the region of the angle of the jaw (Esmarch 1860). Postoperative exercises are carried out to prevent consolidation until a functional pseudarthrosis has formed.

Additional modifications consist of the use of different materials to prevent reankylosis. The stump of the condyle may be covered with a metal cap or self-hardening plastic may be introduced between the glenoid cavity and the end of the stump.

An open bite can be the result of such an implant especially if the implant has been used on both sides. For this reason many authors (Dufourmentel 1959, Trauner 1971, Rehrmann 1967) use an allograft of cartilage or bone.

Leaving the resection cavity empty has also been tried. The cavity fills with granulation tissue which then later forms scar tissue. Depending on the function, a false joint is formed.

Landmarks and Danger Points

In a total ankylosis, a joint cavity is no longer present. The border between the articular face of the tubercle and the condyle is often not visible, so that the vault of the skull can be perforated when the fossa is emptied, particularly if the gouge is used. Since strong adhesion formation around the joint is present, the middle meningeal artery, the deep auricular artery and the anterior tympanic artery, which run medial to the joint, may be damaged (see Fig. 12.174). Lesions of the auriculotemporal nerve and the nerves of the external auditory meatus are less important.

Fig. 12.174 Blood vessels and nerves medial to the joint capsule (part of the infratemporal and retromandibular fossa):

1. Lateral pterygoid muscle
2. Mandibular nerve, lingual nerve and division of the auriculotemporal nerve
3. Maxillary artery, middle meningeal artery and posterior facial vein.

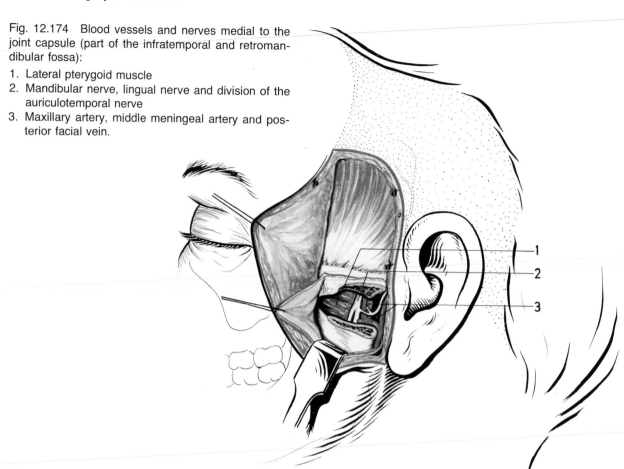

Rules, Hints and Typical Errors

Rules

The resection site should be exposed subperiosteally to avoid damaging the facial nerve.

Hints

The Silastic implant should be introduced with the mouth open.

Errors

Inadequate revision in the direction of the petrous bone and the infratemporal surface of the squamous temporal bone when the history indicates a previous dislocation fracture may result in leaving behind the dislocated medial part of the condyle. Improvement is minimal and trismus recurs.

Postoperative Care

● Antibiotic cover if the operation lasts for more than 2 hours;

● 40 mg prednisolone is given during the operation and 40 mg 4 to 5 hours after the operation;

● Early mobilization of the mandible by passive and active exercises: For the first 3 to 4 weeks a jaw exerciser is used several times a day for 10 to 15 minutes;

● Weekly supervision for the first 6 months.

Functional Sequelae

Since the operation leaves a fairly large defect, there is always the danger of extensive formation of scar tissue which again limits the movement of the mandible and detracts from the postoperative results. For this reason intensive exercises are very important for achieving good results.

Osteotomies on the Upper Jaw

Frontal Displacement Osteotomy

Principle

The anterior part of the upper jaw is completely mobilized in one operation. The blood supply to the fragments is supplied by a vestibular mucosal pedicle (Fig. 12.175). A piece of bone is removed from the appropriate site depending on the extent and direction of the intended fragment displacement.

Indications

Frontal displacement osteotomy is indicated for:

● Overdevelopment of the middle third of the face, whose main features are:
  a) Alveolar and bialveolar protrusion;
  b) Prognathism (maxillary protrusion);

● Too high a lower third of the face, whose main feature is anterior open bite due to thumb sucking;

● Too short a lower third of the face, whose main feature is complete overbite.

The composite term of alveolar and bialveolar protrusion includes:

A narrow jaw with crowded, protruding teeth;

A narrow jaw with protrusion and absent teeth.

As a result of anterior displacement of the front teeth and short upper lip, the teeth and gums are visible when the patient speaks or laughs, which is esthetically disturbing.

This syndrome is usually accompanied by a mandibular distal bite. Since the lower incisors are set back and elongated, they come in contact with the palate when the mouth is closed. In these cases as well as cases of bialveolar protrusion, the alveolar protrusion is corrected simultaneously with a corrective osteotomy of the front of the mandible.

Anterior open bite due to thumb sucking is a vertical superior deflection of the anterior part of the jaw. It

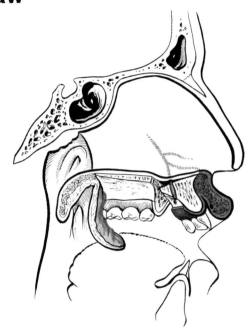

Fig. 12.175

is usually traced back to an anomaly of the deciduous teeth caused by thumb sucking. The anterior dental arch, which is usually protruding, narrow and acute, disappears behind a normal upper lip; the teeth are not visible when the patient speaks or laughs.

Complete overbite indicates a pronounced inclination of the upper front teeth (the opposite of protrusion), which completely cover the lower front teeth. The lower front teeth are usually elongated and make contact with the palate because they cannot occlude with the steeply inclined upper teeth.

Preoperative Diagnosis

The description of the intraoral findings includes first of all the basic type of the anomaly: Alveolar or bialveolar protrusion, open bite, or complete overbite. The need for preliminary orthodontic treatment should be clarified when the teeth are extremely crowded and when teeth are missing. In such cases, the therapy plan should be worked out together with an orthodontist.

During examination of the external appearance, the following questions should be answered:

1. Does the upper lip protrude markedly compared to the lower lip?

2. Is the upper lip normal in length or is it too short?

3. Are the upper teeth visible
   a) at rest,
   b) when speaking,
   c) when laughing?

4. Does the patient have a markedly receding chin?

Finally, the patient is asked to bring his teeth together, so that the mandible glides forward (if there is normal overbite of the front teeth). The profile view is carefully examined during the movement. If the cause of the anomaly lies in the upper jaw, it will now be worse. This is seen on the now markedly protruding and disproportionate lower third of the face. In this case the upper jaw, rather than the mandible, must be corrected.

The clinical picture of the anterior open bite due to thumb sucking is characterized by vertical nonocclusion of the front teeth.

In the diagnosis of complete overbite, it is important to determine whether a fanlike incisor overbite is present. Complete overbite is not an isolated anomaly of occlusion but is part of a particular malformation of the skull. If there is a posterior dis-

placement of the mandible (distal bite), the complete overbite is more pronounced. The abnormal retroclination of the upper front teeth in the presence of marked sagittal development of the middle third of the face with a large nasal profile is even more pronounced. Thus, while the body of the upper jaw is strongly developed, the shortened lower third of the face is conspicuous. It is accentuated by a deep supramental fold.

Teleroentgenograms are crucial for classifying the basic types of anomaly mentioned above:

- Alveolar protrusion (see Fig. 12.139),
- Maxillary prognathism (Fig. 12.176),
- Open bite (Fig. 12.177),
- Complete overbite (Fig. 12.178).

Routine Radiographs

- Occipitodental views,
- Dental views of the upper and lower jaw,
- Orthopantomograms of the upper and lower jaw.

The following points must be clarified:

- Chronic inflammation of the maxillary antrum,
- Periapical inflammation, cysts or other intraosseous disease of the apices,

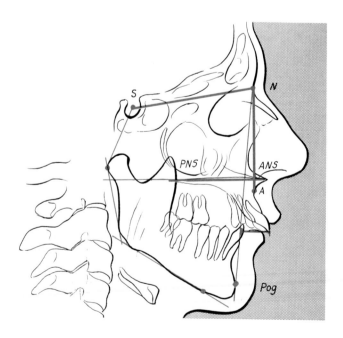

Fig. 12.176 Prognathism: S-N-A and PNS-ANS are large; excessive protrusion of the anterior teeth.

Fig. 12.177 Skeletal open bite: The angle of the horizontal plane (B) and the angle of the jaw Ar-Go-Gn are large. The length of the ascending ramus Ar-Go is small.

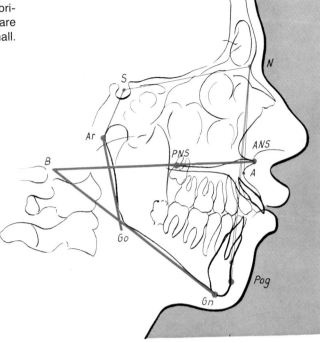

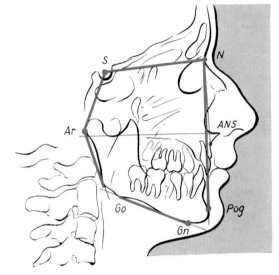

Fig. 12.178 Complete overbite: The lower border of the mandible Go-Gn and the basal prognathia S-N-Pog are small. The angle of the base of the skull N-S-Ar and the angle of the jaw S-Ar-Go are large.

● Periodontal state: Marginal inflammation, pocket formation and the degree to which the teeth are loosened.

The **plaster-of-Paris cast** generally demonstrates whether the anomaly in question is an alveolar protrusion (dentoalveolar anomaly) or a prognathism (skeletal anomaly) and the position of the mandible.

The preoperative findings are documented on the model as a basis for comparison with the later results of surgery.

A **profile photograph** basically assists in the preoperative documentation.

Preparation for Surgery

Out-Patient Preparation

Simulation. Since the displacement osteotomy is basically limited to the alveolar and palatal processes, the usual model of the jaw fixed in a simulator suffices for the simulation. The purpose of the operation is to achieve normal occlusion taking into account the proportions of the mandible (bialveolar protrusion or elevation of the front of the mandible in posterior displacement of the mandible) and the profile line. If necessary, an osteotomy on the mandible is also simulated at the same time.

The desired result of the operation is established and documented by sticking the fragments together. A palatal plate is constructed on the resulting simulation model; the plate serves not only as an occlusal template but also as part of the fixation apparatus. Many authors recommend accurate measuring during adjustment and/or posterior and superior displacement of the fragments. Measurements within a millimeter are of little significance since such a high degree of accuracy cannot be controlled during the operation. Accuracy is, however, important for adapting the position of the fragments to the occlusal overlay and the occlusion to the row of teeth as on the simulated model.

If a marginal gingivitis is present, the patient should be referred for preliminary periodontal treatment.

In patients with protrusion and *absent teeth*, preliminary orthodontic treatment is indicated, for which at least 6 months should be allowed. Filling the gaps can be expedited by weakening the interalveolar septa. The center of the broadened septum is perforated from the palatal to the vestibular side down to the apical base with a fine rose-head burr. We have not found it necessary to divide the cortex on the vestibular side. In view of the later operation in which the fragment will remain pedicled on the vestibular mucosa, the bone is denuded on the palatal side only. The border of the gingiva is preserved for a distance of 5 mm; the alveolar process is perforated under it from the palatal side. The operation is carried out under local anesthesia on an out-patient basis.

In-Patient Preparation

On the day before operation:

The oral cavity is disinfected with 0.5% cetrimide spray. Premedication is given according to the schedule.

On the day of operation:

Immediately before the operation, the patient is placed in the supine position with the head in the neutral position. The oral cavity is sprayed with diluted cetrimide. The lips are smeared with Vaseline.

Special Instruments

- Nasal hooks,
- Rose-head burr,
- Fissure burr,
- Single hook,
- Wide periosteal elevator,
- Curved periosteal elevator,
- Pear burrs,
- Fine rose-head burr,
- Sharp curved scissors.

Anesthesia

A displacement osteotomy of the anterior part of the upper jaw can be performed under local anesthesia. A nerve block is carried out at 5 points: On the left and right sides of the incisive foramen, in the vestibule of the nose and in the angle between the septum and the floor of the nose. The nerve block is carried out with 2% lidocaine (Xylocaine) and norepinephrine, supplemented at the end of the injection by 1% pure lidocaine (Xylocaine).

Usually, however, the operation is carried out under general anesthesia using nasal intubation. The hypopharynx is packed with gauze impregnated with Vaseline; the eyes are held shut with nonirritant adhesive tape and protected with a large pledget.

Operative Technique

We use Wunderer's method (1962) exclusively for the following three reasons:

1. It is suitable for all recognized anomalies. Distinguishing between methods of operations for protrusion with or without deep bite or with open bite or complete overbite is, therefore, unnecessary. Using one surgical principle considerably simplifies the indications and the surgical technique.

2. It is simple and allows the operation to be carried out in one stage.

3. Ideal adjustment of the fragments is possible without supplementary intermaxillary traction by means of rubber bands. If the dental arch is too narrow, the fragment can be split in the center in the same operation.

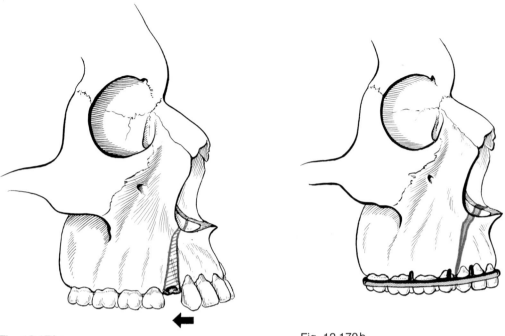

Fig. 12.179a   Fig. 12.179b

The purpose of the osteotomy is:

● In protrusion: Posterior and superior displacement and, if necessary, broadening of the front of the upper jaw;

● In anterior open bite due to thumb sucking: Inferior displacement and possibly internal rotation of the anterior part of the upper jaw;

● In complete overbite: Superior displacement and possibly external rotation of the anterior part of the upper jaw.

The posterior displacement is usually equal to the breadth of a premolar (Fig. 12.179a,b). The operation begins, if necessary, with dental extraction. A laterally placed mouth gag holds the mouth open as wide as possible.

Incision (Fig. 12.180). A paragingival incision is made outlining the palate from tuberosity to tuberosity through the mucosa and periosteum which are elevated with a wide periosteal elevator. Exposure of the bone is begun at the level of the molars because the periosteum can be elevated most easily at this point without damaging the palatine vessels.

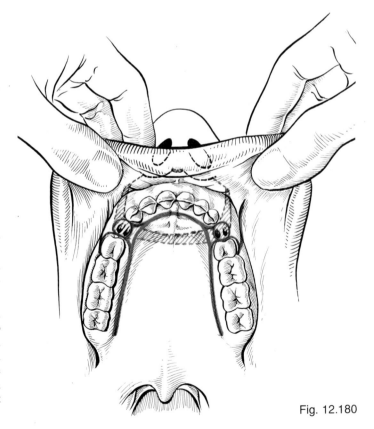

Fig. 12.180

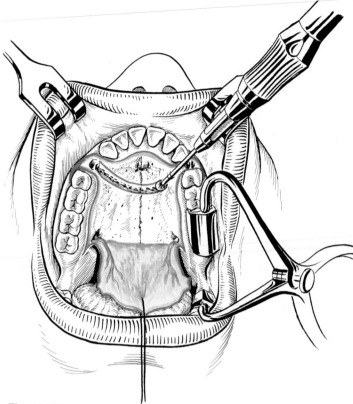

Fig. 12.181

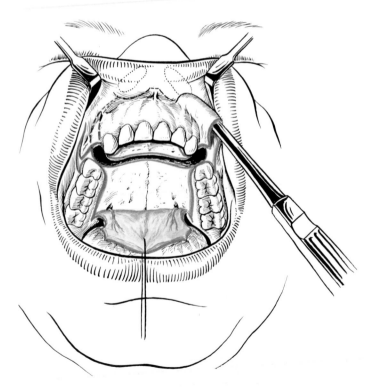

Fig. 12.182

Division of the palatal process and the nasal crest. The hard palate is divided with a thick rose-head burr perpendicular to the alveolus, immediately behind the incisive suture, from one empty alveolar socket to the other (Fig. 12.181). The bone at this point is at least 5 mm thick. The nasal mucosa is protected by using a 3 mm rose-head burr and a strong water jet. The presence of a torus palatinus demands careful drilling in depth since the nasal crest, which runs into the anterior nasal spine (see Fig. 12.179) and in which is enfolded the cartilaginous part of the septum, is located on the nasal side. The narrow edge of the bone to be divided is between 5 and 8 mm thick. The bone is drilled infundibularly until the edge of the cartilage appears.

Division of the alveolar process. The process was partially divided when the lingual wall of the empty alveolar socket was removed (Fig. 12.182).

The gingiva is divided in the vestibule at least the width of a tooth distal to the empty alveolus perpendicular to the sulcus; the gingiva is elevated with a narrow elevator beginning at the alveolar margin (see Figs. 12.180, 12.182). It is important that the elevation be carried out only over the root of the premolars. When the level of the tooth roots is reached, the raspatory is carried obliquely in a superior direction to the edge of the piriform aperture. While the periosteum of the canine fossa is elevated generously, the periosteum remains undisturbed medially in order to preserve an intact pedicle which is as wide as possible. Infraorbitally, there is sufficient space to introduce a narrow nasal hook into the aperture and to drill the base of the alveolar process obliquely under vision at an adequate distance (1 cm) from the root of the canine tooth.

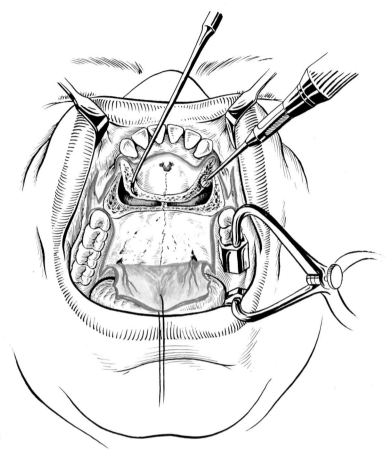

Fig. 12.183

Complete mobilization and realignment of the pedicled fragments. After carrying out the same procedure on the opposite side, the chisel is inserted on both sides through the part of the alveolus which has been removed; the fragment is mobilized with careful leverage. The fragment is now pulled up palatally with a hook anchored in the nasal crest (Fig. 12.183). In this way the mucous membrane on the floor of the nose is put under tension so that it can be elevated safely with a curved raspatory a little distance away from the fragments. Since the fragments are further elevated as a result, a narrow raspatory can be introduced under vision into the groove of the nasal crest and the anchorage of the septum can be carefully freed us far as the nasal spine.

The vestibular pedicled fragment can now be lifted like a trap door (see Fig. 12.183). The exposed surfaces are drilled with a pear burr until the fragments fit together, as on the simulation model and the occlusal overlay.

If the fragment must be displaced nasally because of an existing deep bite, the apical base and the nasal crest are removed successively. In this way 8 additional millime-

ters of height can be required. The septum itself is not shortened.

Realignment of the fragments is easier for anterior open bite due to thumb sucking. Here the anterior dental segment must be displaced inferiorly to achieve the desired overbite. If the resulting bone defect is too large, it is filled with cancellous bone taken from the iliac crest.

Median splitting of the fragments. There are cases of crowded protrusion in the front, in which reconstruction of normal anterior dental relationships is impossible. Posterior displacement of the fragments causes crossbite on the upper canines as a result of crowding of the teeth.

The fragment is split in its center using Heiss's technique (1963). The halves of the fragments are turned outward to widen the arch of the jaw without step formation being necessary.

Median splitting of the fragments (already simulated on the model before operation) follows immediately after the palatal process has been divided transversely while the fragment is still fixed. The hard palate, which along the

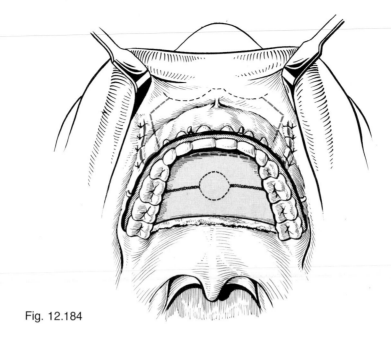

Fig. 12.184

median palatine suture is from 6 to 20 mm thick, is pierced along this line with a rose-head burr. Perforation is carried out most easily at the incisive foramen. Here care must be taken that the burr does not deviate through to the interalveolar septum between both incisor teeth. Farther posteriorly, the perforations do not penetrate through to the anterior edge of the nasal spine because of the increasing thickness of the bone. The weakened bone of the intermaxillary suture is split exactly at the alignment with a thin osteotome.

In a protrusion with gaps and a wide diastema (more than 4 mm), bone is removed centrally, after the intermaxillary suture has been split, until the tooth sockets of the median incisors make close contact. The vestibular mucosa remains intact at this point.

If extensive gaps in the anterior dentition are present, preliminary orthodontic treatment is indicated (Köle 1968). The gaps are closed posteriorly by moving the teeth distally so that a large diastema remains in the center of the maxilla. This is then dealt with in the manner described above, at the same time as the operation for protrusion.

Fixation. An ideal positioning of the fragments can be achieved because the fragments are shaped under vision. The position is controlled with the occlusal template which now becomes a part of the fixation apparatus. First, the palatal flaps are shortened with curved, pointed scissors to fit the reduced bone surfaces. In this way bulging of the mucosa is prevented.

The archbar, which has already been prepared on the simulation model, is introduced and fixed to the occlusal template (Fig. 12.184).

Neither gradual postoperative correction with rubber bands nor intermaxillary fixation is necessary with this operation.

After extubation the inferior part of the nasal cavity is packed with nitrofurazone (Furacin) gauze.

Important Modifications and Surgical Alternatives

There are a large number of modifications which do not differ in method but are different in terms of technical details. The principle of the operation was first described by Cohn-Stock (1921). He was the first to mobilize the protruding section of the jaw with an extensive osteotomy. The fragment was rotated around a transverse axis passing through the anterior nasal spine, usually with the help of an orthopaedic apparatus.

The most difficult part of the mobilization was transverse division of the palate maintaining the mucosal pedicle, particularly in the presence of a highly arched palate. Undermining of the palatal mucosa was facilitated by modifying the incision (Axhausen 1932, Wassmund 1935, Immenkamp 1941).

This does not solve the basic problem of superior transposition of the fragments. In the absence of a method of achieving such a superior displacement, the patient with a simultaneous deep bite could not be treated satisfactorily. Intensive orthodontic aftercare was, therefore, unavoidable, and it was time-consuming and inconvenient for the patient.

Schuchardt (1954), therefore, recommended a two-stage operation. In the first stage, a premolar was extracted on both sides, the palatal mucosa was completely elevated and the palate was divided transversely. At the second stage (6 weeks later), the piriform aperture was exposed together with the spine and the septum; the septum and the base of the alveolar process were divided obliquely from the edge of the piriform aperture to the fundus of the empty alveolus. If the edge of the piriform aperture was in the way when the fragment was displaced superiorly, it was resected.

Although this operation represented a step forward in dealing with deep bite, it was still necessary for the patient to be hospitalized twice. Köle (1968) introduced a one-stage operation in which the palatal mucosa was preserved in the form of 2 bridge flaps.

Compared to Wunderer's (1962) operation, the described operation has the disadvantages that the fragments are formed under difficult circumstances and that realigning and maintaining the position of the fragments are relatively complicated, inconvenient and time-consuming.

Landmarks and Danger Points

Landmarks

For transverse division of the hard palate:

● The median palatal suture,
● The nasal crest which runs anteriorly into the anterior nasal spine (the septum is elevated along this bony ridge and the ridge itself is removed if a superior displacement of the fragment is necessary).

For transverse division of the alveolar process and the apical base:

● The empty alveolar socket of the first and second premolar or the interalveolar septum,
● The canine eminence (the alveolus curves anteriorly),
● The edge of the piriform aperture.

Danger Points

● Damage to the roots of the neighboring teeth when splitting the interalveolar septum, which can be prevented by using a fine rose burr.
● Damage to the mucosa of the floor of the nose, which can be prevented by using a broad rose burr and a water jet under pressure.
● Opening the antral cavity which is inevitable when dividing the apical base of the first and second premolar. Complications usually do not arise.
● Necrosis around the vestibular pedicled fragment (Becker, personal communication). In our experience this complication develops only when the pedicle is narrower than the fragment. This sort of narrowing must be avoided (see under Operative Technique).

If the surgeon prefers to separate the nasal septum from the inferior edge of the aperture, it is preferable to expose the anterior nasal spine intranasally by making an incision at the anterior edge of the cartilaginous septum (Fig. 12.185).

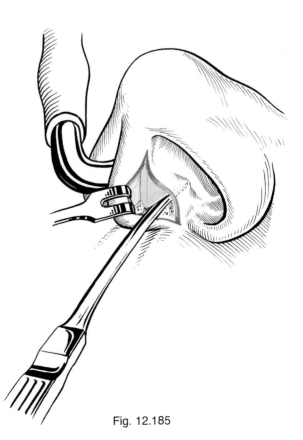

Fig. 12.185

Rules, Hints and Typical Errors

- If bilateral extraction of the premolar is indicated, the operation begins with the extraction.
- On the palatal side, the incision lies along the gingival margin.
- On the vestibular side, the incision lies posterior to the osteotomy line so that the suture line does not lie over the osteotomy.
- The palatal flaps are elevated carefully as far as the palatal foramen with careful preservation of the periosteum.
- The fragments should be everted sufficiently wide anteriorly so that the advantage of this method can be fully utilized.
- The fragment should be held by its posterior edge with sharp bone forceps during drilling. Care should be taken to preserve the mucosal pedicle.
- Division should be carried out, if possible, completely with the drill. Violent breaking of the remaining bony connections leads to splintering
- around the apices of the teeth, which makes realignment of the fragment difficult, especially if the fragment has not been exposed widely enough.

Postoperative Care

- Antibiotic cover is not necessary.
- Thorough cleaning of the oral cavity daily with cetrimide spray.
- Chamomile irrigation every 2 hours.
- Moist dressings on the upper lip and cheek for the first 3 days.
- Puréed diet (tube feeding is not necessary).
- Nasal packing is changed on the second day and is finally removed on the fourth day. If the nasal mucosa has been perforated, the packing is changed again on the fourth day.

Functional Sequelae

Functional narrowing of the lower part of the nasal cavity has not been observed.

Temporary loss of sensation of the teeth in the region of the osteotomy persists for 6 months.

Temporary paresthesia of the vestibular mucosa may occur in the same area.

Lateral Displacement Osteotomy

Principle of the Operation

Complete mobilization of the lateral alveolar process (Fig. 12.186) by a two-stage osteotomy. In the first operation, an osteotomy is done on the vestibular side; the mucosal pedicle is maintained. Three weeks later the palatal side is divided and the fragments are displaced and fixed.

Indications

A lateral displacement osteotomy is indicated:

- If the lower third of the face is too high, the main feature being open bite,
- In crossbite (bilateral or unilateral).

The open bite referred to here is usually caused by rickets. It is also called a true open bite in contrast to anterior open bite due to thumb sucking (see p. 265). Its characteristics are:

- Vertical nonocclusion,
- Deformity of the entire facial skeleton,
- A short upper lip,
- Abnormal height of the mandible with a flattened angle of the jaw.

When the teeth are brought together, a 1.5 cm gap remains anteriorly. In extreme cases, only one molar occludes with its antagonist. As a result of the action of the hyoid musculature on the rachitic mandible, the anterior dental arch characteristically levels off from canine to canine tooth and becomes straight (Schmid-Gussenbauer line). The body of the mandible itself may be bent inferiorly, resulting in excessive height of the lower third of the face.

The infraposition of the anterior part of the upper jaw can be compensated by superior displacement of the lateral alveolar process (Schuchardt 1955) (see Fig. 12.186).

The advantage of this operation is that the original relationship between the upper lip and the teeth is maintained. If the anteriorly curved segment of the jaw was displaced inferiorly to obtain normal occlusion (anterior open bite due to thumb sucking, see p. 271), closure of the lips would be even more difficult and the alveolus, the gingiva and teeth would be visible even when the lips were at rest.

As stated above, both the mandible and the upper jaw are affected in the rachitic open bite. If the mandible is so markedly curved inferiorly that the open bite persists in spite of superior displacement of the lateral alveolar process within the upper jaw, an osteotomy is carried out on the alveolus of the mandible between $\overline{54|45}$ in the same operation. The segment is pushed upward until normal occlusion and overbite is achieved. The defect in the bone is filled with cancellous bone taken from the iliac crest. The fragment is supplied by the lingual mucosa.

Simulation on the model together with analysis of the radiographs is essential for the preoperative assessment of such a two-part operation. Cosmetic considerations are also taken into account. Prosthetic treatment may be indicated rather than operative correction if enamel hypoplasia is present on the anterior teeth (which in any case would have to be crowned) in a moderate open bite.

Crossbite is an anomaly in which the upper and lower teeth cross each other. The unilateral form is considerably more common than the bilateral form. The cause is usually on a unilateral sucking habit and lying on one side during sleep. The crossbite

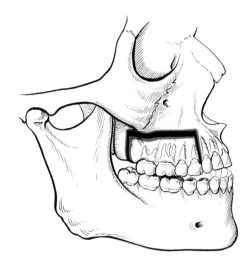

Fig. 12.186

usually occurs as a late result of a cleft of the primary palate. Depending on the type of cleft (unilateral or bilateral), a unilateral or bilateral internal rotation of the alveolar process occurs because of palatal scar contracture. This collapse of the arch can be relieved by tilting or rotating the affected fragment in an outward direction.

Preoperative Diagnosis

The following questions are important in true open bite:

● Is the relation of the upper lip to the front teeth normal or is the upper lip underdeveloped?

● Are the following present:
   a) Marked open bite?
   b) Inferior position of the occlusal plane?
   c) Pronounced degree of underdevelopment of the upper jaw?
   d) High standing molars?
   e) Shallow angle of the jaw and a bend in the mandibular arch?
   f) Excess elevation of the center of the mandible?

In crossbite, only the extreme cases which show a clear-cut transverse asymmetry of the upper jaw are of surgical interest. The most important are the cases with a deformed maxillary arch after previous operations for a cleft of the primary palate.

Teleroentgenograms are useful for analysis of the *true open bite* in terms of other rachitic developmental anomalies of the facial skeleton. They are less important for assessing *crossbite*.

Routine Radiographs

● Occipitodental views of the nasal sinuses;

● Dental films of the upper jaw and also the lower jaw if a simultaneous operation on the mandible is planned.

The following must be assessed:

● The condition of the nasal sinuses;

● The condition of the apices of the teeth, looking for periapical inflammation, cysts or other intraosseous processes;

● The width of the interalveolar septum between the roots of the canine and premolar teeth;

● The position of the upper wisdom teeth.

In true open bite, the **plaster-of-Paris model** helps to estimate and assess accurately:

● The difference in height of the various sections of the arch (oblique position of the occlusal plane, erection of lateral teeth);

● The extent of compression of the upper jaw;

● The part played by the mandible in open bite deformity (opposite bending of the arch).

In crossbite the model demonstrates whether the asymmetry is unilateral or bilateral as well as sagittal or transverse.

Preparation for Surgery

Out-Patient Preparation

The required site of the osteotomy is best determined by simulation using several different positions of the fragments on a simple plaster-of-Paris model.

If wisdom teeth are present, they are extracted 3 months before the first stage of the operation.

In-Patient Preparation

On the day before operation: Cleansing the oral cavity with 0.5% cetrimide spray; premedication according to the schedule.

On the day of operation: The patient is placed in the supine position with his head in the neutral position; the oral cavity is sprayed with dilute cetrimide; the lips are smeared with Vaseline.

Special Instruments

● Nasal hooks,

● Fissure burr,

● Short Lindemann drill,

● Wide periosteal elevator,

● Curved periosteal elevator,

● Finest rose-head burr (for taking down the interalveolar septum),

● Chisel with a wooden handle,

● Lead hammer.

Anesthesia

Although the vestibular osteotomy can be carried out under local anesthesia as a preliminary stage, it is recommended that the second operation be carried out under intubation anesthesia.

Local anesthesia for the vestibular osteotomy is achieved by a nerve block in the infraorbital and tuberosity areas with 2% lidocaine (Xylocaine) and norepinephrine solution. In addition the vestibular mucosa is infiltrated with 1% pure lidocaine; 1 ml of 2% lidocaine with norepinephrine added is injected into the greater palatine foramen and into the incisive foramen.

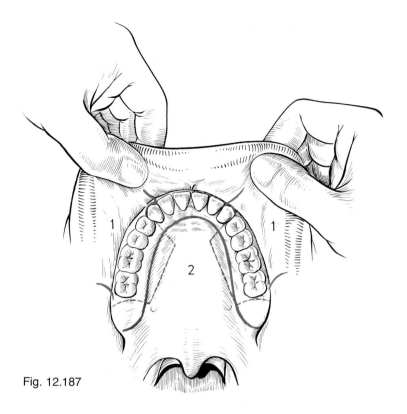

Fig. 12.187

Operative Technique

Due to the danger of necrosis of the fragments, the operation is carried out in 2 stages. The maxillary tuberosity remains in position. The alveolar process is always divided in the molar area. A summary of the plan of the operation is shown in Figure 12.187 (operation 1 vestibular osteotomy; operation 2 palatal osteotomy).

Vestibular Osteotomy

Two incisions are made in the vestibule, perpendicular to the gingival margin. The anterior incision is one width of a tooth medial to the planned osteotomy line. The posterior incision is one width of a molar posterior to the zygomaticoalveolar crest (Fig. 12.188).

The mucoperiosteum around the anterior incision is elevated not only over the roots but also in the canine fossa. The periosteum with the muscular insertions is elevated widely in the direction of the infraorbital foramen and the root of the zygomatic process with preservation of the gingiva until a spacious tunnel has been formed beneath the soft tissue of the cheek. A similar procedure is carried out from the posterior incision in order to expose the infratemporal region and the rounded external surface of the tuberosity subperiosteally.

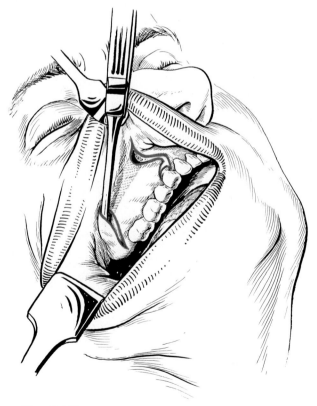

Fig. 12.188

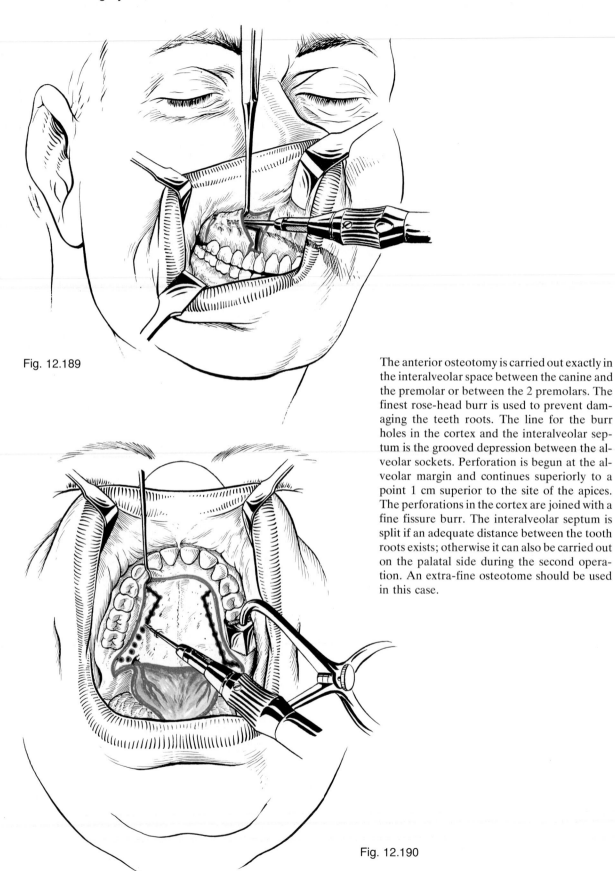

Fig. 12.189

The anterior osteotomy is carried out exactly in the interalveolar space between the canine and the premolar or between the 2 premolars. The finest rose-head burr is used to prevent damaging the teeth roots. The line for the burr holes in the cortex and the interalveolar septum is the grooved depression between the alveolar sockets. Perforation is begun at the alveolar margin and continues superiorly to a point 1 cm superior to the site of the apices. The perforations in the cortex are joined with a fine fissure burr. The interalveolar septum is split if an adequate distance between the tooth roots exists; otherwise it can also be carried out on the palatal side during the second operation. An extra-fine osteotome should be used in this case.

Fig. 12.190

The posterior osteotomy is made with the short Lindemann drill which is introduced perpendicularly to the surface of the tuberosity if possible. At the same time, the cortex on the opposite (palatal) side is also divided. Finally, the vertical incisions are joined with the horizontal one; the mucosal bridge is preserved (Fig. 12.189). The width of the superior bony strip to be resected can be seen on the model. The oral mucosa is closed with continuous 4 × 0 sutures. Opening the maxillary antrum is unavoidable but usually has no sequelae.

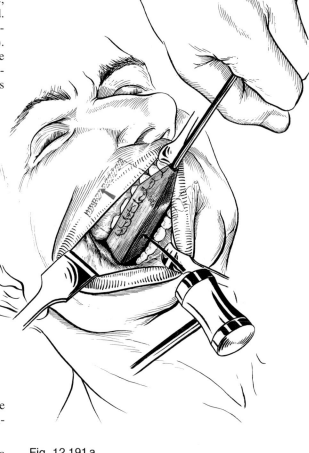

Palatal Osteotomy

This must follow within 3 weeks, at the latest, since the tissue which forms in the osteotomy cleft makes alignment of the fragments increasingly more difficult.

The palatal mucosa is elevated beginning at the gingiva and ending at the maxillary tuberosity; the palatal vessels are preserved (Fig. 12.190). The interalveolar osteotomy which began on the vestibular side is now completed on the palatal side. Since the perforation marks are still visible on the tuberosity, the last remaining bony bridge can be accurately divided along the junction between the palatal surface and the alveolar process. It is important to drill obliquely in the direction of the maxillary antrum and not perpendicular to the palate. The floor of the nose should remain intact. The palatal part of the fragment is shortened depending on the size of the segment resected from the wall of the maxillary antrum.

Fig. 12.191 a

If the osteotomy has been done cleanly, thumb pressure suffices to mobilize the fragment. A light hammer blow is necessary to displace it upward into its final position; the wooden handle of a chisel should be used as a buffer to avoid damaging the teeth (Fig. 12.191 a).

After the same procedure has been carried out on the opposite side and the occlusion has been tested on the simulation model, a rigid wire-Palavit splint is introduced using a palatal plate. Intermaxillary fixation is advisable for 2 weeks to ensure retention of the occlusion (Fig. 12.191 b).

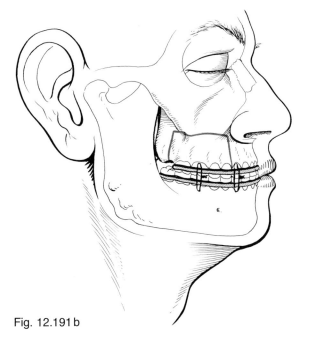

Fig. 12.191 b

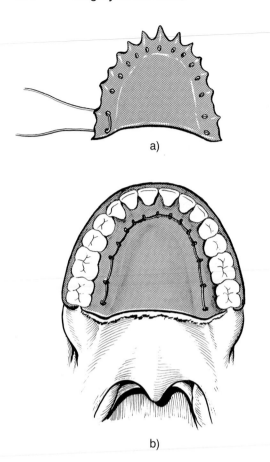

a)

b)

Fig. 12.192

Correction of a crossbite or a too narrow maxillary arch is carried out according to the same principles. In this case the fragments are tilted outward or rotated. This is fairly difficult in patients who have undergone previous surgery for clefts of the primary palate because the palatal mucosa is scarred. The fragments cannot be displaced into the correct position by hand pressure alone. Bone forceps would produce a great deal of trauma. A long lever with a plastic key at the end is used on each side; the key accurately fits the dental crowns of the corresponding fragment. This method provides a large grasping surface and the necessary force is evenly distributed over all of the teeth in order to allow displacement of the fragments into the correct position. Normally, an occlusal template (Fig. 12.192a) is used which is fixed to a vestibular splint (Fig. 12.192b).

Often it is necessary to displace the fragment by more than a centimeter; this results in a secondary cleft in the palate. The defect is usually closed spontaneously only after the fragment has consolidated in position, which generally requires at least 1 year.

Important Modifications and Surgical Alternatives

Schuchardt's osteotomy is unquestionably an advance; Kapovits and Pfeifer (1961) modified the procedure by placing the incision through the molar area. The danger of relapse, particularly emphasized by Köle, is then much lower. If the posterior incision lies behind the maxilla as described by Schuchardt, the distal end of the fragment lacks both support and the necessary contact surface between the tuberosity and the pterygoid process. With functional stress the free end of the fragment moves so that excess callus forms over the remaining surface and pushes the fragment back into its old position before it has had a chance to consolidate.

We have modified the original method even further. Basically, we carry out an osteotomy on the vestibular side during the first operation; a bridge of mucosa and periosteum is maintained. This is important for the second stage because it allows the fragment to be mobilized without the danger of necrosis. The mucoperiosteal pedicle on the vestibular side is significantly more elastic than that on the palatal side which is easily detached during extensive displacement of the fragment. This danger is particularly great during external tilting or rotation.

In this regard, there is an additional problem. Since external tilting or rotation of the fragment produces a secondary defect of the palate and the tendency toward consolidation is reduced, the palate had to be closed at a later date. This was a complicated procedure in terms of the long period of aftercare and the necessity of a second operation. Osteoplasty, therefore, should be carried out immediately, even if closure of the palatal and antral mucosa is impossible. The open cleft is filled with a cancellous bone graft. The bone paste can be adapted to the edges of the bone and closes the bony defect without forming cavities.

Experience shows that the cancellous bone graft revascularizes quickly in spite of its exposed position. An additional advantage of a cancellous bone graft is its resistance to infection. The readapted palatal mucosa and the cancellous graft are covered by a palatal plate supported by a thick layer of nitrofurazone (Furacin) gauze (see Figs. 12.184; 12.192 a, b).

Landmarks and Danger Points

Landmarks

For the anterior and posterior transverse division of the alveolar process:

- The interalveolar septum between the alveolar sockets; the canine tooth and the first premolar or the first and second premolar.
- The molar area between the zygomaticoalveolar crest and the maxillary tuberosity.

For the vestibular incision:

- The base of the superior alveolus and a plane through the inferior edge of the piriform aperture projected inferiorly;
- The zygomaticoalveolar crest;
- The infratemporal area;
- The infraorbital foramen, which forms the superior limit of subperiosteal undermining.

For the palatal incision:

- Osteotomy line: The apex of the angle between the surface of the palate and the alveolar process;
- The greater palatine foramen;
- The pterygomaxillary fissure.

Danger Points

- Damage to the roots of the neighboring teeth when splitting the interalveolar septum, which should be prevented by using the finest rose-head burr;
- Bleeding from the pterygoid plexus, which should be prevented by strict subperiosteal elevation of the posterior infratemporal structures.

Rules and Hints

- The vestibular osteotomy should be carried out first.
- Avoid cutting the vestibular mucosa horizontally.

- Preserve a pedicle on the vestibular side by cutting the mucosa vertically.
- Use the finest rose-head burr for the interalveolar osteotomy but a large rose-head burr, which is most likely to preserve the antral mucosa, for the vestibular and palatal incisions.
- Mobilize the fragment completely (nutrition is maintained by the vestibular mucosal pedicle and the continuity of the antral mucosa).
- Immediate realignment of the fragments. Advantages: Immediate and final fixation of the fragments.
  Intermaxillary fixation is not necessary.
  Gradual secondary realignment of the fragments via intermaxillary traction with rubber wires is not necessary.
  Prolonged aftercare is not necessary.
- Secure the position of the fragments via rigid fixation.
- For difficult external tilting or rotation of the fragments, an individually prepared lever which can be anchored to the dental crowns should be used.
- Secondary defects in the bony palate should be filled with cancellous chips; primary closure of the palate.

Typical Errors

- Lack of clarification of the state of the nasal sinuses. Opening a healthy antrum is harmless, but this is not the case if the mucosa is chronically inflamed.
- Retromaxillary osteotomy requires a long time for consolidation and there is a danger of recurrence.
- Damage to the mucosa of the nose by making the osteotomy perpendicular to the surface of the palate instead of oblique to the alveolar process.
- Carrying out the two-stage osteotomy in the wrong order. If the operation is begun on the palatal side, the palatal pedicle may be torn during the second operation, particularly if external tilting or rotation of the fragment is indicated. (After 3 weeks the palatal flap has not yet regained its original adhesion to the bone.)

Postoperative Care

- Antibiotic cover is not necessary. It should be started only at the first sign of infection. Penicillin (20–40 million I.U. per day) combined with streptomycin (1 gram per day).

- The oral cavity is sprayed thoroughly twice a day with cetrimide spray.

- Chamomile irrigation every 2 hours is advised.

- Moist dressings are applied to the upper lip and the cheek for the first 3 days.

- A soft diet is given.

- Tube feeding is necessary only if an osteoplasty has been carried out at the same time.

- The splint is removed after 6 weeks, at the earliest; if an osteoplasty has been carried out, only after 8 weeks.

Functional Sequelae

Complications in regard to the nasal sinuses have not generally been observed.

There is little danger of relapse if the described method is followed.

Temporary hypoesthesia of the teeth in the region of the osteotomy lasts for about 6 months.

Possibly temporary paresthesia of the vestibular mucosa.

Osteotomy of the Middle Third of the Face

The upper jaw forms the middle part of the facial skeleton. Its trajectory transmits the masticatory forces evenly and almost perpendicularly to the base of the skull (Fig. 12.193). The plane of the base of the skull and the occlusal plane form an angle of approximately 45°; both planes intercept at the level of the foramen magnum. Since the masticatory forces are greater in the molar area than in the incisor area, the bony pillars are sturdier in the molar area than farther forward in the incisor area.

The arterial blood supply is provided by branches of the maxillary artery which run, in part, through a thin-walled bony canal (infraorbital canal). The nerve supply is from branches of the maxillary division of the fifth nerve. Its intracanalicular course increases the danger of damage to the vessels and the nerve during osteotomy and extensive displacement of fragments; but the blood supply is so rich that bone necrosis is seldom observed, even after extensive osteotomies.

Nevertheless, a large palatal or vestibular mucoperiosteal pedicle must remain to ensure blood supply during an extensive osteotomy on the upper jaw. Certain osteotomies must, therefore, be carried out in two stages.

Indications

If cephalometry (see p. 167) shows retroposition of the upper jaw in relation to the mandible accompanied by malocclusion, an osteotomy of the middle third of the face is indicated for the mobilization and anterior displacement of the upper jaw and/or the middle third of the facial complex.

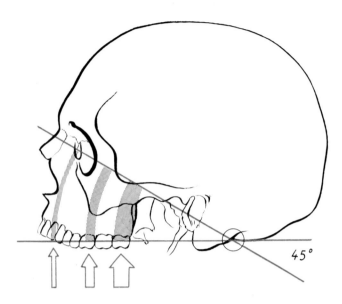

Fig. 12.193

A typical retroposition of the upper jaw is found in:

● A "dishface" after injury;

● Hypoplasia of the upper jaw: After previous operations for cleft of the primary and secondary palates;

● Crouzon's disease: Congenital retroposition and failure of development of the zygomaticomaxillary region.

Crouzon's disease is accompanied by numerous other anomalies such as brachycephaly or oxycephaly, receding frontal bone resulting from premature fusion of the coronoid suture, proptosis, exophoria, exotropia and lateral displacement of the canthus. In such patients a more or less pronounced degree of malocclusion in the form of a socalled pseudoprognathism is present.

The question as to when an extensive osteotomy should be carried out remains unanswered. As previously mentioned, an extensive osteotomy should not be carried out on the growing facial skeleton so that further growth is not disturbed by additional trauma and later contracture of scar tissue. Early surgery, however, is urgently indicated under certain circumstances between the tenth and twelfth year of life (Tessier 1967), e.g., Crouzon's disease in order to allow normal development of the neurocranium and the facial skeleton.

Diagnostic Preoperative Measures

Dental status. Dental views are used to show the position of the upper wisdom teeth, which must be extracted, and the extent of the dental work required before the operation.

Teleroentgenograms are taken (1 : 1 views, with the head in the neutral position) to determine the extent of the required anterior displacement of the upper jaw. The displacement is simulated by drawing the entire complex of the middle third of the face on an unexposed x-ray film and bringing it into the appropriate relationship with the mandible. The extent of the required anterior displacement of the upper jaw is then measured in millimeters.

Simulation of the operation. The best possible occlusion is determined using a simple plaster-of-Paris model. Intervening dental cusps are ground down and marked with a black felt-tip pen.

Photographs. Full frontal and profile views allow measurement of the soft tissues and the interrelationship of the different areas of the face.

Ophthalmological consultation. In extensive osteotomies which must be extended through the orbital area, visual acuity and the ocular movements should be tested before surgery.

Neurological consultation. An assessment should be made of the function of the cranial nerves, particularly the trigeminal and olfactory nerves.

Preparation for Surgery

Since the osteotomy is to be carried out in the molar area, the wisdom teeth must be extracted at least 6 weeks before the operation. The dental splint and palatal plate are inserted before the operation and the teeth are ground down in accordance with the model.

Special Instruments

- Fine chisel and osteotome, partly straight and partly curved, 10–15 mm wide, prefarably with a guide on both sides to protect the septal mucosa;
- Different burrs (round and oval, straight side-cutting, etc.);
- Elevator;
- Awl and hollow needle;
- Rocking forceps;
- Nasal specula;
- Swivel knife;
- Dental splint;
- Georgiade "halo" fixation apparatus.

Anesthesia

Due to the extent of the operation, endotracheal intubation anesthesia is indicated following suitable premedication. Nasal intubation should be used since the occlusion must be realigned after the osteotomy has been carried out and the jaws must be fixed by intermaxillary fixation.

A tracheotomy is seldom indicated and then only for extensive osteotomies of the middle third of the face. Aspiration of blood at the end of the operation is prevented by a throat pack soaked in paraffin. A nasogastric tube is also introduced after intubation.

Principles of the Operation

The purpose of the osteotomy of the middle third of the face is to bring the maxilla or the middle third of the facial complex into harmonic relationship with the remaining parts of the face. Normal occlusion should be restored at the same time as the correction of the external profile. Since, in certain cases, other anomalies (Crouzon's disease or the state after a cleft of the primary palate) may be present, additional operations such as rhinoplasty, correction of the chin or the forehead as well as displacement osteotomy of the mandible may be necessary.

In every osteotomy on the upper jaw, the origins of the masticatory muscles should be preserved so that the mechanism of the masticatory apparatus is not damaged. Furthermore, the muscles of the soft palate and their insertion must remain intact, particularly in those patients operated on for a cleft of the primary palate.

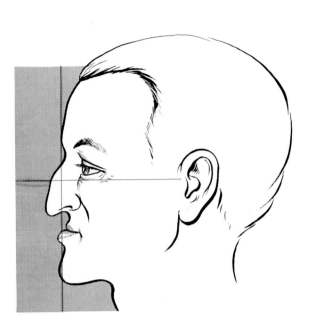

Fig. 12.194

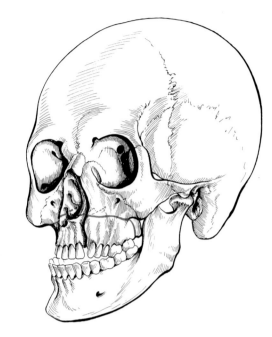

Fig. 12.195

Operative Technique

Le Fort Type I Ostetomy

The original findings are those of hypoplasia of the upper jaw in a patient previously operated on for a cleft of the primary and secondary palates. A typical profile is shown in Figure 12.194.

Vestibular osteotomy. The principle is transverse division of the body of the maxilla and of the septum above the base of the alveolus at the level of the floor of the antrum and the nasal cavitiy (Fig. 12.195).

The maxilla is divided from the piriform sinus to the maxillary tuberosity; a vestibular mucoperiosteal pedicle is preserved. The wall of the antrum is divided first (Fig. 12.196), and then an osteotomy of the lateral nasal wall and

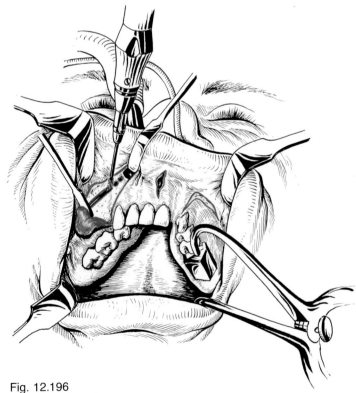

Fig. 12.196

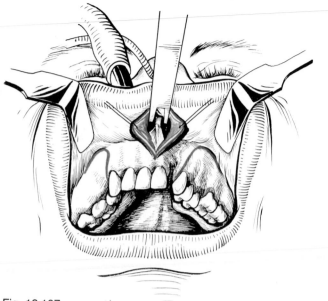

Fig. 12.197

of the nasal septum is carried out (see Fig. 12.197). Finally, the alveolar process is divided with the osteotome transversely in the region of the wisdom tooth (Fig. 12.198).

Palatal osteotomy. At a second stage, 3 weeks later, the palate is divided as far as the previous osteotomy line anterior to the tuberosity by forming a palatal mucosal flap (Fig. 12.199). The inferior part of the upper jaw can now be mobilized en bloc or in segments. Since this osteotomy is particularly indicated in patients who have had previous surgery for clefts of the secondary palate and, therefore, have a preexisting short palate and a more or less pronounced velopharyngeal insufficiency, the palatal osteotomy is carried anterior to the greater palatal foramen through the transverse palatal suture in order to prevent further shortening of the soft palate when anterior displacement is carried out.

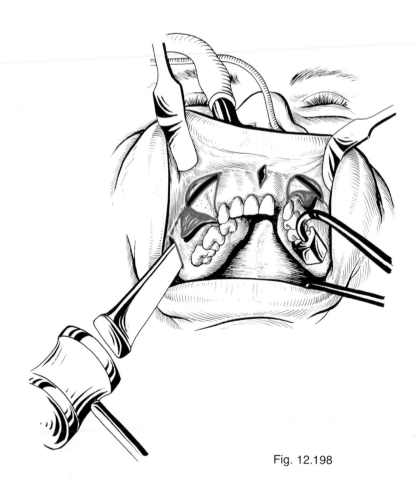

Fig. 12.198

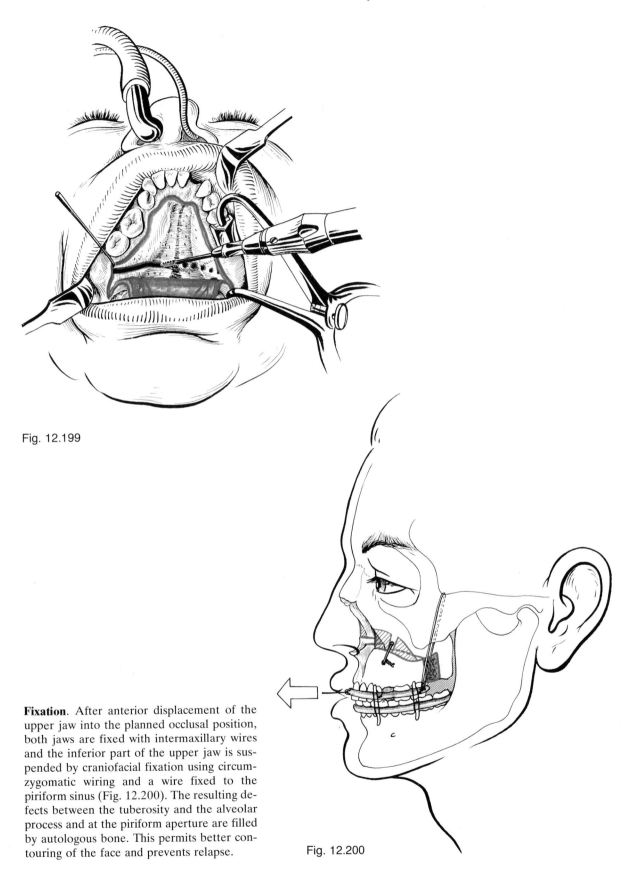

Fig. 12.199

Fixation. After anterior displacement of the upper jaw into the planned occlusal position, both jaws are fixed with intermaxillary wires and the inferior part of the upper jaw is suspended by craniofacial fixation using circumzygomatic wiring and a wire fixed to the piriform sinus (Fig. 12.200). The resulting defects between the tuberosity and the alveolar process and at the piriform aperture are filled by autologous bone. This permits better contouring of the face and prevents relapse.

Fig. 12.200

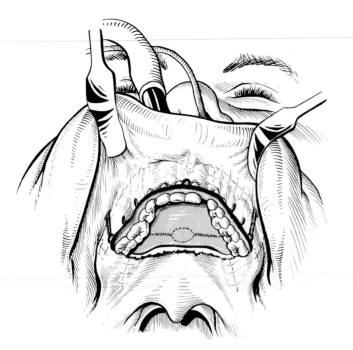

Fig. 12.201

In extensive clefts of the secondary palate, it is worthwhile to use a palatal plate made of self-hardening plastic which not only adapts the palatal mucoperiosteal flap but also stabilizes the position of the fragment (Fig. 12.201). The "halo" fixation apparatus ensures the ventral position of the fragment (Fig. 12.202).

Le Fort Type II Osteotomy

Le Fort Type II osteotomies have not proved useful since the lacrimal apparatus and the canthal ligaments may be damaged and obstruction may develop as can be seen after a Le Fort Type II fracture.

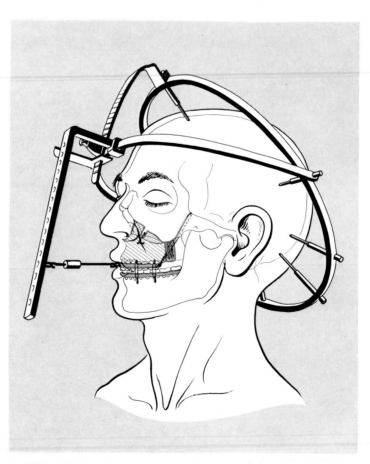

Fig. 12.202

Le Fort Type III Osteotomy

The basic findings are a "dishface" (Fig. 12.203).

Principle: Central and lateral division of the facial skeleton from the base of the skull (Fig. 12.204).

The osteotomy lines run as follows:

- Interorbital: Through the base of the perpendicular plate, the vomer and the ethmoid cells;
- Intraorbital: Through the anterior part of the floor and the lateral wall;
- Periorbital: Through the frontal and zygomatic processes and the body of the zygoma;
- Palatal: Through the transverse palatal suture;
- Infratemporal: Through the alveolar process and the floor of the antrum.

A symmetrical curved incision is made along the facial crease from the infraorbital margin over the root of the nose to the opposite side (Fig. 12.205).

The lateral wall and the bony bridge of the nose are exposed by elevating the periosteum. The root of the nose is divided with an oscillating saw and the osteotomy is then begun with an osteotome on the nasoethmoid complex (see Fig. 12.206). The cut lies superior and posterior to the vault of the lacrimal sac in order to preserve the openings of the lacrimal canaliculi and the origin of the medial palpebral ligament. The osteotomy is continued parallel to the base of the skull through the perpendicular plate of the ethmoid and through the ethmoid cell on both sides as far as the choanae. This must be carried out strictly sub-

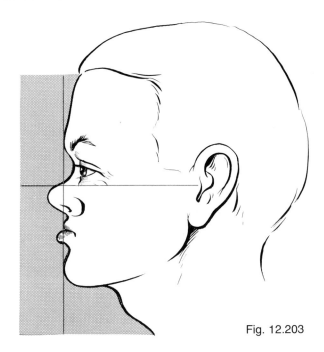

Fig. 12.203

periosteally so that the trochlea of the superior oblique muscle or the infratrochlear nerve is not damaged.

The anterior end of the inferior orbital fissure is sought by elevating the periosteum of the orbital floor; the osteotomy is continued to this point. In the process the orbital contents are retracted with a soft retractor; the anterior part of the floor of the orbit is divided perpendicular to the infraorbital canal; care should be taken to preserve the infraorbital nerve.

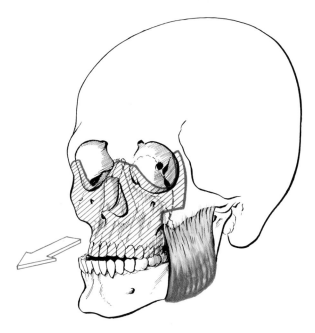

Fig. 12.204

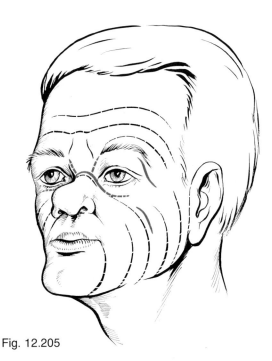

Fig. 12.205

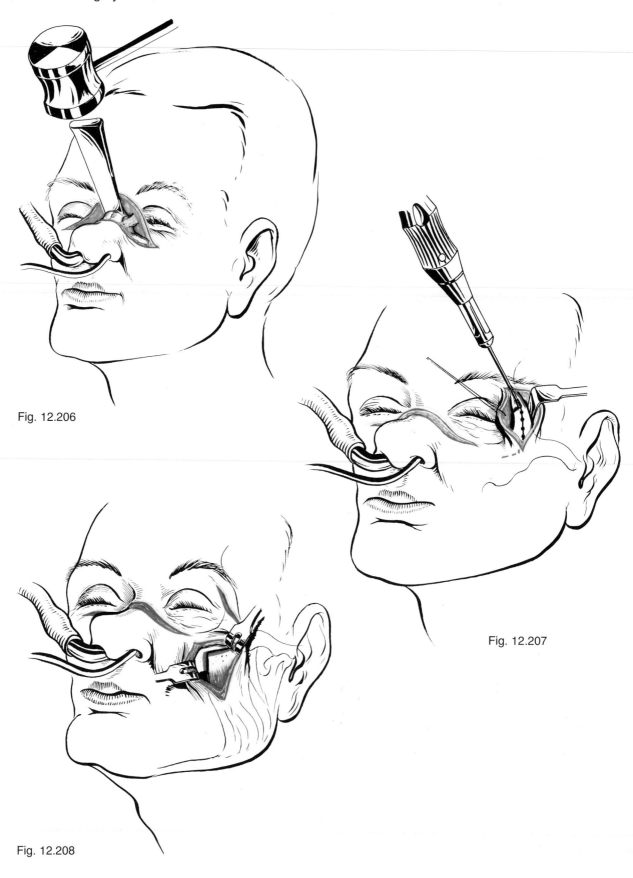

Fig. 12.206

Fig. 12.207

Fig. 12.208

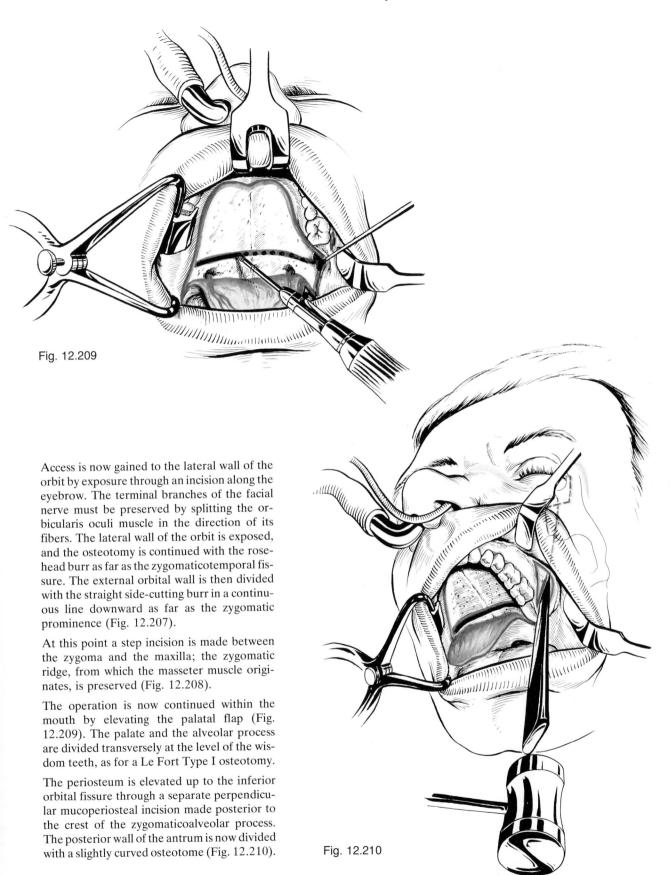

Fig. 12.209

Fig. 12.210

Access is now gained to the lateral wall of the orbit by exposure through an incision along the eyebrow. The terminal branches of the facial nerve must be preserved by splitting the orbicularis oculi muscle in the direction of its fibers. The lateral wall of the orbit is exposed, and the osteotomy is continued with the rose-head burr as far as the zygomaticotemporal fissure. The external orbital wall is then divided with the straight side-cutting burr in a continuous line downward as far as the zygomatic prominence (Fig. 12.207).

At this point a step incision is made between the zygoma and the maxilla; the zygomatic ridge, from which the masseter muscle originates, is preserved (Fig. 12.208).

The operation is now continued within the mouth by elevating the palatal flap (Fig. 12.209). The palate and the alveolar process are divided transversely at the level of the wisdom teeth, as for a Le Fort Type I osteotomy.

The periosteum is elevated up to the inferior orbital fissure through a separate perpendicular mucoperiosteal incision made posterior to the crest of the zygomaticoalveolar process. The posterior wall of the antrum is now divided with a slightly curved osteotome (Fig. 12.210).

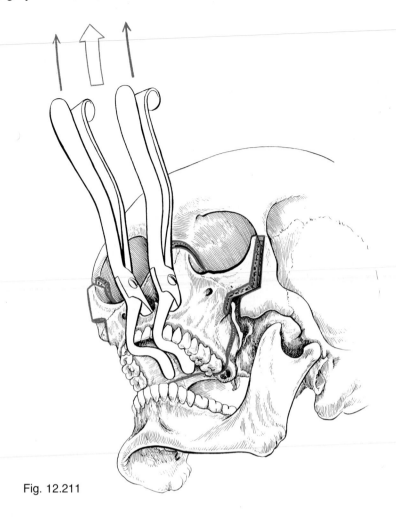

Fig. 12.211

The central middle third of the face is mobilized en bloc with rocking forceps which are engaged both intranasally and intraorally (Fig. 12.211). During the anterior displacement, the intended occlusion should be achieved by careful comparison with the simulation model; attention should be paid to the distance between the frontal bone and the nasal bone.

Distraction demands extreme care in order to avoid damaging nerves and vessels. The position of the fragments is achieved by *intermaxillary fixation* and by *interposition of a bone graft* between the frontal and nasal bones and between the pterygoid tuberosity and the alveolar process.

A bony allograft from the iliac crest is most suitable. A graft of cortical and cancellous bone is introduced and fixed with wire. Any remaining holes are filled with cancellous bone (Fig. 12.212). The palatal flaps are then adapted using an already prepared palatal plate of self-hardening plastic (see Fig. 12.184) with an underlying layer of nitrofurazone (Furacin) gauze.

After the throat pack has been removed and the mouth has been cleaned, intermaxillary fixation with 0.6 mm wire is undertaken. In addition the position of the fragments is secured by craniofacial suspension and by anterior extension using a "halo" apparatus (Fig. 12.213). The facial suspenison wire is removed after 6 weeks, at the latest, by means of a parietal pull out device.

The wound is closed in layers with 4 × 0 Supramid sutures inside the mouth and 5 × 0 Supramid sutures outside.

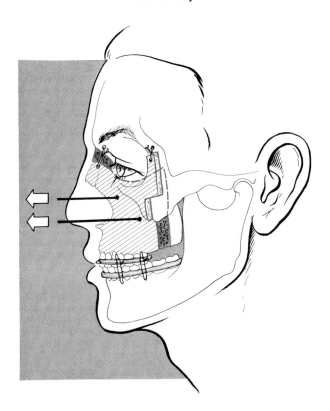

Fig. 12.212

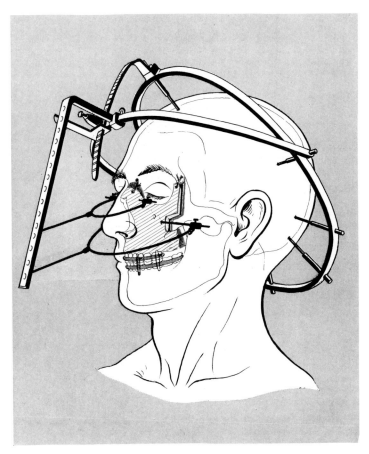

Fig. 12.213

Modifications and Surgical Alternatives

To the Le Fort Type I Osteotomy

It is not so important whether the vestibular osteotomy is carried out before the palatal one; the time interval, however, is important.

It is possible to mobilize the fragments at one sitting; the base of the maxilla is divided from the medial and lateral pterygoid processes to preserve the blood supply of the hard palate from the palate vessels. The disadvantage of this procedure is the danger of fracturing the pterygoid process and the loss of a broad-based buttress for the interposition of the bone graft. Since the blood supply on both sides comes almost completely from the greater palatine artery, there is an advantage to this procedure. When carrying out the vestibular osteotomy, the bone can be divided without forming a mucosal pedicle and the osteotomy can be carried out under better vision.

This operation is not indicated in patients with clefts of the secondary palate since they also have a shortening of the soft palate; the velopharyngeal insufficiency already present is made even worse by anterior displacement of the maxilla.

Another alternative exists for those patients in whom the nasal tip area must be elevated by a rhinoplasty. Access for division of the septum or the vomer is then via the usual intercartilaginous incision which is then extended on both sides in the nasal vestibule to the transfixion incision. The mucoperichondrium is elevated from the cartilage and the entire nasal septum is visualized with the speculum. The septum can then be divided obliquely up to the dorsum using Ballenger's swivel knife. It can be displaced anteriorly later since it is still attached to the osteotomized maxillary segment. The tip of the nose is then elevated at the same time that the maxilla is displaced anteriorly.

To the Le Fort Type III Osteotomy

There are modifications to this operation, particularly in the type of access. According to Tessier (1967), the first part of the operation should be a temporal access with division of the lateral wall of the orbit and sagittal splitting of the zygoma. A step osteotomy is then undertaken on the zygoma, the nasoethmoidal osteotomy is performed and then posterior division of the maxilla is carried out up to the inferior orbital fissure.

Further modifications have been described for the osteotomy on the zygoma. Gillies (1950) divided the zygoma transversely across the zygomaticotemporal fissure and perpendicularly across the zygomatic arch. The disadvantage of this procedure is that the anterior part of the origin of the masseter remains attached to the divided segment and, therefore, must be released. If this is not done, a relapse may easily occur.

An additional modification consists of dividing the maxilla in the region of the tuberosity from the origin of the pterygoid plates so that the entire framework of the roof of the oral cavity is included in the anterior displacement. In this procedure there is danger of breaking the fragile pterygoid process from the base of the skull which can lead to a dural tear (Trauner, personal communication).

Landmarks and Danger Points

● Damage to the cribriform plate, the lacrimal sac and the canthal ligaments which then lead to cerebrospinal rhinorrhea, epiphora and displacement of the canthus.

● Lesions of the trochlea or the infratrochlear nerve which then lead to disorders of ocular movement.

● Lesions of the nerves in the area of the orbital fissure and of the infraorbital nerve.

● Damage to the orbital periosteum. The orbital contents prolapse into the ethmoid cells or to the maxillary sinus causing enophthalmos or ophthalmoplegia if incarceration of the inferior oblique muscle is also present.

● Tearing of the lateral palpebral ligament in osteotomy of the orbital rim.

● Division of the zygomatic branches of the facial nerve which leads to lagophthalmos and corneal ulceration.

- Damage to the nasal turbinates or shattering of the perpendicular plate of the vomer which may be followed by nasal obstruction.

- Damage to the internal maxillary artery during infratemporal osteotomy in the region of the inferior orbital fissure.

- A secondary oronasal fistula in a previously operated cleft of the secondary palate.

Rules, Hints and Typical Errors

- In osteotomy of the central middle third of the face, the extraoral operation is usually carried out first; then the osteotomy is completed from within the mouth.

- Because of the extent of the operation and as a bone graft must be inserted partially in communication with the ethmoidal cells or the maxillary sinus, treatment with antibiotics is indicated.

- The most important bone graft is that lying between the pterygoid tuberosity and the alveolus. It should consist of 1 large piece of cortical and cancellous bone. The second most important bone graft is that lying between the frontal and nasal bones. There is a danger of producing a socalled Grecian nose in which the natural nasofrontal step is filled out with the graft.

- Overcorrection should be achieved anteriorly, particularly in the naso-frontal area, because of the danger of retrodisplacement. This danger is not so great in the oral area because interdigitation of the cusps provides good retention during intermaxillary fixation.

- The face must be lengthened in Crouzon's disease by wedging a suitable thick bone graft between the orbits. This graft serves as a fulcrum and, at the same time, forms the medial wall of the orbit.

Functional Sequelae

- There is danger of retrodisplacement if dentition is incomplete and the graft does not provide adequate support and if the anterior origin of the masseter is left attached to the zygoma in Gillies' modified osteotomy.

- Scarring, scar contractures, hypertrophic scars and keloid formation, e.g., scar contracture in the infraorbital area which then leads to ectropion of the lower lid.

- Temporary or permanent loss of the sense of smell.

- Nasal obstruction.

- Ethmoidal or maxillary sinusitis if fragments of the bone graft are located within the maxillary or ethmoidal cavities.

Bibliography

Aller, T. G.: Operative treatment of prognathism. Dent. Cosmos 59: 394, 1917

Angle, E. H.: Double resection for treatment of mandibular protrusion. Dent. Cosmos Nr. 8, 1898/99; 45: 268, 1903

Axhausen, G.: Beiträge zur Mund- und Kieferchirurgie. Dtsch. Zahnheilk. 82, 1932

Barrow, G. V., R. O. Dingman: Orthodontic consideration in the surgical management of developmental deformities of the mandible. Am. J. Orthodont. 36: 121, 1950

Böhler, L.: Technik der Knochenbruchbehandlung, 12th–13th Edn. Maudrich, Vienna 1957

Boyne, P. J.: Osseous healing after oblique osteotomy of the mandibular ramus. J. Oral Surg. 25: 125, 1966

Caldwell, J. B., G. S. Lettermann: Vertical osteotomy in the mandibular rami for correction of prognathism. J.Oral Surg. 12: 185, 1954

Cohn-Stock, G.: Die chirurgische Immediatregulierung der Kiefer, speziell die chirurgische Behandlung der Prognathie. Vjschr. Zahnheilk., Berlin 37: 320, 1921

Converse, J. M.: Restoration of facial contour by bone grafts introduced through the oral cavity. Plast. Reconstr. Surg. 6: 295, 1950

Converse, J. M.: Technique of bone grafting for contour restoration of the face. Plast. Reconstr. Surg. 14: 332, 1954

Converse, J. M., H. H. Shapiro: Treatment of developmental malformations of the jaws. Plast. Reconstr. Surg. 10: 473, 1952

Dal Pont, G.: L'osteotomia retromolare per la correzione della progenia. Minerva Chir. 1, 1958

Dal Pont, G.: Retromolar osteotomy for the correction of prognathism. J. Oral Surg. Anesth. 19: 42, 1961

Dieffenbach, J. F.: Operative Chirurgie, Vol. 2. Brockhaus, Leipzig 1848, p. 47.

Dingman, R. O.: Surgical correction of mandibular prognathism, an improved method. Am. J. Orthodont, 683, 1944

Dingman, R. O.: Surgical correction of developmental deformities of the mandible. Plast. Reconstr. Surg. 3: 124, 1948

Dingman, R. O.: Ostectomy of the mandible in cleft lip and palate habilitation. Plast. Reconstr. Surg. 25: 213, 1960

Dufourmentel, C., R. Mouly: Chirurgie plastique. Paris 1959

Eggers, G. W. N., W. H. Ainsworth, T. O. Shindler, C. M. Pomerat: Clinical significance of the contact-compression factor in bone surgery. Arch. Surg. 62: 467, 1951

von Eiselsberg, A.: Über Plastik bei Ektropium des Unterkiefers. Münch. Med. Wochenschr. 54:36, 1907

Ernst, F.: in: Die Chirurgie, Vol. IV, Part 1, ed. by M. Kirschner, O. Nordmann. Urban & Schwarzenberg, Berlin 1927, p. 807

Esmarch, F.: Traitement du resserrement cicatriciel des machoires par la formation d'une fausse articulation dans la continuité de l'os maxillaire inférieure. Arch. Gén. Med. V, Serie 44, 1860

Farr, H. W., B. Jean-Gilles, A. Die: Cervical island skin flap repair of oral and pharyngeal defects in the composite operation for cancer. Am. J. Surg. 118: 759, 1969

Gabka, J.: Zur Progenie-Operation am horizontalen Unterkieferast. Zbl. Chir. 86: 1196, 1961

Gillies, H., S. H. Harrison: Operative correction by osteotomy of recessed malar maxillary compound in a case of oxycephaly. Br. J. Plast. Surg. 2: 123, 1950

Ginestet, G., L. Merville: Recueil périodique de l'encyclopédie médico-chirurgicale. Rev. Stomat. (Paris) 37: 27, 1966 special issue

Heiss, J.: Eine neue Modifikation der operativen Prognathiebehandlung. Zahnärztl. Prax. 14: 220, 1963

Hofer, O.: Die osteoplastische Verlängerung des Unterkiefers nach v. Eiselsberg bei Mikrogenie. Dtsch. Zahn-, Mund-, Kieferheilk. 27: 81, 1957

Immenkamp, A.: Die chirurgisch-orthopädische Behandlung der Progenie: Zahnaerztl. Rundsch. 50: 1439: 1509, 1941

Immenkamp, A.: Chirurgische Kieferorthopädie. In: Die Zahn-, Mund- und Kieferheilkunde, ed. by K. Häupl, W. Meyer, K. Schuchardt; Vol. III, Part 1. Urban & Schwarzenberg, Munich 1957

Kapovits, M., G. Pfeifer: Die chirurgische Behandlung des offenen Bisses nach Schuchardt. Dtsch. Zahn-, Mund-, Kieferheilk. 36: 268, 1961

Kapovits, M., G. Pfeifer: Die chirurgische Korrektur der Progenie und des offenen Bisses durch einzeitige Operation am horizontalen Unterkieferast. Dtsch. Zahnaerztl. Z. 17: 282, 1962

Kazanjian, V. H.: Surgical correction of mandibular prognathism. Internat. J. Orthodont. 18: 1224, 1932

Kazanjian, V. H.: The treatment of mandibular prognathism with special reference to edentulous patients. Oral Surg. 4: 680 1951

Kazanjian, V. H.: Bone transplanting to the mandible. Am. J. Surg. 83: 633, 1952

Kiehn, C. L., J. D. Desprez: Malignant tumours of the oral cavity. In: Modern Trends in Plastic Surgery, ed. by T. Gibson. Butterworths, London 1964

Köle, H.: Zur operativen Behandlung der Progenie. Öst. Z. Stomat. 58: 25, 1961

Köle, H.: Aesthetische Operationen im Mund- und Kieferbereich. In: Handbuch der plastischen Chirurgie, ed. by E. Gohrbandt, J. Gabka, A. Berndorfer, Vol. 2, Lfg. 11. de Gruyter, Berlin 1968

Neuner, O.: Operationen bei posttraumatischen Unterkiefer-Asymmetrien. Fortschr. Kiefer-, Gesichtschir. 12: 232, 1967

Obwegeser, H.: Vorteile und Möglichkeiten des intraoralen Vorgehens bei der Korrektur von Unterkiefer-Anomalien. Fortschr. Kiefer- u. Gesichtschir. 7: 159, 1961

Obwegeser, H.: cited after Reichenbach, E., H. Köle, H. Brückl: Chirurgische Kieferorthopädie. Barth, Leipzig 1965, p. 7

Obwegeser, H.: Simultaneous resection and reconstruction of part of the mandible via the intraoral route. Oral Surg. 21: 693, 1966

Obwegeser, H.: in: Plastic Surgery in Infancy and Childhood, ed. by J. C. Mustardé. Livingstone, Edinburgh 1971, p. 54

Pichler, H.: Doppelte Unterkieferresektion in einem Fall von Progenie. Vjschr. Zahnheilk. 35: 1, 1919

Pichler, H., R. Trauner: Mund- und Kieferchirurgie. Urban & Schwarzenberg, Vienna 1948

Rehrmann, A.: Eine Methode zur operativen Beseitigung der doppelseitigen Ankylose der Kiefergelenke durch breite Knochenresektion, temporäre Implantation von Palavitkörpern und autogene Knochentransplantation. Fortschr. Kiefer-, Gesichtschir. 12: 64, 1967

Robinson, M.: Micrognathism corrected by vertical osteotomy of ascending ramus and iliac bone graft: a new technique. Oral Surg. 10: 1125, 1957

Rowe, N. L.: The etiology, clinical features and treatment of mandibular deformity. Br. Dent. J. 108: 45, 1960

Schmuziger, P.: Die funktionelle und ästhetische Indikation der Progenie-Operation bei Akromegalie. Fortschr. Kiefer- u. Geschichtschir. 7: 155, 1961

Schuchardt, K.: in: Bier-Braun-Kümmel (eds.): Chirurgische Operationslehre, Vol. II. Barth, Leipzig 1954

Schuchardt, K.: Formen des offenen Bisses und ihre operativen Behandlungsmöglichkeiten. Fortschr. Kiefer- u. Gesichtschir. 1: 222, 1955

Schuchardt, K.: Erfahrungen bei der Behandlung der Mikrogenie. Langenbecks Arch. Klin. Chir. 289: 651, 1958

Schuchardt, K.: Experiences with the surgical treatment of some deformities of the jaws: prognathia, micrognathia and open bite. In: Transactions of the International Society of Plastic Surgeons, ed. by A. B. Wallaće. Livingstone, Edinburgh 1960

Spiessl, B.: Das Plattenepithelcarcinom der Mundhöhle. Thieme, Stuttgart 1966

Spiessl, B.: Probleme der Wiederherstellung nach Tumoroperationen im Kiefer-Gesichtsbereich. Therapiewoche 23: 1917, 1972

Spiessl, B. et al.: Eine klinische Untersuchung zur Wertbestimmung der TNM-Klassifikation des Mundhöhlenkarzinoms. Dtsch. Zahnaerztl. Z. 28: 844, 1973

Tessier, P.: Ostéotomies totales de la face: syndrome de Crouzon; syndrome d'Apert, oxycéphalies, scaphocéphalies, turricéphalies. Ann. Chir. Plast. 12: 273, 1967

Tessier, P.: The definitive plastic surgical treatment of the severe facial deformities of craniofacial dysostosis. Plast. Reconstr. Surg. 48: 419, 1971

Thoma, K. H.: Deformities of the jaws. A comparison of two methods of treating apertognathia. Am. J. Orthodont. 31: 248, 1945

Thoma, K. H.: Oral Surgery. 3rd Edn., Mosby, St. Louis 1958

Thoma, K. H.: Oblique osteotomy of the mandibular ramus. Oral Surg. 14: Suppl. 1, 1961

Trauner, R.: Die retrocondyläre Implantation, eine Operationsmethode zum Vorbringen des Unterkiefers beim Distalbiß. Dtsch. Zahn-, Mund-, Kieferheilk. 20: 391, 1954

Trauner, R.: Operationen am Kiefergelenk. Dtsch. Zahn-, Mund-, Kieferheilk. 57: 327, 1971

Trauner, R.: Kiefer- und Gesichtschirurgie, Vol. II, 2nd edn. Urban & Schwarzenberg, Munich, 1973, p. 274

Trauner, R., H. Obwegeser: Zur Operationstechnik bei der Progenie. Dtsch. Zahn-, Mund- Kieferheilk. 23: 1, 1955/56

Trauner, R., H. Obwegeser: The surgical correction of mandibular prognathism and retrognathia with consideration of genioplasty. Oral Surg. 10: 677, 1957

UICC (Union Internationale Contre le Cancer): TNM-Classification of Malignant Tumors, 3rd edn. Geneva 1978

UICC/AJC (Union Internationale Contre le Cancer/American Joint Committee on Cancer Staging and End Results Reporting): Supplement to TNM-Classification of Malignant Tumours. Geneva 1973

Wassmund, M.: Lehrbuch der praktischen Chirurgie des Mundes und der Kiefer. Heusser, Leipzig 1935, p. 245

Wassmund, M.: Zur Chirurgie des Kiefergelenks. Suom. Hammastääk. Toim. 48: 95, 1952

Wunderer, S.: Die Prognathieoperation mittels frontal gestieltem Maxillafragment. Oesterr. Z. Stomatol. 59: 98, 1962

13 Surgery of Malignant Tumors of the Tongue and the Floor of the Mouth

By R. M. Rankow

The floor of the mouth and the oral part of the tongue (the anterior two-thirds) differ in morphology and pathology compared to the base of the tongue (posterior one-third). The vast majority of malignant tumors of the floor of the mouth and of the tongue are squamous carcinomas. These tumors usually behave in a similar fashion and can be regarded as homogeneous for the purpose of diagnosis and treatment. Approximately 70% of all tumors of the tongue are moderately to well differentiated squamous carcinomas. Most of these patients use tobacco or alcohol.

Malignant tumors of the floor of the mouth and of the oral part of the tongue larger than 2 cm in diameter or arising in an area of chronic mucosal irritation or leukoplakia which are very firm on palpation and appear to be penetrating the underlying muscles behave in a very malignant fashion and tend to metastasize early to the lymph nodes of the neck (Fig. 13.1a).

In contrast, tumors of the base of the tongue are histologically less well differentiated or anaplastic and usually found only when they have reached a considerable size. Often there are unilateral (70%) or even bilateral (15%) metastases in the upper cervical nodes. Such a metastasis is often the first symptom of the tumor (Fig. 13.1b). Tumors of the base of the tongue often involve the neighboring structures of the mesopharynx, i. e. the tonsil, the pharyngeal walls and the laryngeal inlet.

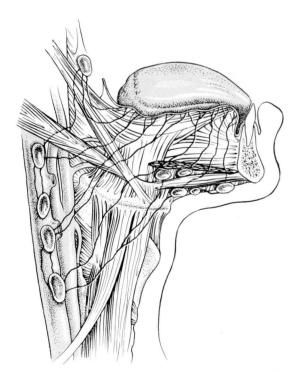

Fig. 13.1a Lymphatic drainage of the tongue and the floor of the mouth.

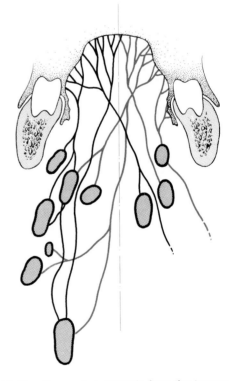

Fig. 13.1b Crossed metastasis from the tongue.

Tumors of the Floor of the Mouth and the Oral Part of the Tongue

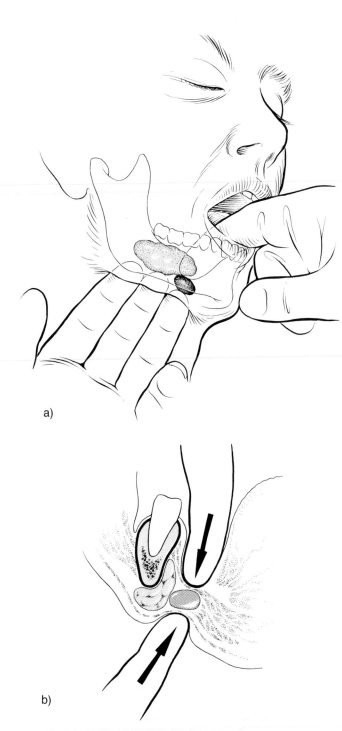

a)

b)

Fig. 13.2 a, b   Bimanual palpation of the floor of the mouth.

Partial Resection of the Tongue

Indications

Under certain circumstances small, noninvasive and superficial tumors of the tongue can be excised by a purely local procedure:

● The tumor must not be more than 2 cm in diameter.

● The tumor must be freely mobile and not fixed to underlying structures.

● No palpable lymph nodes should be present in the neck.

Diagnostic Preoperative Procedures

The diagnosis is confirmed by inspection, palpation and a punch or incisional biopsy from the suspected area taken under topical or infiltration anesthesia.

Palpation. The lymph glands of the medial and lateral triangles of the neck, the jugular chain and the submandibular and submental region must be palpated. The floor of the mouth is palpated bimanually with one finger inside and one finger of the other hand pressing the soft tissues of the submandibular and the submental region from outside. This allows suspect lymph nodes to be differentiated more easily from normal connective tissue structures (Fig. 13.2 a, b).

Biopsy. As described above, the neck should be examined before a biopsy is taken; suspicious lymph nodes should be documented. This allows an inflammatory lymphadenopathy appearing later as a result of the biopsy to be differentiated from an already existing lymph node enlargement. This is important in determining whether a simple partial excision of the tongue will suffice rather than an extensive resection of the tongue with simultaneous neck dissection.

Principles of the Operation

The tumor must be excised with a margin of at least 1.5 to 2 cm of macroscopically healthy tissue on each side of the specimen and in depth (Fig. 13.3).

Preparation for Surgery

Premedication is given on the evening before the operation and 1 hour before the operation.

The patient is placed on the operating table in such a **position** that the mandible runs horizontally (Fig. 13.4).

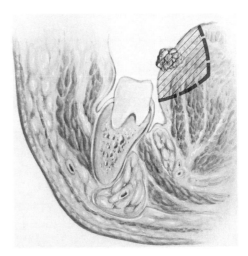

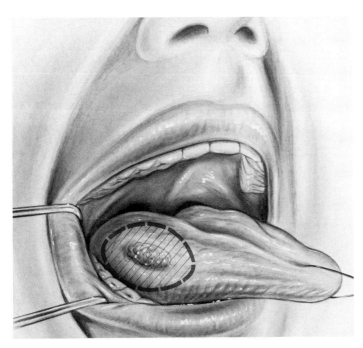

Fig. 13.3   Margins of excision in all three dimensions.

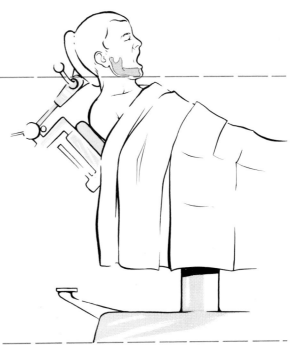

Fig. 13.4   Position of the patient.

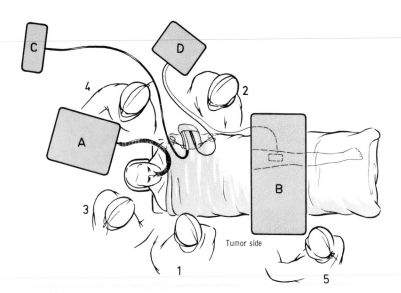

Fig. 13.5   Location of the operation team
1 = Surgeon
2 = First assistant
3 = Second assistant
4 = Anesthetist
5 = Scrub nurse
A = Anesthetic apparatus
B = Instrument table
C = Suction apparatus
D = Diathermy

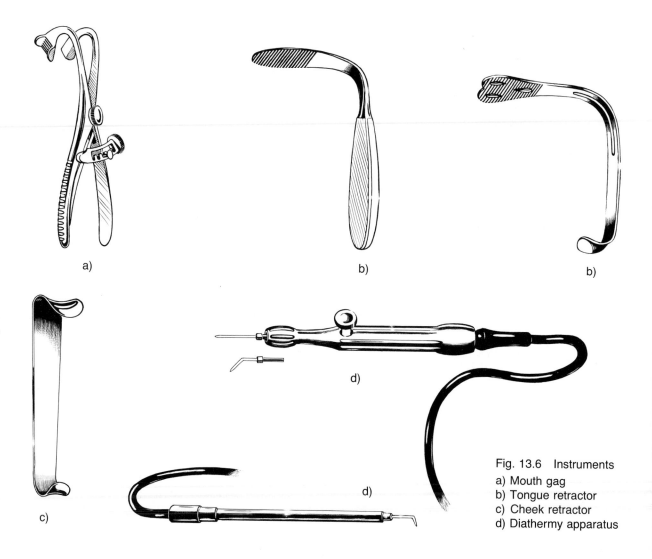

a)

b)

b)

c)

d)

d)

Fig. 13.6   Instruments
a) Mouth gag
b) Tongue retractor
c) Cheek retractor
d) Diathermy apparatus

Preparation of the operative area of the nose, lips, face and neck must ensure a sterile area around the mouth. It is not necessary to disinfect the oral cavity itself, but the usual sterile precautions must be taken to ensure that pathogenic microorganisms do not penetrate from outside into the oral cavity.

Location of the operative team. The anesthetist sits at the head of the operating table. Location of the operative team and important equipment can be seen in Figure 13.5.

Special Instruments

The following instruments are useful in addition to the general set:

● A mouth gag to hold the jaws apart (Fig. 13.6a).

● Tongue and cheek retractors (Figs. 13.6b, c).

● Several angled and straight cutting diathermy knives which facilitate hemostasis, particularly during resection of the tongue and the floor of the mouth (Fig. 13.6d).

Anesthesia

The choice of general or local anesthesia depends on the physical and psychological condition of the patient. If local anesthesia is preferred, a lingual nerve block is preferable to topical superficial or infiltration anesthesia. Blocking the lingual nerve anesthetizes half of the tongue and the floor of the mouth on the same side so that the surgeon may excise the tumor with a healthy margin without repeated injections and infiltration in the immediate neighborhood of the tumor (Figs. 13.7a, b).

If the operation is carried out under general anesthesia, *nasotracheal* intubation is preferred, but orotracheal intubation can be used.

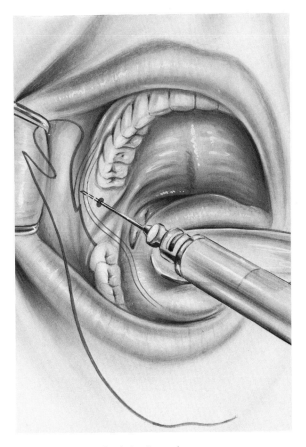

Fig. 13.7a   Block of the lingual nerve.

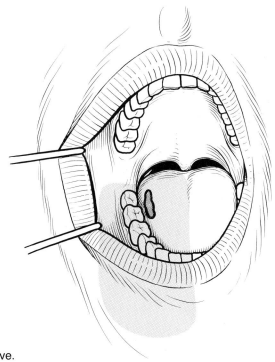

Fig. 13.7b   Area of anesthesia after blocking the lingual nerve.

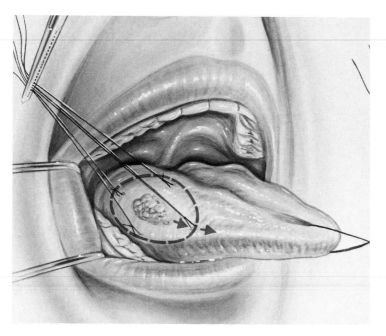

Fig. 13.8 a

Operative Technique

After introducing a mouth gag, a thick silk stay suture is passed through the tip of the tongue. Additional silk stay sutures are introduced on each side of the tumor, 1.5 to 2 cm from its edge. Excision is then carried out with cutting diathermy or with a scalpel immediately outside the sutures. The sutures act as landmarks and are used for traction. The operative specimen must be surrounded on all sides by macroscopically healthy tissue. The 4 stay sutures are left on the specimen and mark the anterior, posterior, medial and lateral edges of the excision for the pathologist (Figs. 13.8 a, b).

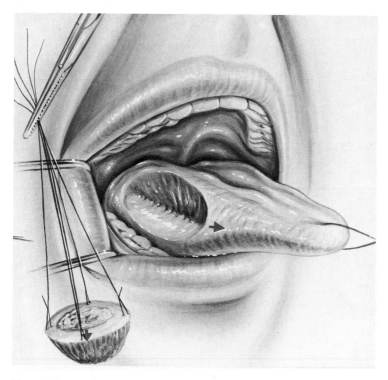

Fig. 13.8 b

Bleeding points are grasped with fine forceps and ligated or coagulated. The resulting defect is closed with alternate simple and mattress sutures of 3 × 0 chromic catgut or silk. A drain is not used (Fig. 13.9).

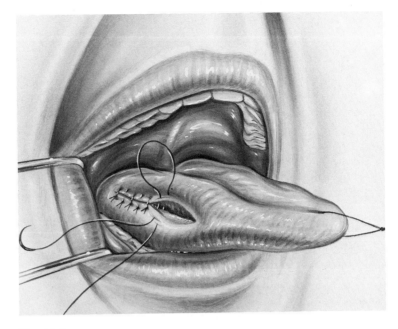

Fig. 13.9

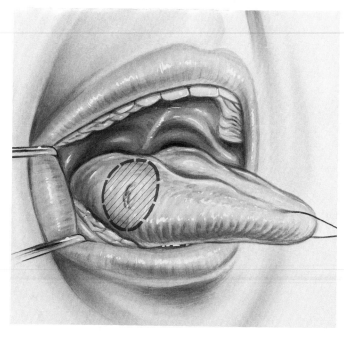

a)

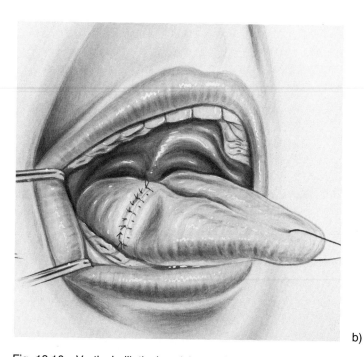

b)

Fig. 13.10   Vertical elliptical excision and closure.

Modifications and Surgical Alternatives

The lateral elliptical incision may occasionally be placed vertically if the position of the tumor requires it (Fig. 13.10).

A tumor of the tip of the tongue is dealt with by a wedged-shaped excision through all layers of the tongue (Fig. 13.11).

Rules, Hints and Typical Errors

If the surgeon is not certain whether all edges of the operative specimen are free of tumor in all dimensions, a frozen section should be done. Tissue can also be taken for this examination from the edges of the wound to ensure that the excision has been carried out through healthy tissue.

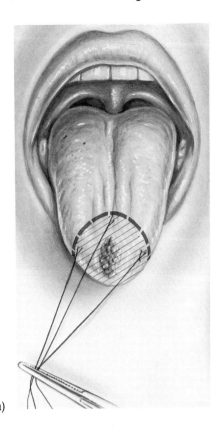

a)

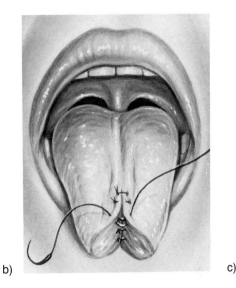

b)

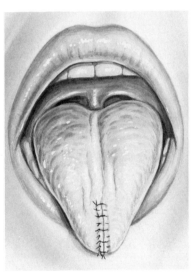

c)

Fig. 13.11   Excision of the tip of the tongue and closure.

Postoperative Care

● Antibiotic cover is usually not necessary.

● In the first 12 hours, pronounced edema of the tongue can occur, but this gradually subsides. A tracheotomy tray should be ready at the bedside, but it is seldom necessary.

● The patient should be in the half-sitting position and should be asked to breathe through his nose.

● A severe reactionary hemorrhage must be dealt with by reopening the wound. The bleeding point must be grasped with forceps. The muscles of the tongue are transfixed or the lingual artery is ligated.

Functional Sequelae

Partial resection of the tongue for tumors less than 2 cm in diameter has very satisfactory cosmetic and functional results.

Excision of the Floor of the Mouth with Simultaneous Marginal Mandibulectomy

Indications

Small superficial malignant tumors of the floor of the mouth located near the mandible can be excised by a local, limited resection including a part of the neighboring mandible.

● The tumor must not be fixed to or penetrating the periosteum of the neighboring mandible.

● The tumor must be freely mobile over the mylohyoid muscle.

● There must be no palpable lymph nodes in the neck.

Principles of the Operation

The edge of the operative specimen must include at least 1.5 to 2 cm of healthy soft tissue and a piece of the neighboring mandible with its lingual periosteum (Fig. 13.12).

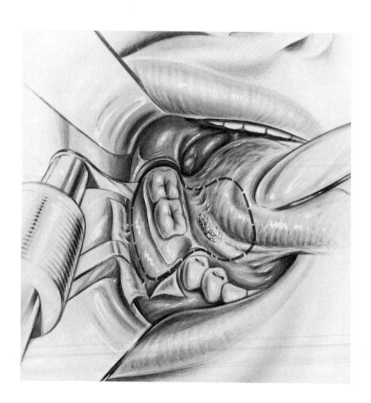

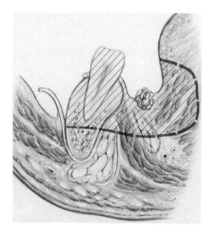

Fig. 13.12   Plan of the resection.

Preparation for Surgery

The immediate preoperative procedures are the same as those described above for partial resection of the tongue (see Fig. 13.5), but a donor site must also be prepared for taking a split skin graft (Fig. 13.13).

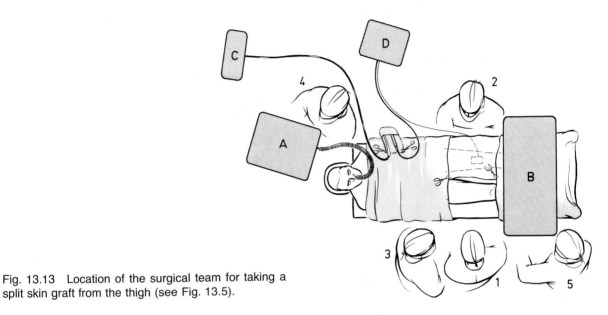

Fig. 13.13 Location of the surgical team for taking a split skin graft from the thigh (see Fig. 13.5).

Special Instruments

In addition to the general set, the following instruments are useful:

- A narrow periosteal elevator for the mucoperiosteum of the mandible (Fig. 13.14a).

- A Stryker electrical unit with a small bone saw for the marginal mandibulectomy (Fig. 13.14b).

- A thin, 10 mm osteotome for completing the marginal mandibulectomy after making the saw cuts (Fig. 13.14c).

- Dental elevators and forceps for extracting teeth from the lower jaw in the area of the planned marginal mandibulectomy (Fig. 13.14d).

- A dermatome, (e.g. Brown's electric dermatome) for removing a split skin graft (Fig. 13.14d).

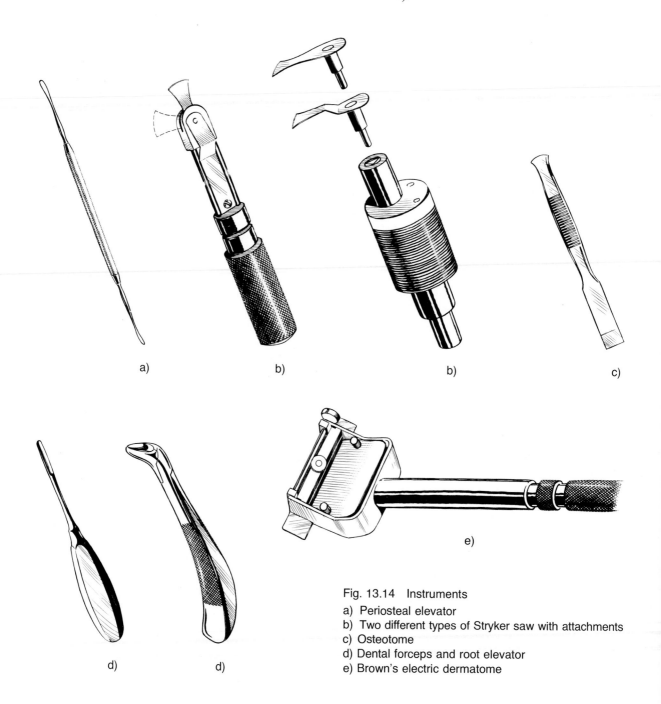

a)   b)   b)   c)

d)   d)

e)

Fig. 13.14   Instruments
a) Periosteal elevator
b) Two different types of Stryker saw with attachments
c) Osteotome
d) Dental forceps and root elevator
e) Brown's electric dermatome

Anesthesia

General anesthesia with nasotracheal intubation is preferable to a nerve block. 2 % lidocaine (Xylocaine) with epinephrine 1 : 100,000 can possibly be used in addition to an endotracheal anesthetic to block the dental and lingual nerves and to reduce bleeding. A prophylactic tracheostomy can be carried out either before or at the end of the operation. If the tracheostomy is done before the operation, it is carried out under local anesthesia. The endotracheal tube is introduced through the tracheostomy so that the operation itself is carried out under general anesthesia.

Operative Technique

Division of the lip in the midline is usually not necessary, but if access to the segment of the mandible containing the posterior molar teeth is too narrow, it may be required. A vertical mucoperiosteal flap is defined on the buccal surface of the mandible and is mobilized; the teeth in the area of the planned resection are extracted.

The mucoperiosteum is now divided by a transverse incision along the edge of the alveolus so that this incision joins the previous vertical incision (Fig. 13.15). The flap formed is turned back off the mandible (Fig. 13.16a).

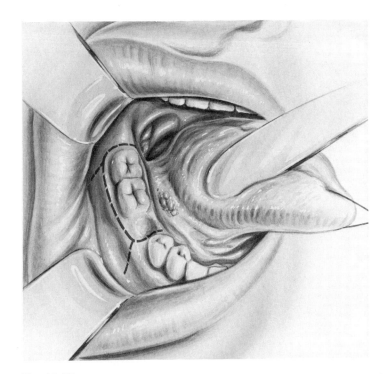

Fig. 13.15a

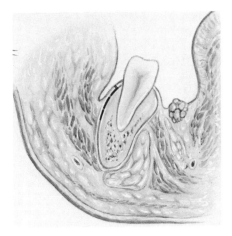

Fig. 13.15b

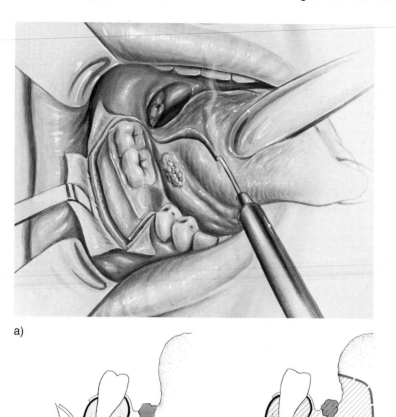

a)

A strip of bone of suitable width is now divided from the mandible in the neighborhood of the tumor with the Stryker saw. It is then carefully turned upward with a thin osteotome and finally divided from the remaining bone (Figs. 13.16a, b). During this part of the procedure, it must be ensured that the lingual mucoperiosteum of the mandible is not divided but remains intact on the specimen (Fig. 13.16b). The lateral edge of the tongue and the posterior and anterior part of the floor of the mouth are now divided by cutting diathermy or a scalpel; the incision must always be at least 1.5 to 2 cm from the edge of the tumor and within healthy tissue, superficially and also in depth. Excision proceeds down as far as the mylohyoid muscle (Figs. 13.16a; 13.17).

After removing the operative specimen, the buccal mucoperiosteal flap is sutured to the alveolar mucosa and to the edges of the incision in the floor of the mouth or the tongue (Figs. 13.18a, b).

b)

Fig. 13.16

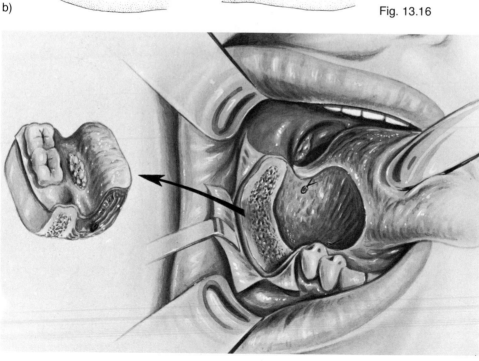

Fig. 13.17

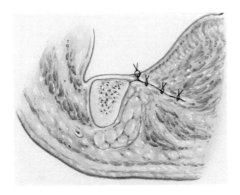

Fig. 13.18a

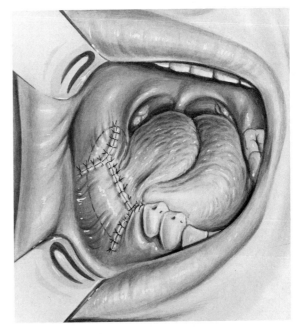

Fig. 13.18b

Modifications and Surgical Alternatives

The defect of the floor of the mouth can also be covered with a 0.4 mm thick split-skin graft from the thigh (Fig. 13.19); the 3×0 silk sutures are left long and are knotted over a gauze pad for compression and fixation of the graft (Figs. 13.20, 13.21).

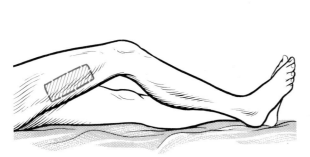

Fig. 13.19   Donor site of split skin graft.

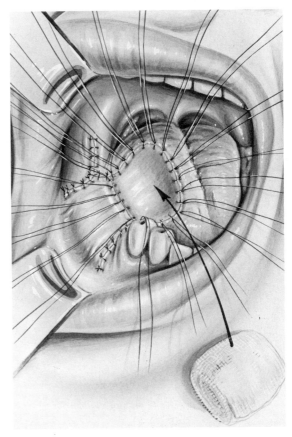

Fig. 13.20   Split skin graft sewn in the defect with sutures left long.

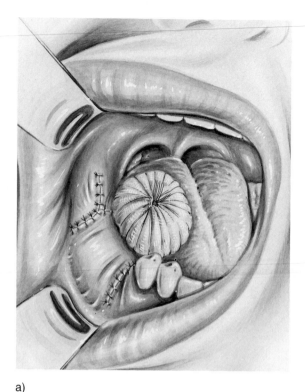

a)

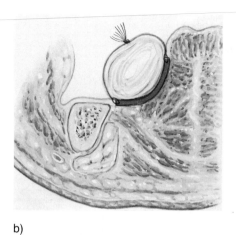

b)

Fig. 13.21 a, b   Split skin graft fixed with stay sutures knotted over a gauze pad.

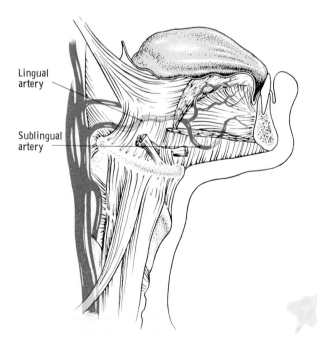

Lingual
artery

Sublingual
artery

Fig. 13.22   Course of the lingual artery.

Danger Points

Potential sources of hemorrhage: The lingual artery and its branches are the principal sources of excessive intraoperative and postoperative bleeding. The artery lies behind the greater horn of the hyoid bone after its point of origin from the external carotid artery. From here it runs behind the hyoglossus muscle and, at the anterior border of this muscle, reappears to enter the body of the tongue where it ends as the deep artery of the tongue. An important branch of this artery in the region of the floor of the mouth is the *sublingual artery*. It pierces the mylohyoid muscle to supply the sublingual gland (Fig. 13.22). This artery is a common site of bleeding after resection of the floor of the mouth, and therefore should be sought during the operation and ligated.

Rules, Hints and Typical Errors

● *Extraction of teeth* should be restricted to the area of resection. Teeth in the immediate neighborhood of the tumor must not be removed since malignant cells can then implant in the alveolar socket. In cases of doubt, it is better not to extract the tooth before the operation. The electric saw may divide the roots of the teeth, but these roots remain in the block of bone so that implantation of malignant cells cannot occur. After the specimen has been removed, the remaining parts of the roots can be easily removed with a suitable root elevator.

● The *external orifice of the submandibular gland* is often divided. The proximal end of the duct should then be identified and fixed in the corner of the wound to ensure drainage of the saliva. This prevents postoperative swelling of the submandibular gland caused by damage to the duct.

● A *nasogastric tube* can be introduced through the nose, either during the operation or on the following day, to permit feeding without disturbing the healing wound.

● An *atrophic edentulous mandible* must not be fractured because of excessive resection of bone. If a large amount of bone must be removed, the saw cut is beveled from above and outward to below and inward in the direction of the mylohyoid muscle in order to preserve as

much bone is possible without compromising the excision (Fig. 13.23). If the mandible fractures despite this, the fracture must be fixed by intraosseous fixation with stainless steel wire introduced through burr holes. The nasogastric feeding is then continued for a longer period of time and is later replaced by a fluid diet to put the fracture at rest until the bone has healed.

Functional Sequelae

Excision of the floor of the mouth with a marginal mandibulectomy for a small carcinoma of the floor of the mouth situated near the mandible is an effective operative treatment. Disturbances of movement and function of the tongue can be corrected by a split-skin graft. If the tongue is stitched to the alveolar mucosa in this operation, its function can be restored by a second operation 3 or 4 months later when a split-skin graft is introduced.

Postoperative Care

● Antibiotic cover is essential.

● The tracheotomy can be plugged and then removed as soon as the edema of the tongue settles and the upper airway is secure.

● The gauze pad sewn over the split-skin graft is removed between the sixth and seventh day after operation.

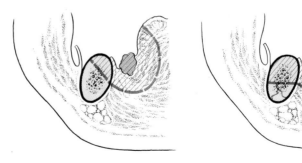

Fig. 13.23   Direction of the incision for an atrophic mandible
a) oblique incision (recommended),
b) horizontal incision (dangerous)

a)   b)

Combined Operation

(Composite Operation, Block Resection)

Indications

A carcinoma of the floor of the mouth or of the tongue which is no longer moveable over the mandible or underlying soft tissues or which has penetrated these tissues is excised by an en bloc resection of the primary tumor together with the neighboring structures of the mouth, the neighboring part of the mandible and the regional lymph nodes. This composite resection must be radical enough at the first operation since further operations for local recurrence are rarely successful.

A lymph node metastasis in the neck is present in 60 % of these tumors. They have the highest frequency of lymph node metastases of all carcinomas of the mouth. The operation must begin in the upper part of the neck so that the lymph vessels are inevitably divided by an adequate resection of the primary tumor. For this reason it is logical and necessary that a neck dissection always be carried out with this operation.

Principle of the Operation

The anatomical situation of the primary tumor and the incision for en bloc excision including a segment of the mandible in continuity with a neck dissection are illustrated in Figures 13.24 and 13.25.

A homolateral neck dissection is first carried out leaving the specimen attached to the nonexcised tissue of the submandibular space. Next, the mandibular segment to be resected is divided anteriorly and posteriorly, the primary tumor is resected with a wide margin. The anterior and posterior limits of the segmental resection of the mandible are determined by the position of the tumor.

A clearance of 1.5 to 2 cm around the border of the tumor must always be maintained. Finally, the deep muscles of the tongue are divided from their insertion on the hyoid bone so that the entire specimen can be removed in one block.

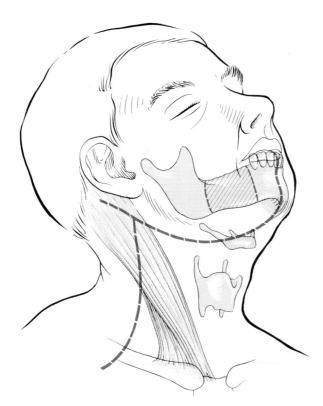

Fig. 13.24   Incision for composite resection.

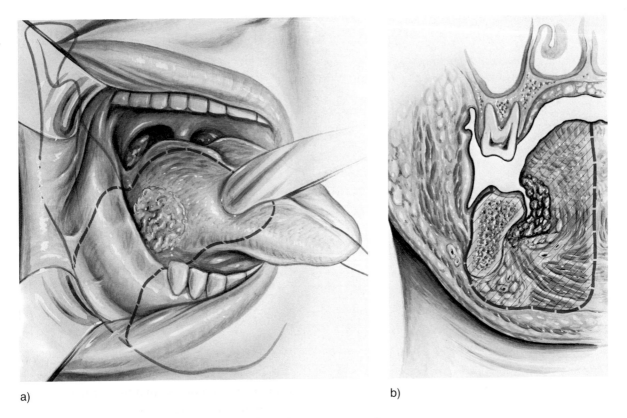

a)   b)

Fig. 13.25   a) Area of resection.   b) Resection scheme, cross section.

Preparation for Surgery

Premedication is given on the evening before and shortly before the operation. The position of the patient on the operating table is the usual one for a neck dissection (Fig. 13.26); good access to the face must also be provided.

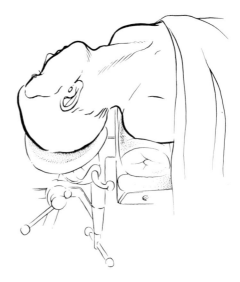

Fig. 13.26   Position of the head and neck.

The location of the surgical team is shown in Figure 13.27.

The eyes are protected with a suitable eye ointment and the eyelids are closed with adhesive tape.

A nasogastric tube for postoperative feeding should be introduced and fixed.

The forehead and the chest must be included in the usual skin preparation if reconstruction by pedicled flaps is anticipated. A thigh should also be prepared for taking a split-skin graft (Fig. 13.27).

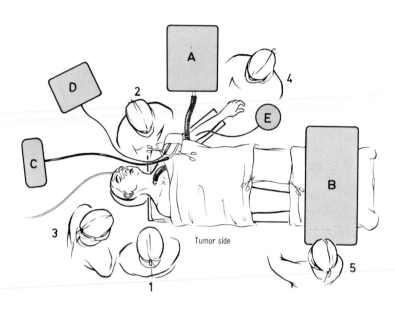

Fig. 13.27   Location of the surgical team (see Fig. 13.5).

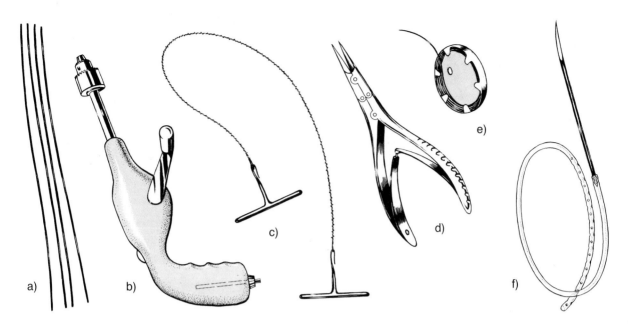

Fig. 13.28 Instruments
a) Kirschner wire   d) Double action bone shears
b) Hand drill   e) Stainless steel wire
c) Gigli saw   f) Tube and needle for introduction of suction drainage

Special Instruments

In addition to the instruments necessary for a neck dissection and a marginal mandibulectomy, the following instruments are also useful:

● Kirschner wires (Fig. 13.28a) and a hand drill (Fig. 13.28b).

● Gigli saw (Fig. 13.28c).

● Simple and double action shears (Fig. 13.28d). Stainless steel wire, 0.4 mm thick. Wire for intermaxillary fixation in case it should be necessary (Fig. 13.28e).

● Suction drain (Figure 13.28f).

Anesthesia

A tracheostomy is done under local anesthesia before the operation, and the tube is introduced through the tracheostomy for general endotracheal anesthesia.

Blood loss during the composite operation is about 1,500 to 2,000 ml. This amount can be reduced by artificial hypotension. The blood loss for neck dissection is about 500 ml, but increases significantly as soon as the resection is extended to the deep muscles of the tongue. The surgeon should warn the anesthetist of this before or during the operation.

Operative Technique

The incision for splitting the lip in the midline is a continuation of the transverse limb of the trifurcate incision used for the neck dissection. The transverse limb of the incision runs from the mastoid process over the hyoid bone to the centre of the chin. The vertical limb of the trifurcate incision extends from a point on the transverse incision along the lateral border of the sternocleidomastoid muscle down to the clavicle (see. Fig. 13.24). The platysma is maintained on the skin flaps if the lymph nodes have not been invaded.

Vertical flaps are elevated anteriorly and posteriorly from the underlying tissue, thus defining the borders of the neck dissection.

Later in the neck dissection, the lingual artery and the facial artery should be ligated to reduce bleeding during resection within the mouth. Ligation and division of the internal jugular vein at the base of the skull is carried out before the operation in the mouth (Fig. 13.29).

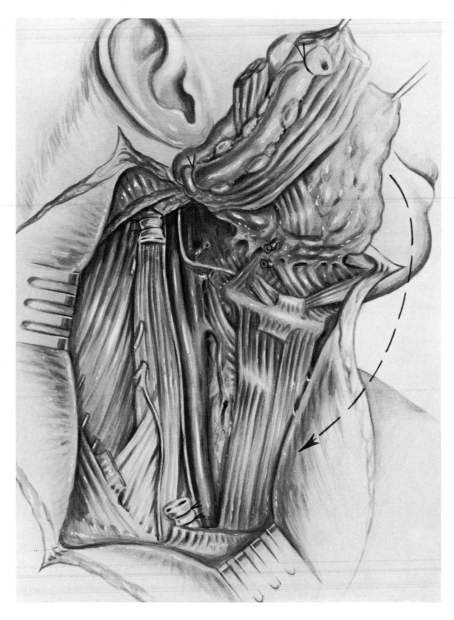

Fig. 13.29

The lip is now split in the midline and the superior flap is developed laterally so that the platysma and the bucco-gingival mucoperiosteum are included in the flap (Fig. 13.30). This is achieved by elevating the buccogingival mucoperiosteum with a periosteal elevator to expose the buccal surface of the mandible. After division and ligature of the mental artery and vein, the chin flap is mobilized as far as the anterior border of the masseter muscle (Fig. 13.31).

The facial artery and vein are ligated and divided inferior to the buccal branch of the facial nerve which is preserved if it does not run in the immediate nieghborhood of suspect prevascular lymph nodes (Fig. 13.32).

The neck dissection is now finished and the specimen is divided from the inferior edge of the anterior part of the mandible and from the mastoid process. The portion situated directly inferior to the primary tumor and to the surrounding healthy tissue to be excised with it is left attached.

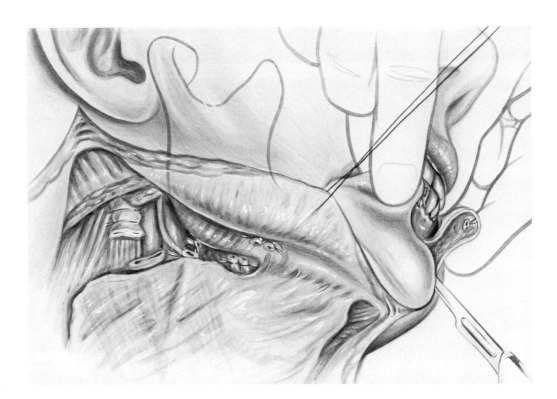

Fig. 13.30

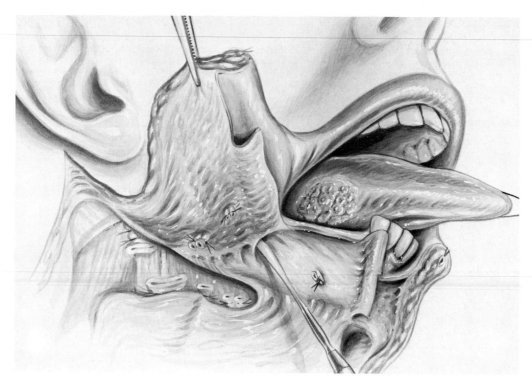

Fig. 13.31

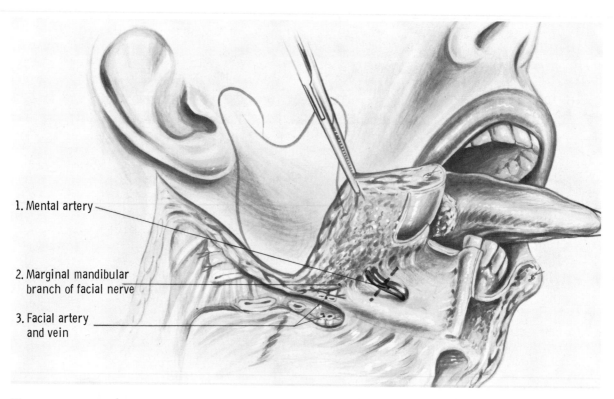

1. Mental artery

2. Marginal mandibular branch of facial nerve

3. Facial artery and vein

Fig. 13.32

The *anterior resection border* of the mandibular segment for lateral tumors of the floor of the mouth and the tongue usually coincides with the anterior border of the submandibular space. The buccogingival periosteum is divided perpendicularly along the anterior edge of resection of the mandible and is turned anteriorly in a mucope-riosteal flap to expose the buccal surface of the mandible. If a tooth is present in the anterior resection line, it is removed. A Gigli saw is introduced around the lingual surface of the mandible and used to complete the anterior division of the mandibular segment (Fig. 13.33).

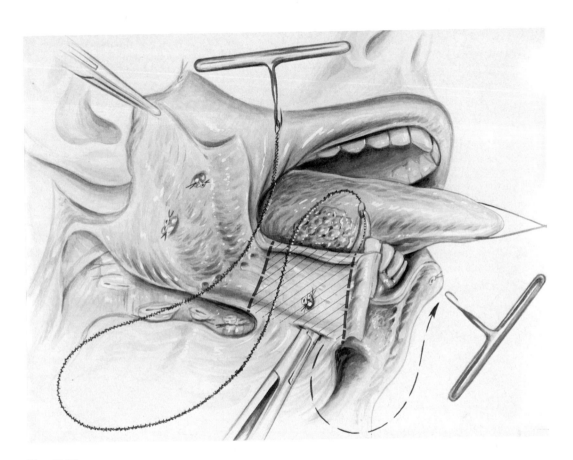

Fig. 13.33

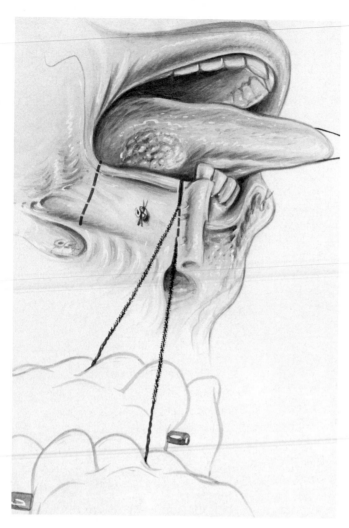

The *posterior limit* of the mandibular segment to be removed is also determined by the position and extent of the primary tumor (Fig. 13.34).

After dividing the bony segment at its anterior and posterior borders, strong stay sutures are introduced through the tongue, 2 cm from the visible border of the tumor. A hemiglossectomy or partial glossectomy is carried out with cutting diathermy. During the excision sparing the lingual or hypoglossal nerves should not be considered. Excision now proceeds as far as the insertion of the musculature to the superior edge of the hyoid bone (Fig. 13.35).

The mylohyoid, digastric, stylohyoid, hyoglossus and genioglossus muscles are then divided (Fig. 13.36).

The specimen can now be removed en bloc (Fig. 13.37) and final hemostasis can be secured (Fig. 13.38).

Fig. 13.34

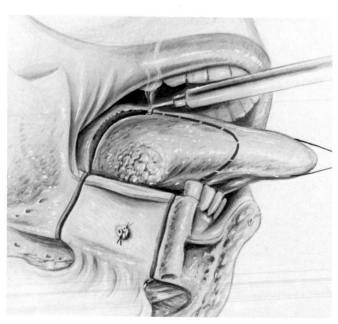

Fig. 13.35

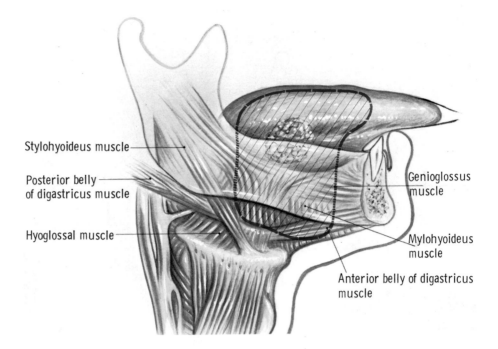

Stylohyoideus muscle

Posterior belly
of digastricus muscle

Hyoglossal muscle

Genioglossus
muscle

Mylohyoideus
muscle

Anterior belly of digastricus
muscle

Fig. 13.36

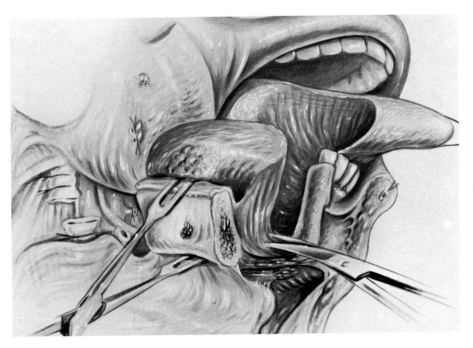

Fig. 13.37

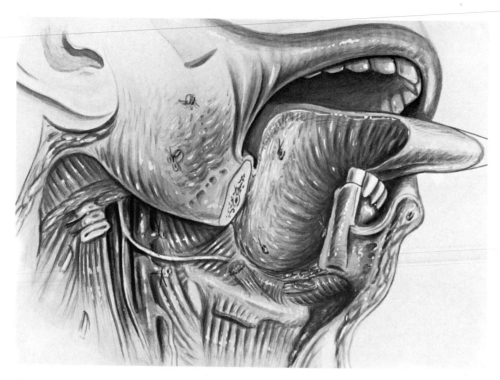

Fig. 13.38

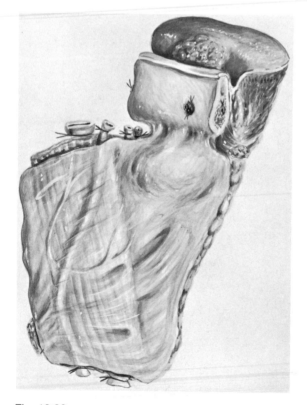

Fig. 13.39

Reconstruction

If the removed mandibular segment lies within the body of the mandible (Fig. 13.39), a 1.5 mm thick Kirschner wire is introduced into the bony stumps to hold the fragments in correct alignment and thus the occlusal surfaces of the teeth in the correct position (Figs. 13.40; 13.41 a, b).

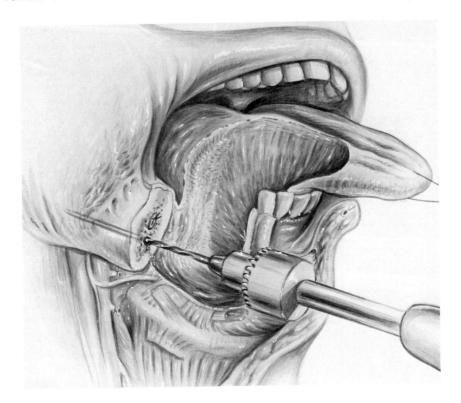

Fig. 13.40

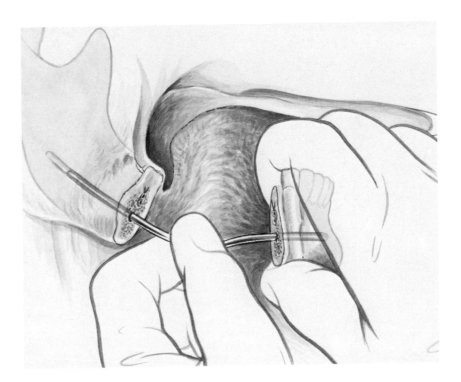

Fig. 13.41 a

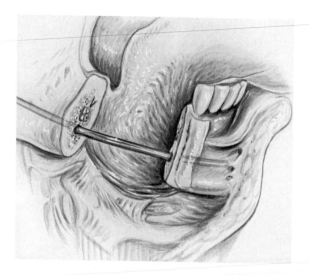

Closure of the wound in the oral cavity then begins at the posterior end of the wound. The wound is closed in layers over the exposed stumps of the bone and the intervening Kirschner wire (Figs. 13.42; 13.43).

Fig. 13.41 b

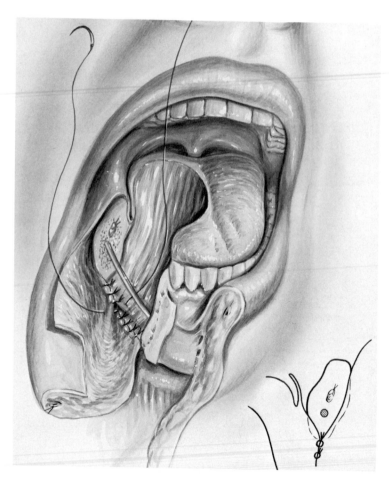

Fig. 13.42

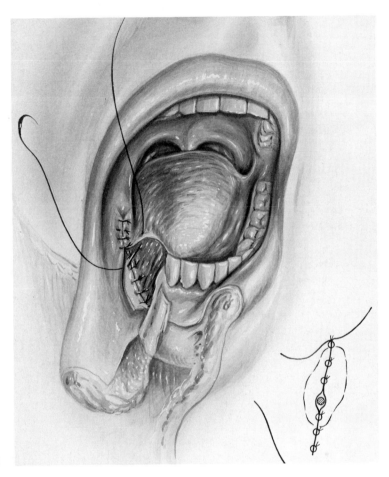

Fig. 13.43

Composite Resection with Hemimandibulectomy

If the carcinoma extends into the *base of the tongue* or infiltrates into the *tonsil* and the *lateral wall of the pharynx*, the entire affected area together with the medial pterygoid muscle must be removed in one piece (Fig. 13.44).

Resection of the bone is then carried out further posteriorly and, for adequate treatment, demands a subcondylar resection or a hemimandibulectomy (Fig. 13.45).

Technique. The masseter muscle is divided from its insertion on the mandible (Fig. 13.46).

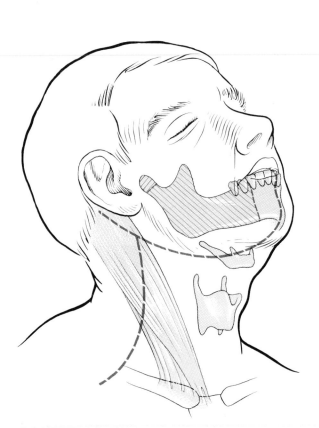

Fig. 13.44   Incision for a composite operation with hemimandibulectomy.

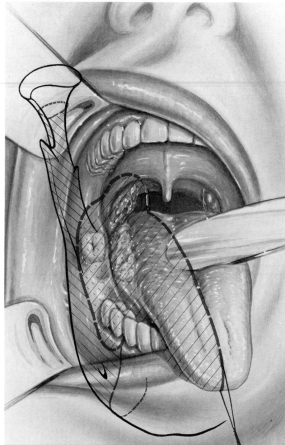

Fig. 13.45   Plan of the resection.

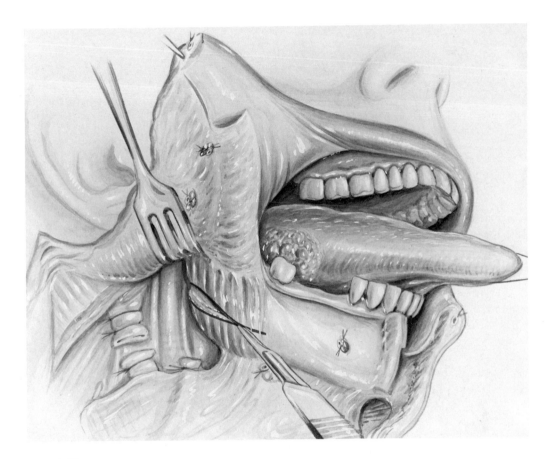

Fig. 13.46

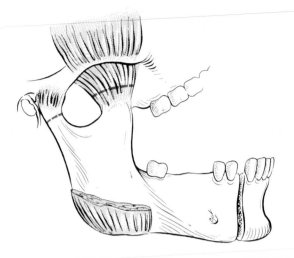

The temporalis muscle is divided from the coronoid process and the subcondylar resection is then carried out inferior to the temporomandibular joint with heavy bone shears (Figs. 13.47; 13.48).

Fig. 13.47

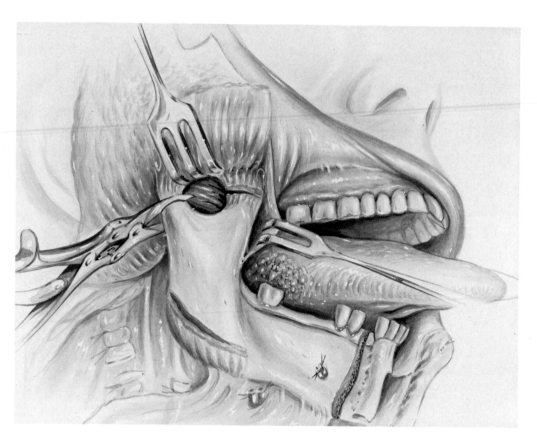

Fig. 13.48

If there is extensive infiltration of the tumor into the mandible, a complete hemimandibulectomy is preferred (Fig. 13.49).

The mandible is rotated externally and the mandibular neurovascular pedicle, the sphenomandibular ligament and the medial pterygoid muscle are divided (Figs. 13.50; 13.51).

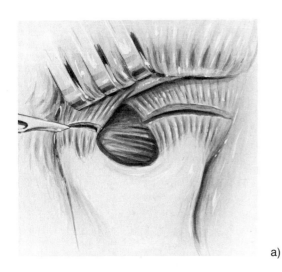

a)

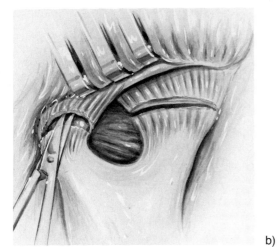

b)

Fig. 13.49

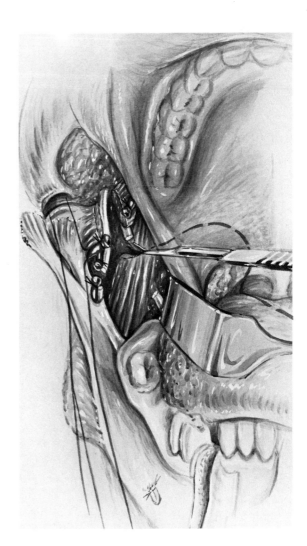

Fig. 13.50

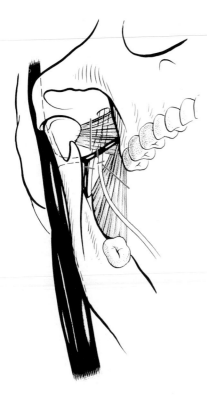

Fig. 13.51

A hemiglossectomy is then carried out with cutting diathermy (Fig. 13.52).

The major vessel in this area is IMA, it should be ligated.

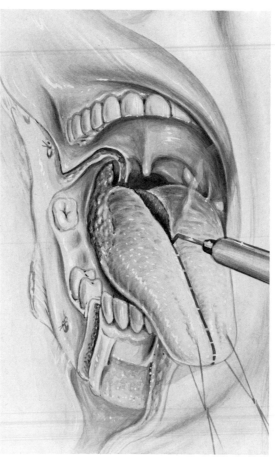

Fig. 13.52

The primary tumor, the resected half of the mandible and the neck dissection remain in one piece (Fig. 13.53). The stumps of the divided masseter and the medial pterygoid muscle are sutured to each other with 3×0 chromic catgut to prevent the formation of a space and to cover the stump of the condyle if this has been preserved (Fig. 13.54).

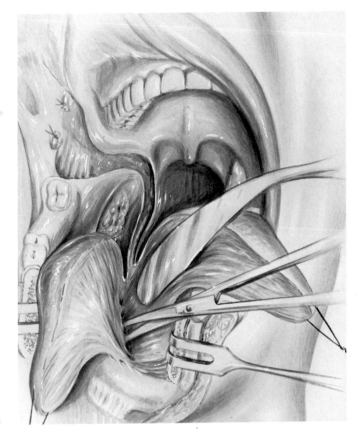

Fig. 13.53

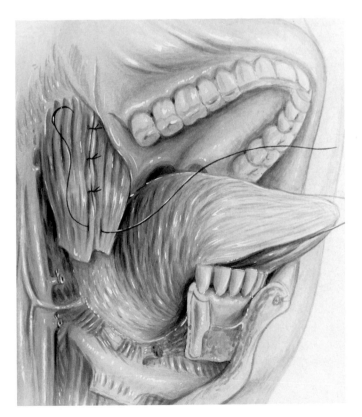

Fig. 13.54

The mucosa of the cheek, the palate and the pharynx are sutured. The base of the tongue is fixed to the lateral wall of the pharynx (Fig. 13.55); the tongue is carefully sutured in layers to the soft tissues and the mucosa of the cheek (Fig. 13.56).

An attempt must be made to achieve watertight closure of the mucosa with alternate interrupted and mattress sutures of 3 × 0 chromic catgut (Fig. 13.57). Next, a small functioning tip of the tongue must be formed (Fig. 13.58).

The lower lip is now closed on the oral side with catgut (Fig. 13.59). The vermilion and the skin of the chin are carefully adapted with fine silk or nylon sutures (Fig. 13.60), and the skin flaps of the neck are then sutured.

Before the lower lip is approximated, 1-2 cm is excised from the cheek flap. This tends to tighten the lower lip reconstruction and helps prevent drooling.

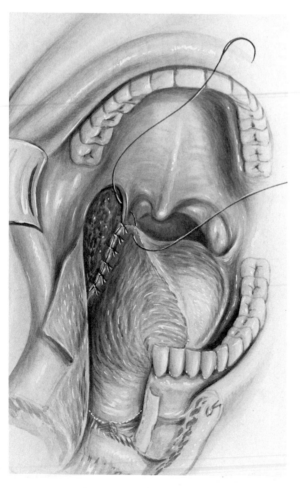

Fig. 13.55

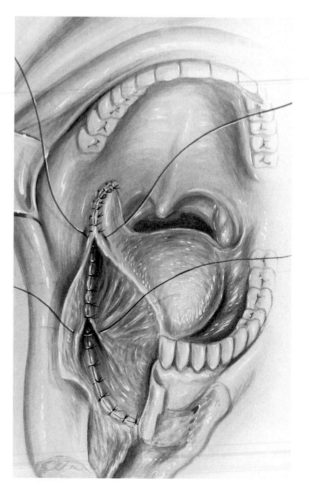

Fig. 13.56

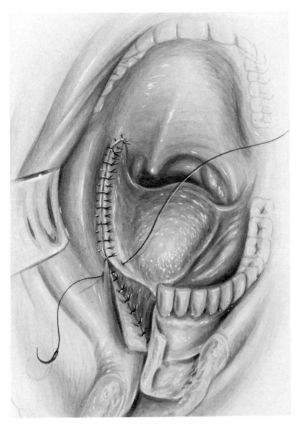

Fig. 13.57

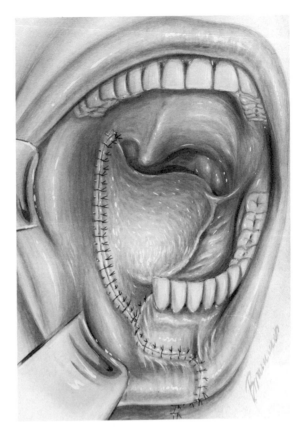

Fig. 13.58

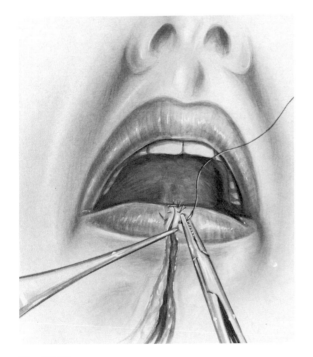

Fig. 13.59

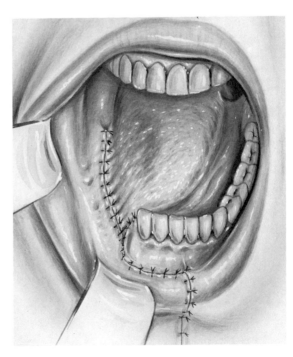

Fig. 13.60

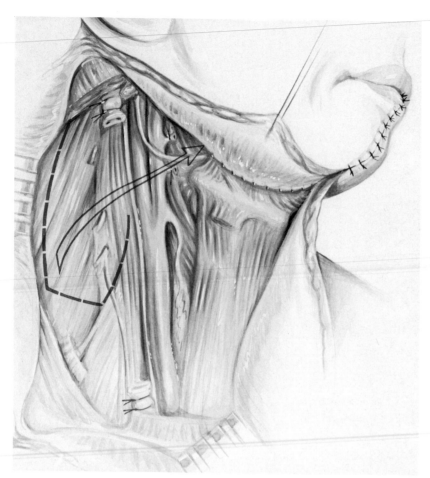

Fig. 13.61

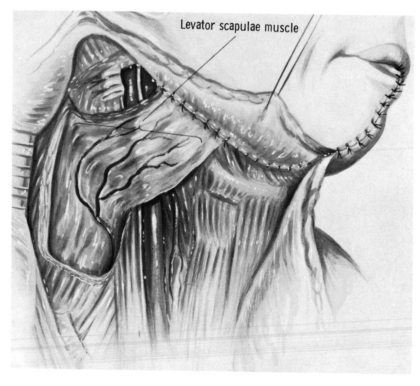

Levator scapulae muscle

Fig. 13.62

Protection of the Carotid System with a Levator Scapulae Muscle

If the carotid artery lies in a heavily irradiated area or may become exposed in the postoperative period as a result of an oropharyngeal fistula or a skin defect, it is advisable to cover it as early as possible. Protection by a levator scapulae muscle flap is particularly suitable (Fig. 13.61). The vessels supplying the muscle enter by the medial edge and must be preserved.

Technique. The inferior insertion of the muscle is exposed and divided. The posterior border is then exposed, rotated anteriorly 90° and fixed to the prevertebral fascia. The carotid sheath is thus effectively covered and protected (Fig. 13.62).

Closure after the composite resection. Suction drainage is used for the wound cavity. The soft tissues are closed with subcutaneous catgut sutures (4×0), and the skin is then closed with fine silk or nylon sutures. A light but secure circular neck dressing is then applied.

A nasogastric tube is introduced either at this time or 24 hours later. Finally, the endotracheal tube is replaced by a tracheostomy tube with an inflatable cuff (Figs. 13.63 a, b).

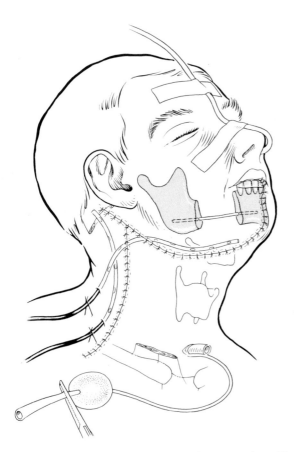

Fig. 13.63 a   Situation after a composite operation with partial mandibulectomy.

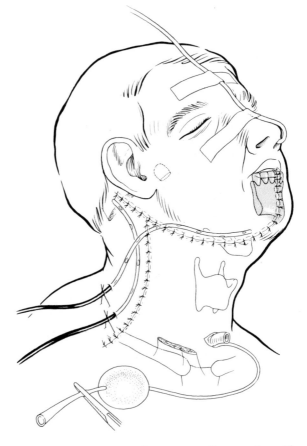

Fig. 13.63 b   Situation after a composite operation with total hemimandibulectomy.

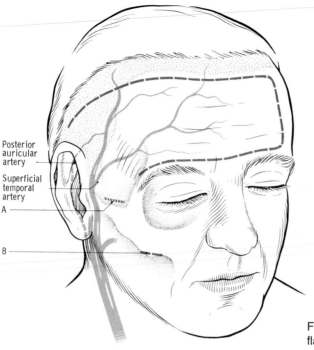

Posterior
auricular
artery

Superficial
temporal
artery

A

B

Immediate Plastic Reconstruction by a Temporal Flap

The surgical defect produced by the resection of a tumor of the tongue, the floor of the mouth and the mandible can be filled at the same sitting by a transposition flap from the forehead. Replacement of the soft tissues to the midline or beyond requires a large and complete forehead flap. The pedicle of such a flap includes not only the temporal but also the retroauricular vessels.

Fig. 13.64   Tunnels for the introduction of the forehead flap

A = Access to the mouth superior to the zygomatic arch
B = Access to the mouth through the cheek

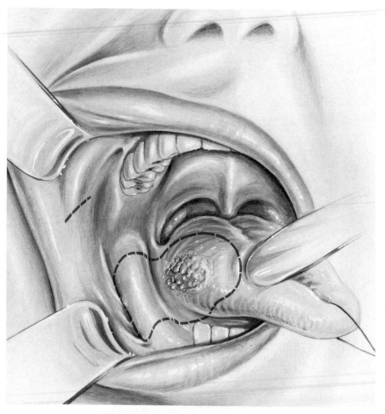

Fig. 13.65

Technique. The tunnel through which the pedicle is introduced into the oral cavity lies either over the zygoma or through the cheek (Fig. 13.64). The incision and the soft tissue defect are shown in Figures 13.64 and 13.65. A forehead flap consisting of the entire width of the forehead is esthetically and functionally preferred to a flap only half the width of the forehead. The external carotid artery should not be ligated during the neck dissection if mobilization of a forehead flap is intended. Otherwise the flap must be applied later. It is preferable to raise the forehead flap off the deep fascia. It contains the frontal belly of the occipital frontalis which provides the flap with a favorable consistency and versatility.

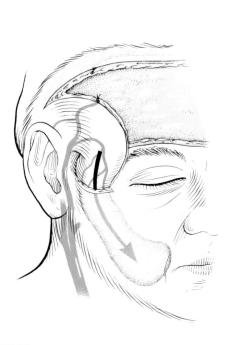

Fig. 13.66

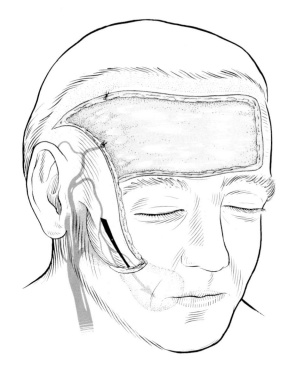

Fig. 13.67

The flap is introduced through a tunnel superficial to or behind the zygoma (Fig. 13.66) or
directly through the cheek into the oral cavity
(Fig. 13.67).

The skin surface lies superiorly to provide internal lining for the resected area (Fig. 13.68).
The tunnel is developed by blunt dissection to
avoid damaging the facial nerve.

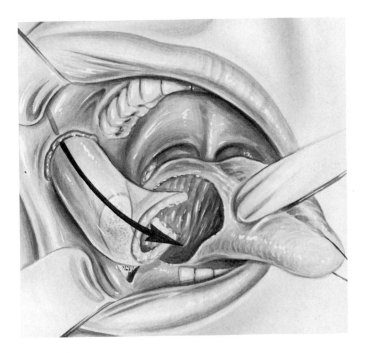

Fig. 13.68

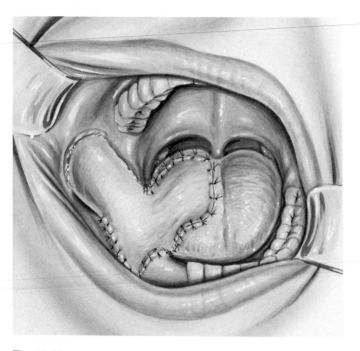

Closure of the wound is then easy, but the soft tissues must not be closed too tightly around the tunnel as this can compromise the blood supply to the flap (Fig. 13.69).

Any remaining soft tissue defect can be covered after the pedicle of the flap has been divided. A *bony mandibular graft should not be carried out at this time.*

A split-skin graft is introduced over the donor area of the forehead, stitched in place (Fig. 13.70a) and adapted by a gauze pad over which the silk sutures are knotted (Fig. 13.70b).

Fig. 13.69

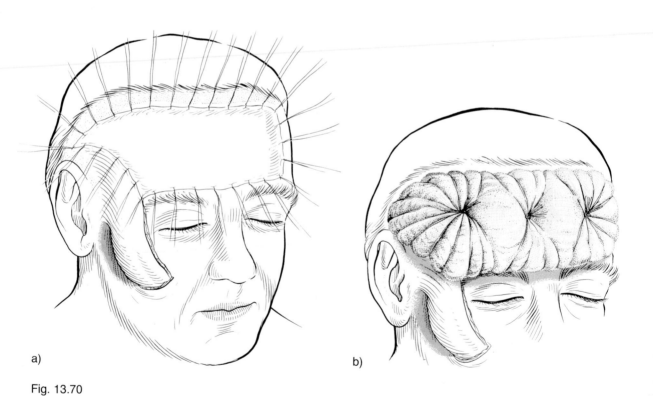

a)

b)

Fig. 13.70

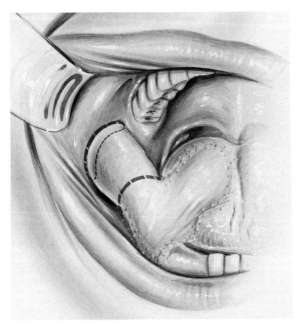

Fig. 13.71

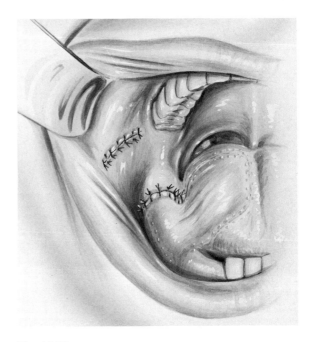

Fig. 13.72

After 3 weeks the pedicle is divided in the mouth through the soft tissues of the cheek at the level of the incision and is withdrawn from the tunnel (Fig. 13.71).

The external wound and the mucosal defect in the oral end of the tunnel are closed (Fig. 13.72).

The remaining part of the pedicle is returned to the forehead after excising the split-skin graft from the appropriate part of the forehead. The remaining part of the split-skin graft remains permanently in place; the skin incision is closed (Fig. 13.73).

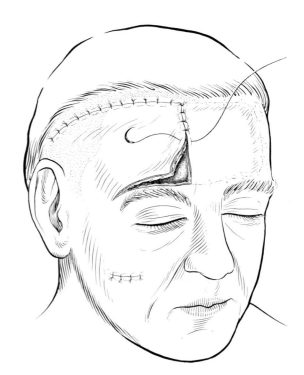

Fig. 13.73

Important Modifications and Surgical Alternatives

Different operative procedures have been described for dealing with carcinomas of the anterolateral part of the tongue and the floor of the mouth with simultaneous neck dissection but with preservation of the mandible, and for small carcinomas of the base of the tongue without neck dissection. Although there is little evidence that the lymph vessels of the tongue pass through the periosteum of the mandible, these operations should be considered with reservation. In most cases it is preferable to sacrifice the part of the mandible in the region of the tumor by a carefully planned en bloc dissection under good visual control. Such an operation prevents complications such as fistulae and delayed bone healing.

Alternate operations with preservation of the mandible are:

1. The *"pull-through" technique for resection* of a carcinoma of the anterolateral part of the tongue and the floor of the mouth;

2. *Median pharyngotomy* in which the *lower lip*, the *mandible* and the *tongue* are split in the midline, for the treatment of a carcinoma of the base of the tongue.

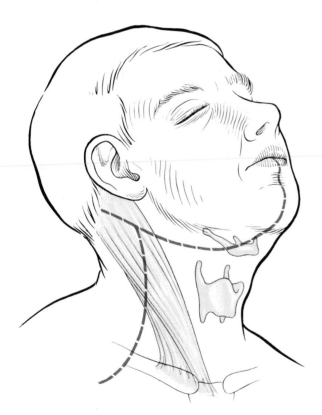

The **"pull-through" procedure** proceeds as for the composite resection as far as median splitting of the lower lip.

Technique. The labial mucoperiosteum is divided vertically (Figs. 13.74; 13.75) and is elevated 1 cm laterally on each side.

Fig. 13.74   Incision for the "pull-through" technique.

The mandible is divided with a Gigli or electric saw in the midline (Fig. 13.75), and an incision is then made along the medial edge of the alveolus in the linguoalveolar mucosa from the midline anteriorly back to the anterior faucial pillar (Fig. 13.76).

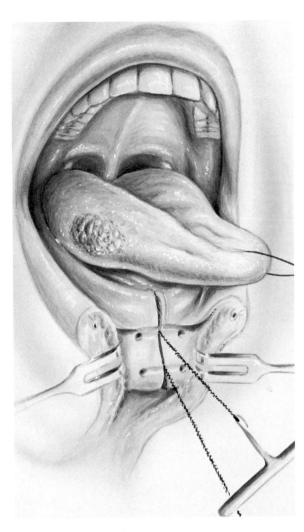

Fig. 13.75

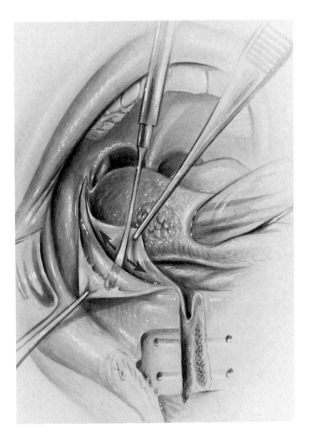

Fig. 13.76

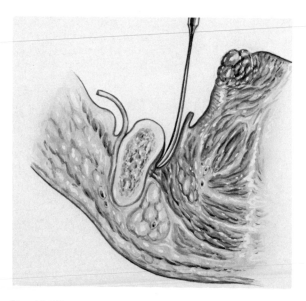

Fig. 13.77

The mucoperiosteum and the mylohyoid muscle are divided from the internal surface of the mandible (Fig. 13.77).

The ramus of the mandible is retracted laterally and the insertions of the genioglossus, the hyoglossus muscles and anterior belly of the digastric muscle are divided by sharp dissection from the mandible (Fig. 13.78).

The resection through the tongue proceeds in an antero-posterior direction approximately in the midline, but at least 2 cm from the edge, of the tumor (Fig. 13.79).

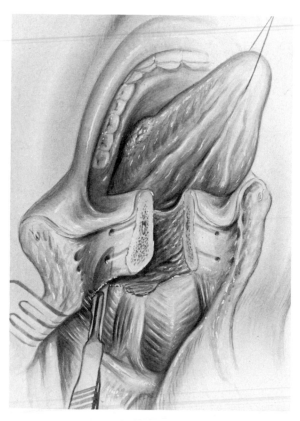

Fig. 13.78

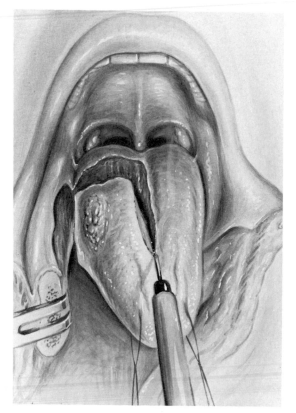

Fig. 13.79

This incision is carried as far posteriorly as the extent of the tumor demands (Fig. 13.80).

The insertion of the tongue muscles into the superior edge of the hyoid bone are exposed (Fig. 13.81) and freed (Fig. 13.82). Figure 13.83 shows the extent of the margin around the tumor in cross section.

The resection then concludes as for the composite resection with the removal of the contents of the neck dissection en bloc.

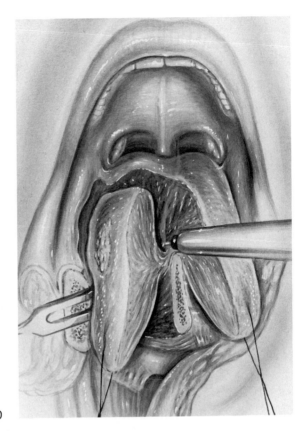

Fig. 13.80

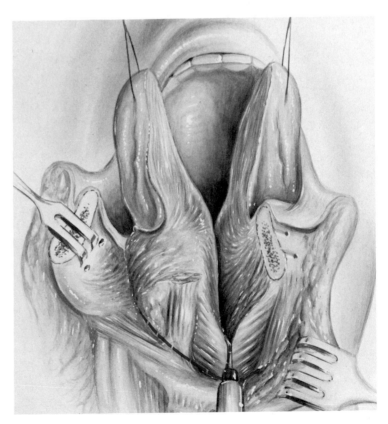

Fig. 13.81

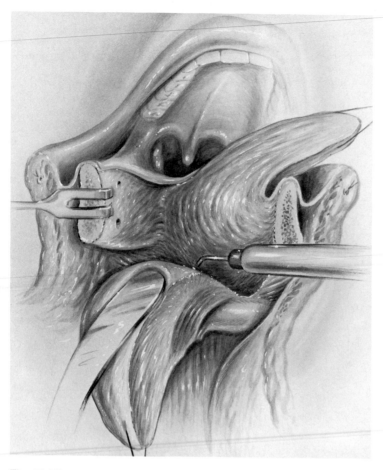

Fig. 13.82

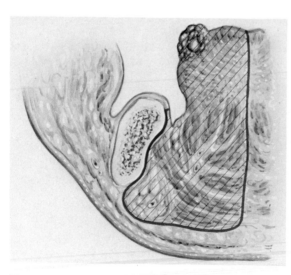

Fig. 13.83

The oral cavity is covered by uniting the mucosa of the dorsum of the tongue to the free edge of the mucoperichondrium of the edge of the alveolus (Fig. 13.84 a). Strong silk sutures are introduced around the mandible to support the fixation of the soft tissues of the tongue to the inner surface of the mandible (Fig. 13.84 b).

The mandible is united in its former anatomical position by 2 wire sutures introduced through burr holes (Fig. 13.85).

The lower lip and the soft tissues of the neck are now sutured as described for the composite procedure (Fig. 13.86). If the patient has teeth, the mandible should be splinted for 4 to 6 weeks.

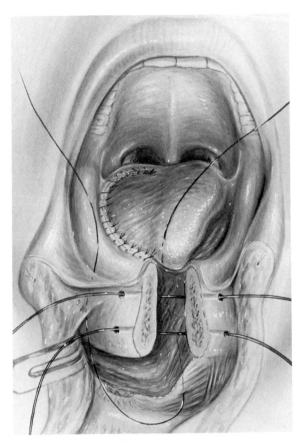

Fig. 13.84 a

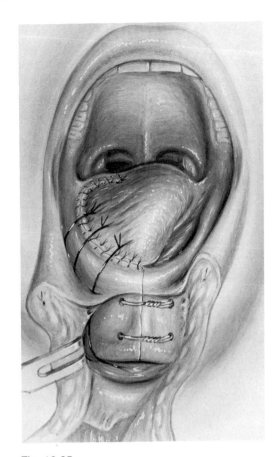

Fig. 13.85

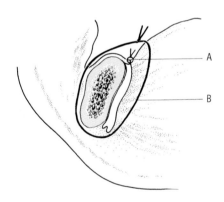

Fig. 13.84 b   Sutures for the closure

A = Suture between the labial mucosa and the muco-
     perichondrium
B = Retention suture around the mandible and through
     the soft tissues

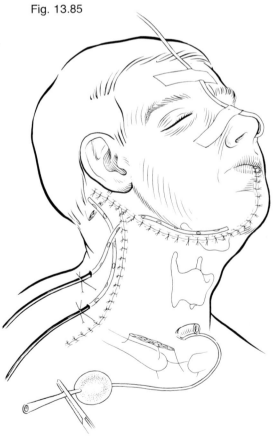

Fig. 13.86

The **procedure using a median split of the lower lip, mandible and tongue** is limited to excision of moderately malignant, noninfiltrating tumors of the central part of the tongue. Extensive or anaplastic carcinomas or epidermoid tumors with palpable cervical metastases should *not* be treated by this procedure.

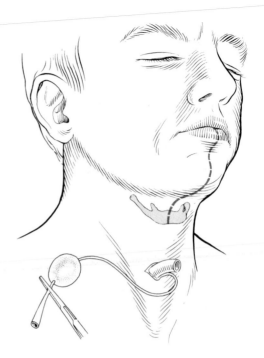

Fig. 13.87   Incision for splitting the lip, the mandible and the tongue.

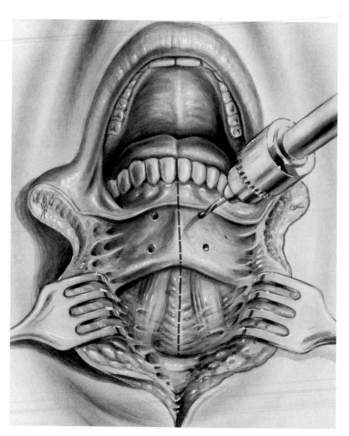

Technique. After a preliminary tracheostomy has been carried out, the lower lip is divided down to the level of the hyoid bone under general anesthesia (Fig. 13.87). The incision is carried down to the periosteum.

Burr holes are then made in the mandible on both sides of the symphysis (Fig. 13.88). The mandible is divided between the burr holes and the two halves are retracted. After dividing the mylohyoid and genioglossus muscles in the midline, the tongue is drawn anteriorly by stay sutures (Fig. 13.89).

Fig. 13.88

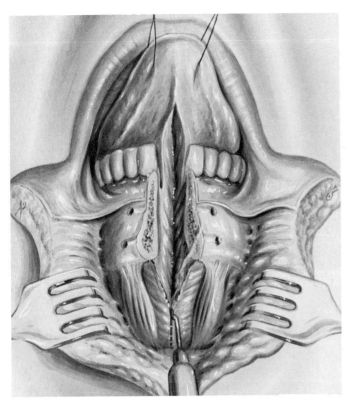

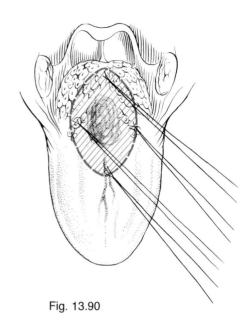

Fig. 13.90

Fig. 13.89

Stay sutures are introduced through
healthy lingual tissue about 1.5 to 2 cm
from the edge of the tumor (Fig. 13.90).
The tongue is divided through its avas-
cular central septum back to a point 2
cm anterior to the anterior edge of the
tumor; the incision is carried in depth
down to the floor of the mouth (Fig.
13.91).

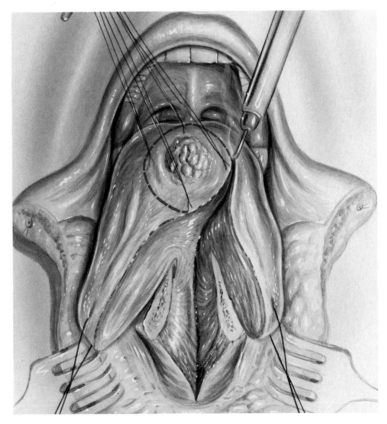

Fig. 13.91

The incision is then carried around the tumor along the stay sutures with cutting diathermy (Fig. 13.92). After removing the tumor en bloc, the halves of the tongue are reunited in layers from

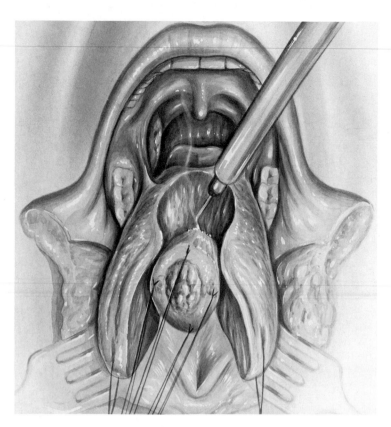

Fig. 13.92

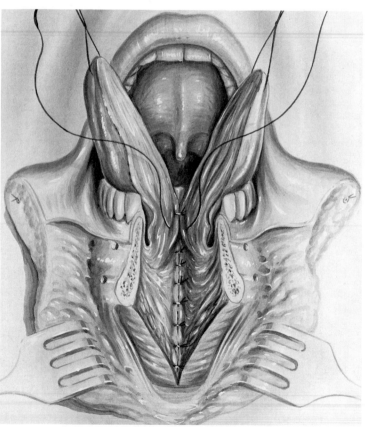

Fig. 13.93

behind forward with 3 × 0 catgut sutures
(Fig. 13.93), until the tip of the tongue
has been reunited (Fig. 13.94). The anterior part of the floor of the mouth is
sutured similarly (Fig. 13.95).

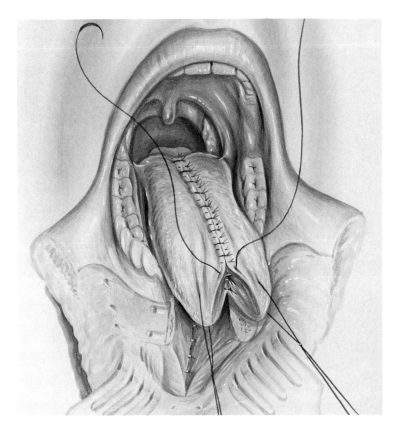

Fig. 13.94

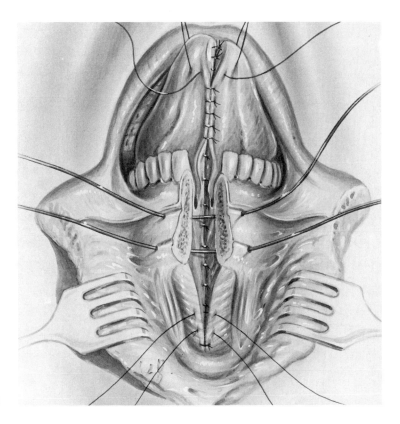

Fig. 13.95

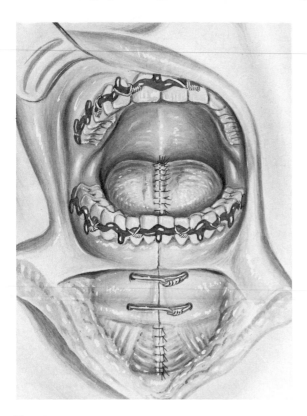

Fig. 13.96

Finally the mandible is reunited with steel wires. The mouths of the ducts of the submandibular glands are carefully preserved (Fig. 13.96).

If the patient has teeth, a dental splint is introduced to allow intermaxillary fixation with elastic bands for 4 to 6 weeks (Fig. 13.97). The lip and external skin are closed in the usual manner as described for the composite operation (see p. 336). Finally a nasogastric tube is introduced for 10 days so that the patient need nut be fed orally during the healing period (Fig. 13.98).

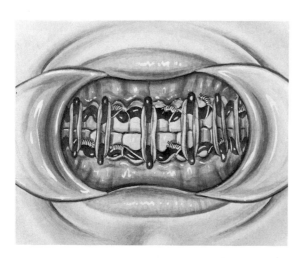

Fig. 13.97

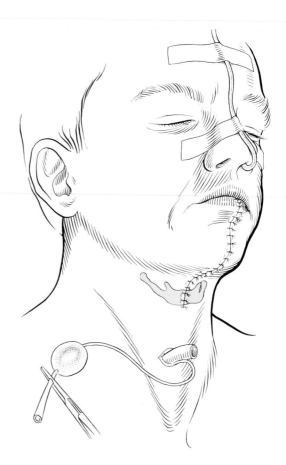

Fig. 13.98

Rules, Hints and Typical Errors

● The bone of the mandible is not, as a rule, preserved if the carcinoma has already extended to the periosteum.

● Immediate replacement of the resected mandible with bone grafts or plastic implants should not be attempted.

● The healing phase can be expedited and displacement of the mandibular stumps can be prevented by using intermaxillary fixation after a partial resection of the mandible.

● If for any reason during the resection of a tumor of the tongue or the floor of the mouth the lateral part of the neck must be opened, a radical neck dissection must always be carried out.

● In the presence of a carcinoma of the tongue or the floor of the mouth, any suspicious enlargement of a lymph node must be regarded as a metastasis and must always be removed together with the primary tumor by radical neck dissection.

Postoperative Care

● It is important to give antibiotics until the wound has healed on the seventh to tenth day.

● Suction drainage of the wound is necessary. The drain should be checked during the first 72 hours to eliminate the possibility of changes of position which could result in hematoma formation.

● The tracheostomy tube should be left in place longer than the feeding tube to prevent aspiration. It should be left in as long as the patient cannot swallow perfectly. This phase may be prolonged if part of the base of the tongue and the lateral wall of the pharynx were also resected.

Functional Sequelae

Swallowing and speech disturbances depend on the extent and localization of the tumor resection. The further the resection extends posteriorly, the more severe the difficulties.

The retained parts of the mandible function satisfactorily for several months if the fragments are united by a well-covered Kirschner wire until bone grafts (preferably of autogenous material) can be used to restore continuity of the mandible. The most favorable time for a bony graft is 3 to 4 months after the wound has healed.

Plastic reconstruction of the soft tissues can be carried out at the time of the excisional surgery by using pedicled flaps from the chest or the forehead or by a split-skin graft. In this way speaking and swallowing after the operation are often improved. Careful reconstruction of the mobility of the retained part of the tongue by pedicled soft tissue flaps and skin grafts can improve the functional results of surgery for carcinoma of the tongue and the floor of the mouth.

Resection of the Lateral Border of the Tongue

Indications

Considerable enlargement of the tongue (*macroglossia*) can occur due to a generalized, nonspecific, congenital *hypertrophy* of the lingual musculature. Occasionally macroglossia may be due to specific disorders such as a *hemangioma*, a *lymphangioma* (also combined in a *hemangiolymphangioma*) or a *neurofibroma*. The tongue then protrudes from the mouth and is visible when the patient speaks and eats; it is often injured during chewing (Fig. 13.99). This benign congenital or secondary enlargement of the tongue can be reduced surgically.

Principles of the Operation

The edges of the protruding tongue are symmetrically reduced until the tongue fits easily into the mouth (Fig. 13.100).

Preparation for Surgery

The preoperative preparation is the same as for a partial resection of the tongue (see p. 301).

Anesthesia

Endonasal intubation is generally preferred.

Operative Technique

The mouth is held open with a mouth gag or a lateral prop. The tongue is pulled forward over the teeth using a strong silk suture introduced through the tip of the tongue. The excess part of the tongue is then removed with cutting diathermy or a scalpel (Fig. 13.101).

Bleeding points are transfixed or ligated. The resulting defect is closed by uniting the mucosa of the dorsal and ventral surfaces of the tongue with interrupted and mattress sutures of 3×0 chromic catgut (Fig. 13.102). A drain is not necessary.

Rules, Hints and Typical Errors

- It is not necessary to remove all the excess tissue at one sitting. This is particularly true for children where sufficient space for the tongue may develop as the jaws grow.

- A nasogastric tube can be introduced during the operation or on the following day. The feeding tube permits feeding without disturbing the healing wound of the tongue.

- Postoperative care is the same as for partial tongue resection (see p. 308).

Functional Sequelae

Resection of the edges of the tongue yields good results for the treatment of benign, pronounced enlargement of the tongue.

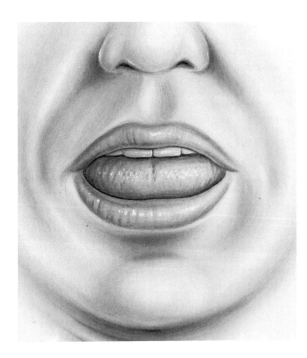

Fig. 13.99   Macroglossia.

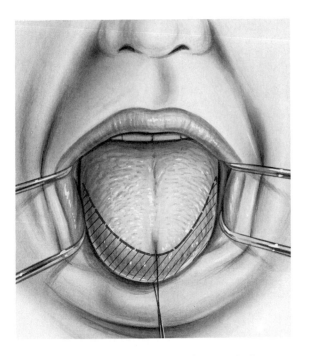

Fig. 13.100   Incision and area to be resected.

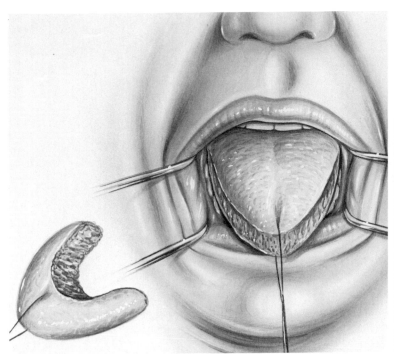

Fig. 13.101

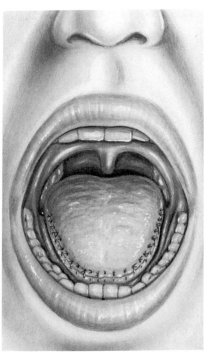

Fig. 13.102

Bibliography

Conley, J. J.: A technique of skin grafting to the tongue and case report. Plast. Reconstr. Surg. 5: 450, 1950

Harrold, C. C.: Surgical treatment of cancer of the base of the tongue. Am. J. Surg. 114: 493, 1967

Harrold, C. C.: Management of cancer of the floor of the mouth. Am. J. Surg. 122: 487, 1971

Helfrich, G. B., M. E. Nickels, A. El-Domeiri, T. K. Dasgupta: Management of cancer of the floor of the mouth. Am. J. Surg. 124: 559, 1972

Hoopes, J. E., M. T. Edgerton: Immediate forehead flap repair in resection for oropharyngeal cancer. Am. J. Surg. 112: 527, 1966

Kremen, A. J.: Cancer of the tongue – A surgical technique for a primary combined en block resection of tongue, floor of mouth, and cervical lymphatics. Surgery 30: 227, 1951

MacComb, W. S., G. H. Fletcher: Cancer of the Head and Neck. Williams & Wilkins, Baltimore 1967

Martin, H.: Surgery of Head and Neck Tumors. Hoeber-Harper, New York 1957

Martin, H., H. R. Tollefsen, F. P. Gerold: Median labiomandibular glossotomy. Am. J. Surg. 102: 753, 1961

McGregor, I. A.: The temporal flap in intra-oral cancer: its use in repairing the post-excisional defect. Br. J. Plast. Surg. 16: 318, 1963

Pack, G. T., I. M. Ariel: Tumors of the Head and Neck. Hoeber-Harper, New York 1959

Rankow, R. M.: Conservative local operations for cancer of the floor of mouth, alveolus and gingiva. In: Cancer of the Head and Neck, ed. by J. Conley. Butterworth, Washington 1967

Rankow, R. M.: Atlas of Surgery of the Face, Mouth and Neck. Saunders, Philadelphia 1968

Schobinger, R.: The use of a long anterior skin flap in radical neck resections. Ann. Surg. 146: 221, 1957

Slanetz, C. A., R. M. Rankow: The intraoral use of split thickness skin grafts in head and neck surgery. Am. J. Surg. 104: 721, 1962

Staley, C. A.: A muscle cover for the carotid artery after radical neck dissection. Am. J. Surg. 102: 815, 1961

Trotter, W.: Operation for malignant disease of the pharynx. Br. J. Surg. 16: 485, 1929

14 Surgery of the Oropharynx and of the Tonsils

By G. Theissing

Tonsillectomy

The tonsils are part of Waldeyer's ring of lymphatic tissue which forms part of the lymph drainage system of the head and neck. The tonsils should only be removed for the strictest indications. The significance of tonsillar diseases is the danger of local and general complications which may be not only acute but may also arise from an exacerbation of a chronic inflammation.

Diagnostic Preoperative Measures

Acute diseases can be recognized on the basis of inspection alone. Inspection may be supplemented by bacteriological examination (in diphtheria and streptococcal or pneumococcal pharyngitis) and hematological examination (leukemias and agranulocytosis) if necessary. Chronic tonsillitis, however, can only be diagnosed by a thorough clinical examination.

- The tonsils may be *palpated* for consistency and mobility (Zange 1926), for tenderness to pressure of the tonsils and the tonsillar bed. The contents of the crypts produced by pressure on the anterior faucial pillar may be examined. Palpation of the lymph nodes is important, particularly the node at the angle of the jaw and the deep cervical chain.

- *Mirror examination*. Laryngoscopy must always be carried out to exclude inflammation extending to the base of the tongue, the lateral wall of the pharynx and the lingual surface of the epiglottis.

- *Aspiration* is carried out using a fairly thick, long cannula introduced in the supratonsillar area if a paratonsillar abscess is suspected.

- *Biopsy* may be needed and is easily carried out under local anesthetic if there is any suspicion of malignancy.

Indications

In children:

- Excessive hyperplasia causing difficulties in breathing, swallowing and speech.

- Recurrent infection, particularly if it pursues a prolonged course with swelling of the regional lymph nodes, decreased resistance to infection, loss of appetite, facial pallor and general debility; routine physical examination should be normal in this case.

- Acute rheumatic fever and nephritis, in a disease-free interval, if the tonsils are suspected to be the source of infection.

Timing of the tonsillectomy in children is generally after the age of 4, but no rigid schedule can be laid down. Tonsillectomy may be indicated earlier if the child's general condition demands it, but the opinion of a pediatrician should be sought.

In adolescents and adults:

- Recurrent tonsillitis.

- Chronic tonsillitis with recurrent exacerbations and particularly in pronounced formation of debris with halitosis and swelling of the regional lymph nodes.

- Recurrent inflammation of the eustachian tube and sinusitis.

- Localized tumors of the tonsil.

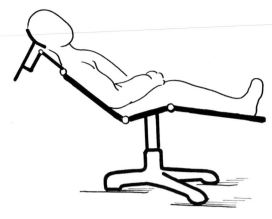

Fig. 14.1   Half-lying position on the operating table for tonsillectomy under local anesthesia.

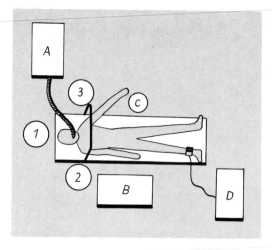

Fig. 14.2   Location of the surgical team for tonsillectomy under general anesthesia:

1 = Surgeon	A = Anesthetic apparatus
2 = Scrub nurse	B = Instrument table
3 = Anesthetist	C = Infusion stand
	D = Diathermy

- Local and general complications: inflammatory edema extending to the base of the tongue and the epiglottis causing inflammatory edema of the vestibule of the larynx; suppurative lymphadenitis and ascending or descending parapharyngeal abscesses. In the presence of sepsis, the vascular spaces of the neck must generally be exposed, the jugular vein may need to be ligated and the tissue spaces drained via an external incision.

- Occasionally in mononucleosis with signs of chronic inflammation and if the hypertrophied tonsils make breathing difficult or if the disease has been present more than 8 to 10 days. In such cases antibiotics and steroid cover are necessary.

Contraindications

These include cardiopulmonary insufficiency, blood disorders, disorders of coagulation, arteriosclerosis, acute infection, etc. Tonsillectomy can be carried out today on hemophiliacs if there are good reasons for doing so. Suitable substitution treatment must be carried out in cooperation with an expert in this field.

Note: During the summer months children should only be operated on if they have had a poliomyelitis vaccination. It has been established that there is an increased risk of bulbar poliomyelitis after a tonsillectomy. Antibiotic cover should be given begin-

ning two to three days before the operation in patients with rheumatic heart disease, nephritis or carditis.

Principles of the Operation

The lymphatic tissue of the tonsil with its capsule must be removed completely. No remnants should be left as this can easily lead to recurrence.

Preparation for Surgery

Premedication is given the evening before the operation and immediately before surgery.

Position. If the operation is carried out under *local anesthesia*, the patient must be placed on the operating table in the half-sitting position, due to the premedication (Fig. 14.1). The surgeon stands on the right side of the patient; and the scrub nurse opposite him.

If the operation is carried out under general anesthesia, the patient is laid flat with his head extended. At the beginning of the operation, the operating table is tilted slightly in the head-down position.

The **location of the surgical team** for tonsillectomy under general anesthesia is shown in Figure 14.2.

The area surrounding the mouth is cleaned in the usual way.

Special Instruments

Suitable instruments for tonsillectomy are shown in Figure 14.3. The following should be noted in particular:

- Haymann's nasal scissors with an offset joint and fine blades (Fig. 14.3e). The first incision can be made easily and exactly with these scissors or with the fine Vetter's knife with a long handle (Fig. 14.3h).

- Long tonsil scissors curved on the flat (Fig. 14.3f, g) for freeing the posterior faucial pillar and dividing capsular and pericapsular adhesions.

- Henke's elevator with fine serrations (Fig. 14.3i) facilitates freeing of the capsule of the tonsil from its surroundings.

- Brüning's tonsil snare (Fig. 14.3j) for dividing the lower pole.

- Schmitt's and Eadle's long, fine forceps for hemostasis (Fig. 14.3l, m).

- Hurd's tonsil needle (Fig. 14.3n).

- For tonsillectomy under *general anesthesia*: bipolar coagulation forceps (Fig. 14.3o), Stierlen's suction elevator (Fig. 14.3k) and a special mouth gag (Fig. 14.3q).

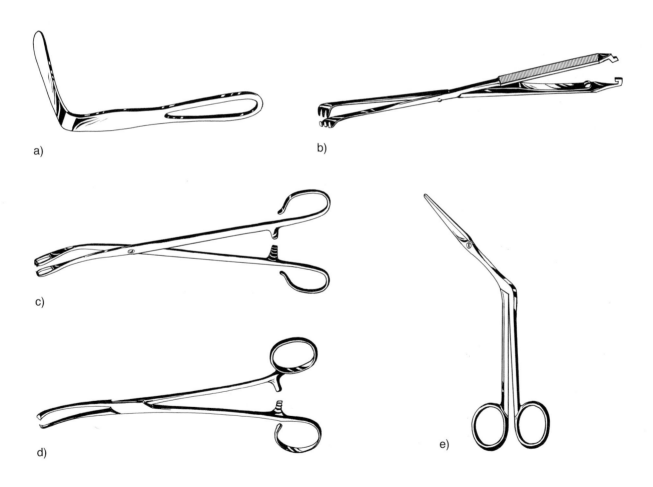

a)

b)

c)

d)

e)

Fig. 14.3 Legend see p. 363.

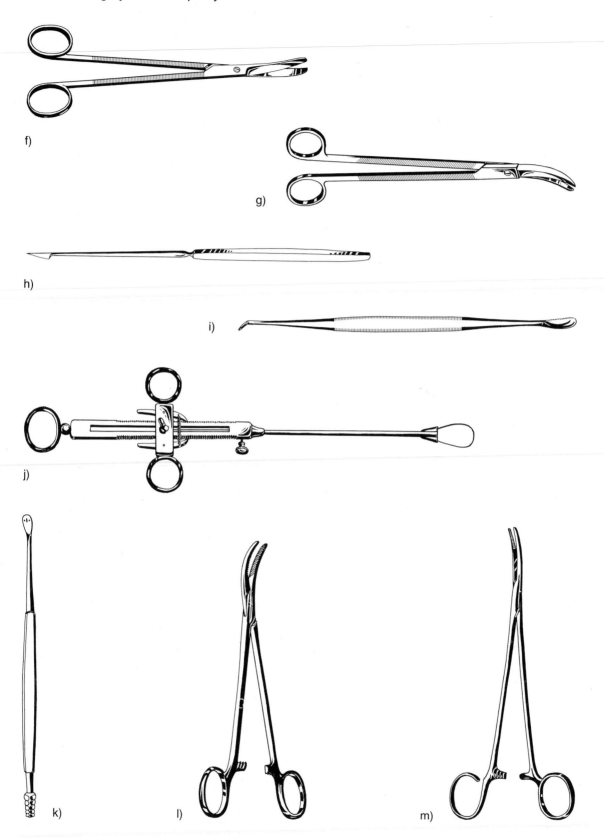

f)

g)

h)

i)

j)

k)   l)   m)

Fig. 14.3

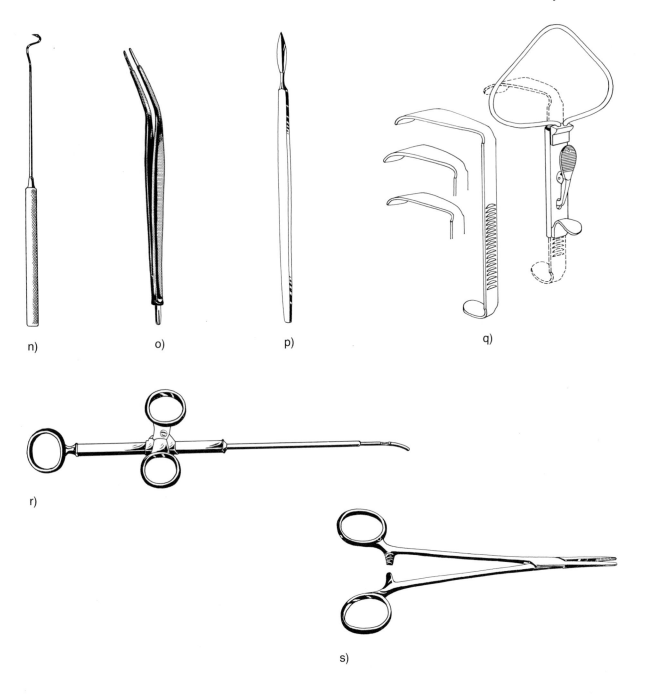

Fig. 14.3 Special instruments for operations on the tonsil:

a) = Hartmann's mouth gag
b) = Special tonsil forceps
c) = Blohmke's tonsil forceps
d) = Colver's tonsil forceps
e) = Curved Haymann's nasal scissors
f) = Tonsil scissors, slightly curved on the flat
g) = Tonsil scissors, strongly curved on the flat
h) = Vetter's fine knife, with long handle
i) = Henke's tonsil elevator, with fine serrations
j) = Brüning's tonsil snare
k) = Stierlen's tonsil suction elevator
l) = Schmitt's tonsil forceps
m) = Eadle's tonsil forceps
n) = Hurd's tonsil needle
o) = Bipolar coagulation forceps
p) = Double-sided tonsil knife
q) = McIvor's mouth gag
r) = Roeder's ligation instrument
s) = Long, fine, special ligature forceps

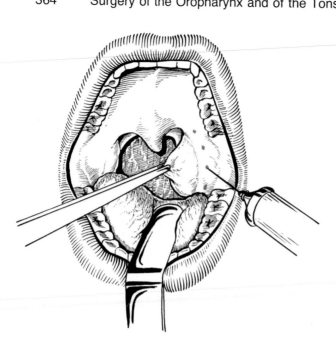

Fig. 14.4   Local anesthesia for tonsillectomy.

Anesthesia

In adults and adolescents, local infiltration anesthesia is unquestionably the most suitable. In children up to 10 or 12 years of age, however, the operation should definitely be carried out under general anesthesia. Local infiltration anesthesia can be used to supplement general anesthesia for reducing the brisk bleeding. It should not be used if a halothane anesthetic is to be administered. Premedication is necessary for the operation under local or under general anesthetic. If there is severe local inflammation such as in a paratonsillar abscess or cellulitis, a local anesthetic should not be used. It should also not be used for patients with epilepsy (because of the interaction between the local anesthetic and the anticonvulsants) or for psychologically disturbed patients.

Ether *insufflation* can also be used as an *anesthetic* for tonsillectomy so that the operator can control the anesthetic himself. If endotracheal *intubation anesthetic* is used, as we do *exclusively*, an anesthetist is necessary.

Infiltration anesthesia is given with the patient in the sitting position. The faucial pillars and the posterior pharyngeal wall are sprayed with a 1% tetracaine (Pontocaine) solution with the tongue depressed;

the patient spits out excess anesthetic after gargling briefly. Several minutes later the infiltration begins with the object of infiltrating the area surrounding the tonsillar bed. We use 1% lidocaine (Xylocaine) solution with norepinephrine (levarterenol) or epinephrine (3 drops of 1% solution to 20 ml of Xylocaine). Since Xylocaine acts more rapidly than procaine (Novocain), the operation can begin shortly after the injection. Despite this, a short delay of several minutes should be observed to achieve better hemostasis. The injection is carried out with a 5 ml syringe; 2 ml of 1% lidocaine (Xylocaine) is injected on each side just above the upper pole of the tonsil (Fig. 14.4). Next, the right and then the left tonsil is drawn medially with forceps in order to demonstrate the margins of the tonsillar bed via the slight depression of the anterior faucial pillar and to stay behind the capsule. Injection through the tonsil to the tonsillar bed should be avoided to prevent spread of bacteria and subsequent wound infection. Two ml of 1% lidocaine (Xylocaine) is injected at 3 sites on both sides behind the capsule of the tonsil (Fig. 14.4). Finally, 1 to 2 ml of anesthetic solution is injected directly into the tissue of the tonsil on each side immediately above the lower pole in order to achieve complete anesthesia. The total amount of 1% lidocaine (Xylocaine) solution with norepinephrine required is 18 to 20 ml.

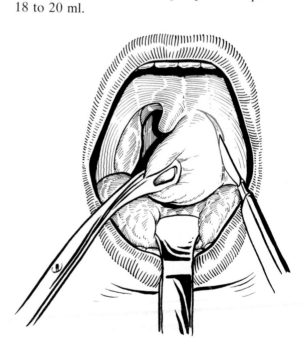

Fig. 14.5   Incision for tonsillectomy.

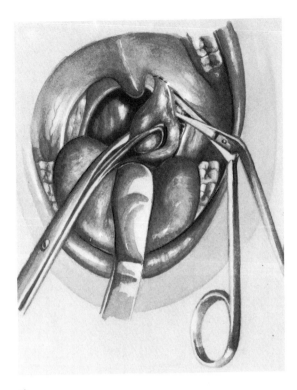

a)

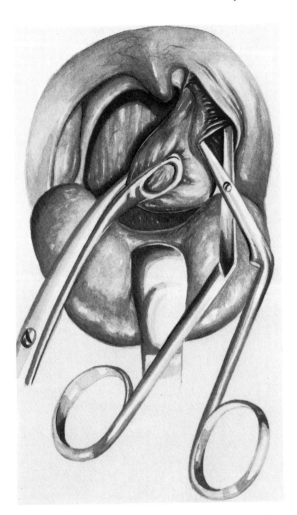

Fig. 14.7

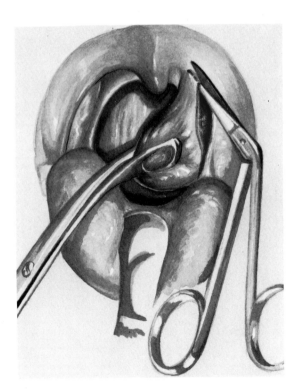

b)

Fig. 14.6

Operative Technique

Usually the right tonsil is enucleated first and then the left. In inflammatory processes such as a paratonsillar abscess, the tonsil on the nonaffected side is removed first. The tonsil is grasped with forceps and retracted medially. Slight pressure on the base of the tongue keeps the triangular fold under tension; the anterior edge of the faucial pillar can be easily recognized.

The incision in the anterior faucial pillar is usually made with a knife (Fig. 14.5), but we prefer scissors with an offset handle. A superficial incision is made down to the tonsillar capsule along the stretched anterior pillar and the scissors are spread to expose the tonsillar capsule from above downward. In this way the correct plane is immediately displayed (Fig. 14.6).

The scissors are now turned at a right angle in order to detach the faucial pillar and are spread again, carefully elevating the whole breadth of the anterior faucial pillar (Fig. 14.7).

The faucial pillar is detached from the upper pole by spreading the scissors obliquely in a superior direction (Fig. 14.8).

Further mobilization is carried out posteroinferiorly by spreading movements of the scissors; the upper pole is exposed after the supratonsillar cleft has been slit (Fig. 14.9).

Henke's elevator is now introduced over the upper pole which is displaced outward and grasped with forceps.

The posterior faucial pillar is now divided from the posterior surface of the tonsil with Cooper's scissors curved on the flat (Fig. 14.10).

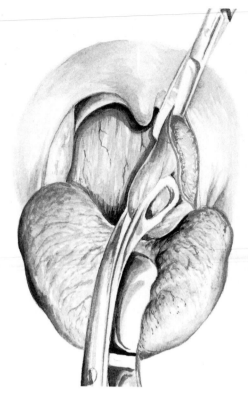

Fig. 14.9

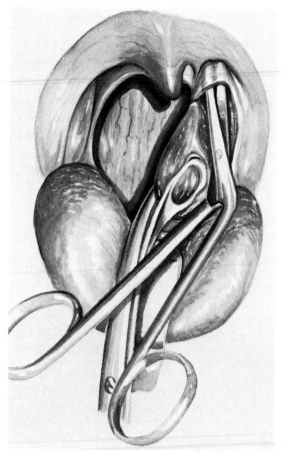

Fig. 14.8

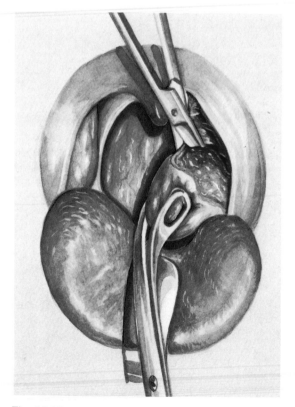

Fig. 14.10

The lateral and posterior parts of the capsule are stripped with the elevator down to the lower pole (Fig. 14.11). The pressure of the elevator must be directed away from the tonsil toward the surrounding tissue to prevent muscle tissue remaining attached to the tonsil.

When the tonsil has been completely mobilized, the lower pole is divided with the Brüning's snare (Fig. 14.12).

After removing one tonsil a tagged swab is introduced and the other tonsil is removed in a similar fashion. A tagged swab is again introduced and must be held by an assistant standing behind the patient. The first swab is now removed and hemostasis is achieved by grasping bleeding points with forceps and transfixing them (Fig. 14.13). This can be done with a patent needle and transfixion forceps or with Roeder's instrument (Figs. 14.3r, s). The needle should not be carried too deeply through the tissues to prevent unnecessary wound infection. Bleeding is controlled considerably by introducing the swab and may often cease spontaneously.

The operation concludes with the insufflation of hemostatic powder into the wound bed.

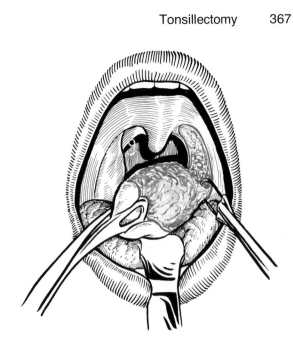

Fig. 14.12

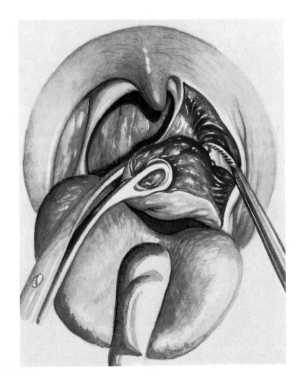

Fig. 14.11

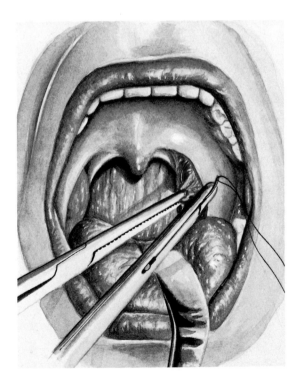

Fig. 14.13

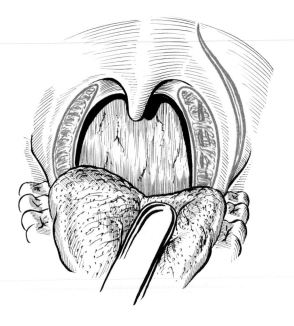

Fig. 14.14   Incision for a bipedicled flap from the anterior faucial pillar.

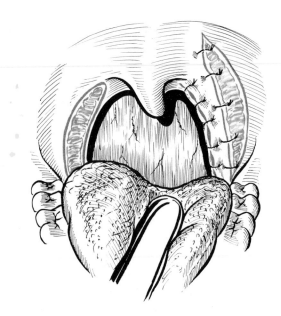

Fig. 14.15   Suturing of the bipedicled flap.

Landmarks and Danger Points

● The first incision should lie immediately next to the edge of the anterior faucial pillar. This is best recognized by putting pressure on the base of the tongue and, at the same time, medial traction on the tonsil. This puts the triangular fold under tension.

● A further landmark is the capsule of the tonsil. It should not be incised, otherwise the correct layer (i.e., the external surface of the tonsillar capsule) is missed and it may become impossible to enucleate the entire tonsillar tissue accurately.

● The next landmark is the upper pole of the tonsil which must be retracted from above downward and medially without damaging the capsule.

Danger points include the neighboring large vessels (internal carotid artery and ascending pharyngeal artery) and the glossopharyngeal nerve which runs just beneath the mucosa of the lower part of the wound bed and breaks up here into its terminal branches. Damage to the nerve can cause disturbance of taste. Damage is prevented by dividing the lower pole of the tonsil with the Brüning's snare.

An abnormally placed artery, particularly the ascending pharyngeal artery, may be exposed in the bed of the wound where it can be recognized by its pulsation. The artery should be protected from secondary erosion by a bipedicled flap from the anterior faucial pillar which can easily be drawn over the vessel (Fig. 14.14). The posterior suture line of this flap lies along the edge of the posterior faucial pillar; the anterior edge of the flap must be sutured with chromic catgut directly anterior to the vessel in the wound bed (Fig. 14.15).

If necessary, a transposition flap can be formed from the posterior pharyngeal wall (Herrmann 1968) and sutured in position in the same way (Fig. 14.16). Damage to an abnormally located internal carotid artery is rare. If damage does occur, the artery should be ligated immediately from an external approach. If necessary, the vessel should be repaired by using the external carotid artery to bridge the defect in the internal carotid artery.

Diffuse bleeding from the lower part of the wound bed seldom occurs and rarely needs to be dealt with by ligating the facial artery or the external carotid artery.

Rules, Hints and Typical Errors

● The chief rule is to maintain the correct layer during the entire operation so that enucleation is carried out immediately outside the tonsillar capsule. This is particularly difficult laterally and posteriorly because the muscle layers frequently intermingle in this area. The elevator must, therefore, always be carried away from the tonsillar capsule so that no muscle tissue remains on the capsule. If firm scar tissue is encountered, it must be divided with Cooper's scissors since blunt dissection easily damages the surrounding tissue. The posterior faucial pillar should be carefully preserved. When the upper pole of the tonsil has been dissected free, it is carefully retracted in an anterior direction to preserve a narrow strip of mucosa along the posterior pillar. This maneuver puts the mucosa of the posterior pillar under tension and the mucosa can then be divided with Cooper's scissors from above downward.

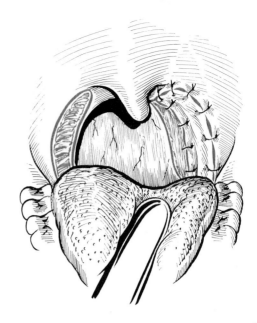

Fig. 14.16   Transposition flap from the posterior pharyngeal wall and position of the sutures.

● If the incision in the anterior faucial pillar is not carried down to the base of the tongue, the triangular fold can be easily left behind. Since tissue containing crypts is found here, the fold must be divided carefully and removed with the snare.

● Careful hemostasis must always be achieved at the end of the operation. Overlooking a small bleeding point can easily lead to a considerable reactionary hemorrhage.

Important Modifications and Surgical Alternatives

Tonsillectomy carried out under general anesthesia is less damaging for a child psychologically and, therefore, is preferred by pediatricians. It is also preferred for adults when the operation is to be carried out during an acute inflammatory process such as an abscess.

Tonsillectomy under General Anesthesia

Since there is no danger of aspiration with endotracheal intubation, each stage of the operation can be carried out accurately. The advantages of intubation anesthesia over other methods such as insufflation are clearly recognized by most authors.

The patient is *positioned* flat on the operating table which is provided with a harness for attaching the anesthetic mouth gag. The head itself rests on the head support in an extended position and should not "hang" from the mouth gag (Fig. 14.17).

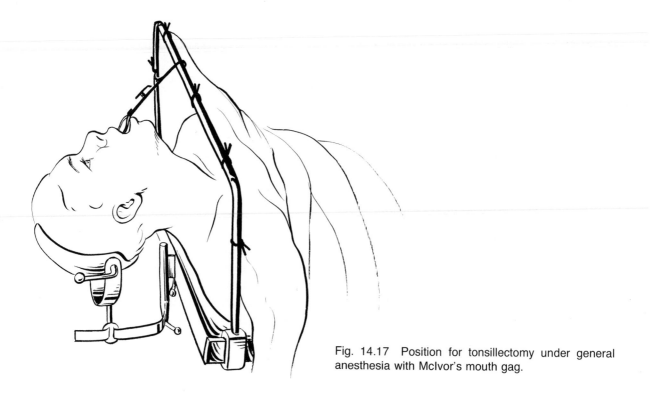

Fig. 14.17   Position for tonsillectomy under general anesthesia with McIvor's mouth gag.

Technique. The technique is the same as under local anesthesia, but the position of the surgeon is different because the patient's head is extended (see Fig. 14.2). Since bleeding is always more pronounced when the operation is done under general anesthesia, local infiltration can also be carried out. This, however, is not necessary. The incidence of postoperative hemorrhage is even lower if the solution used does not contain vasoconstrictors. The operation with the head in the extended position is shown in Figures 14.18 to 14.21.

The use of a tongue blade with a suction attachment or simultaneous suction by an assistant permits the individual steps of the operation to be carried out calmly, under good vision.

The left tonsil is usually removed first and then the right. Exposure of the tonsillar capsule and careful release of the upper pole is carried out in the same way as when the operation is carried out with the head upright (Figs. 14.18, 14.19). In children the operation is not any more difficult since the upper pole of the tonsil can be very easily displaced with the elevator.

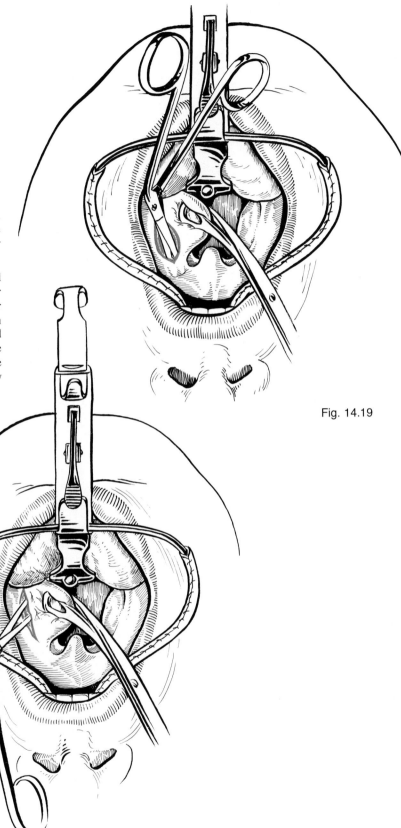

Fig. 14.19

Fig. 14.18

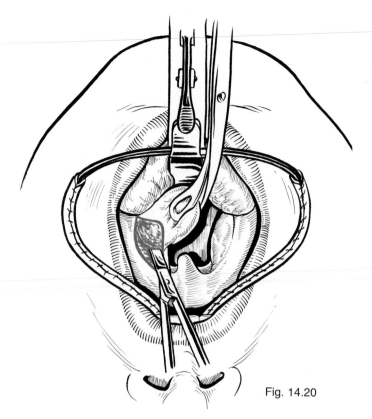

The incision is continued along the posterior faucial pillar with Cooper's scissors (Fig. 14.20); the tonsil with its capsule is then separated from the surrounding tissue. After dividing the lower pole with the snare (Fig. 14.21), careful hemostasis is achieved, preferably with diathermy forceps. Only large spurting vessels must be transfixed.

The endotracheal tube is removed only after complete hemostasis has been achieved. Postoperative supervision is essential.

Fig. 14.20

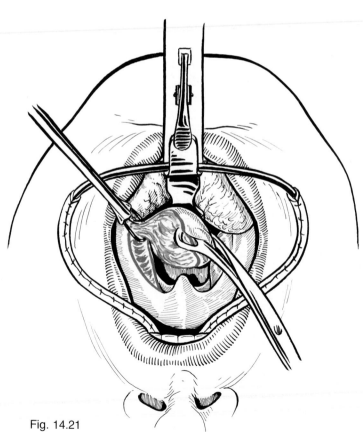

Fig. 14.21

Sluder's Operation

Although tonsillotomy has been generally abandoned, the tonsils are still sometimes removed by Sluder's method. In contrast to tonsillotomy, this operation permits the tonsil to be removed completely. However, if hypertrophy of the lymphatoid tissue is confined to the nonprojecting parts of the tonsil, complete removal is not always possible. Tonsillar remnants can remain behind despite a good technique. We feel therefore that the principle of Sluder's method is unsatisfactory, and we do not recommend this technique.

The **technique** for Sluder's operation is shown in Figures 14.22 to 14.24.

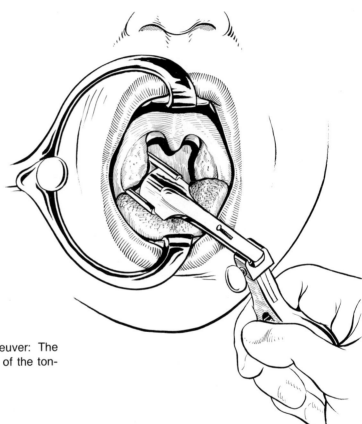

Fig. 14.22 Sluder's operation, first maneuver: The tonsil is engaged from beneath in the ring of the tonsillotome.

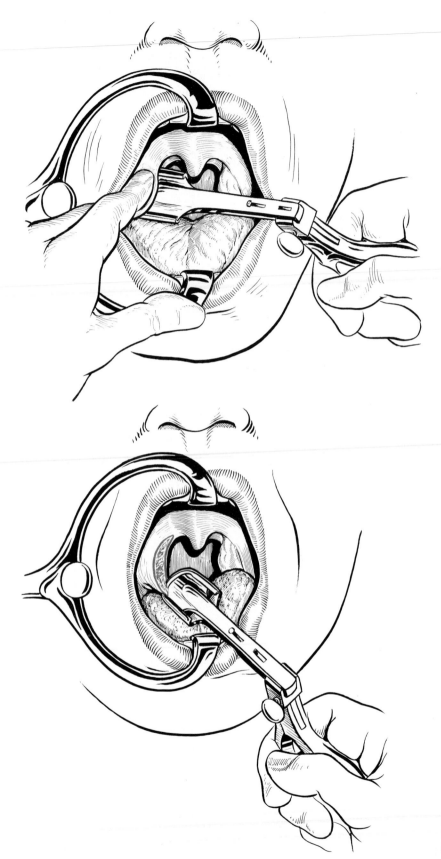

Fig. 14.23 Sluder's operation, second maneuver: The tonsil is pressed completely through the ring of the tonsillotome with the index finger of the left hand.

Fig. 14.24 Sluder's operation, third maneuver: The knife of the Sluder tonsillotome is closed.

Uvulaplasty

Tonsillectomy under endotracheal intubation permits the surgeon to work so carefully that undesirable injuries such as an accidental resection of the uvula almost never occur. If an accidental resection should occur, it can be managed by a simple plastic procedure.

Technique. A 1 cm incision is made through all layers of the soft palate transversely above the defect of the uvula. This incision must be positioned in such a way as to preserve a sufficiently large pedicle medial to the faucial pillars to guarantee a satisfactory blood supply. The lower edge of the bridge flap is drawn downward with a stay suture in its center and fixed to the posterior pharyngeal wall (Fig. 14.25). The defect is sutured in all three layers (Fig. 14.26): first, with an inverting suture to the pharyngeal wall; second, with chromic catgut to the muscle layers; third the oral mucosa with 4×0 nylon (Fig. 14.27). The reconstructed uvula is shorter than the original one, but it is cosmetically and functionally satisfactory.

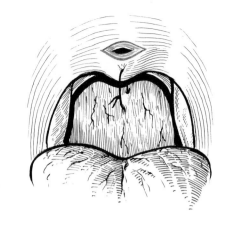

Fig. 14.25

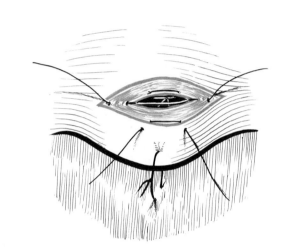

Fig. 14.26

Postoperative Care

The patient should be kept in bed for 2 to 3 days and in the hospital for 5 to 7 days whether the operation was carried out under local or general anesthesia. Pyrexia is treated with antibiotics which are started 2 to 3 days before the operation if there seems to be any a danger of a flare-up. Ice packs are applied to the neck and analgesics are given (morphine derivatives are seldom necessary).

A fluid diet is given on the first day and a soft diet on the second or third day. Fruit and fruit juices are to be avoided since they produce a burning sensation.

After the scabs have dropped off, the wound bed can be swabbed with 3–10% silver nitrate solution (in increasing concentrations).

Heavy manual, labor, sport and gymnastics should be avoided for 8 to 14 days after discharge from the hospital.

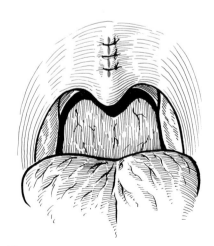

Fig. 14.27

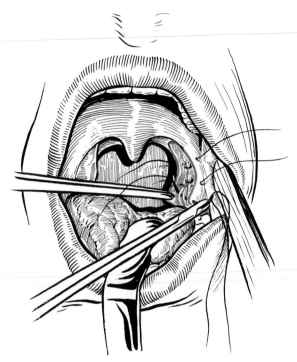

Fig. 14.28   Suturing of the tonsillar bed in diffuse postoperative hemorrhage.

Postoperative Complications

The chief danger is *secondary hemorrhage* which generally occurs within 24 to 48 hours and occasionally on the fifth to sixth day or later. If the bleeding occurs from spurting vessels, the vessels are transfixed after infiltration with 1% lidocaine (Xylocaine) after epinephrine. Minor bleeding ceases after infiltration of this anesthetic solution supplemented by simultaneous administration of hemostatics. Suturing the wound bed for diffuse bleeding is seldom necessary.

Suturing of the wound bed of the tonsil in diffuse bleeding. A silk or nylon suture is introduced through the anterior faucial pillar with a strong curved needle, the muscle layer of the wound bed is picked up at several points with fine forceps and included in the suture. The needle is then brought out through the posterior faucial pillar (Fig. 14.28). Usually only 3 or 4 such transfixion sutures are necessary to secure hemostasis. Tying all knots only after having introduced all transfixion sutures facilitates the positioning of the last sutures, which can otherwise be difficult. Endotracheal anesthesia makes the necessary manipulations easier.

Arterial bleeding occurring after the operation is described on page 367. Sewing of tagged pledgets into the wound bed for diffuse bleeding from the tonsil should be necessary only on rare occasions. (The tags should be fixed to the cheek in such cases.)

Longer aspiration of blood requires suction of the entire bronchial tree via a bronchoscope or endotracheal tube. Sedatives should, of course, not be given because of the danger of unnoticed aspiration of blood. Severe loss of blood should always be treated with a blood transfusion.

Infection of the wound bed seldom occurs today. It is usually controlled by antibiotics. Occasional suppuration of the regional lymph nodes requires wide incision via an external approach. Infection spreading along the great vessels occasionally accompanied by thrombosis of the jugular vein also requires wide exposure via an external incision (see p. 382).

Retropharyngeal and parapharyngeal abscesses as well as cellulitis are seldom observed after tonsillectomy. They are usually the result of persisting tonsillar remnants. After diagnostic aspiration has been carried out a wide exposure is necessary. The initially severe symptoms resolve rapidly under high antibiotic cover and regular opening of the wound with sinus forceps. Severe complications are very rare.

Functional Sequelae

Mild disturbances of taste occasionally occur after tonsillectomy but generally resolve quickly and spontaneously. Persistent disturbances of taste are uncommon and are very disturbing to the patient. They often have a psychological basis.

- In small children rhinolalia aperta occurs because of immobility of the soft palate, but this usually resolves spontaneously and rapidly. There is no organic cause for this.

- Formation of scar tissue on the soft palate sometimes extending across the soft palate is caused by a poor technique. These scars are cosmetically disturbing but usually of no practical significance.

Abscess Tonsillectomy

Local complications during and after tonsillitis are usually caused by acute exacerbation of chronic tonsillitis and, on rare occasions, by quinsy. Either an intratonsillar or peritonsillar abscess or peritonsillar cellulitis is produced. Extension to the parapharyngeal space (see Fig. 14.32) with inevitable extension to the base of the skull or the mediastinum occurs only occasionally today because on antibiotics. Surgery, however, is mandatory if it does occur. The same is also true of the once feared tonsillogenic septicemia syndrome which is seldom seen today.

There are several sites for a peritonsillar abscess. The most common are a supratonsillar abscess in the loose connective tissue of the supratonsillar fossa arising from a crypt near to the capsule or a paratonsillar abscess spreading laterally from the tonsil. Retrotonsillar and infratonsillar abscesses are less common (Fig. 14.29). The position of the abscess determines the treatment.

Although abscess tonsillectomy is the *method of choice*, simple incision (Fig. 14.30) with daily spreading of the wound edges usually suffices in un-complicated paratonsillar or supratonsillar abscess formation. Tonsillectomy is carried out within 3 to 5 days, or later if the general condition is not good.

Immediate abscess tonsillectomy in the common supratonsillar and paratonsillar abscess is often difficult because of simultaneous trismus. It is also a greater strain for the already debilitated patient.

In retrotonsillar and infratonsillar abscesses, immediate abscess tonsillectomy is always indicated since a search for a retrotonsillar or infratonsillar loculus of pus is difficult and often not successful. Cellulitis also requires urgent tonsillectomy under antibiotic cover.

Tonsillectomy carried out in a disease-free interval is often difficult because of the scar tissue which has formed in the meantime. Today it is preferable to carry out the operation a few days after the incision.

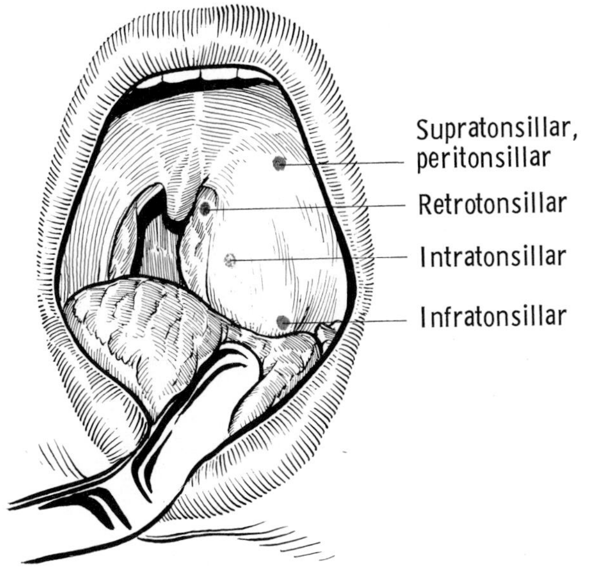

Supratonsillar, peritonsillar

Retrotonsillar

Intratonsillar

Infratonsillar

Fig. 14.29   Sites of peritonsillar abscess formation.

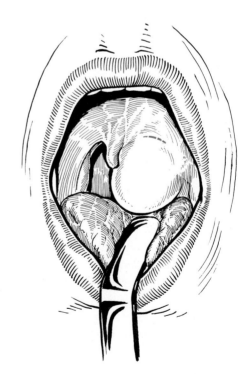

Fig. 14.30   Direction of the incision for incising a peritonsillar abscess (a supratonsillar abscess).

Indications

- If the site of the abscess is concealed, in retro-tonsillar and infratonsillar abscesses;

- Extension of inflammation to the base of the tongue and the epiglottis, inflammatory edema of the epiglottis and in actual or impending parapharyngeal abscess;

- In tonsillogenic septicemia (together with further exploration from without);

- If the healing of a paratonsillar or supratonsillar abscess is delayed, despite a previous incision and daily spreading of the wound edges;

- In recurrence of an abscess (Since the paratonsillar abscess usually arises in an already chronically inflamed tonsil, there is a tendency toward recurrence. Tonsillectomy then is indicated after the first abscess).

Principles of the Operation

Removal of the tonsil which is the origin of an abscess or cellulitis not only provides complete drainage of the inflammatory process but also prevents local and general complications or recurrence.

Preparation for Surgery

Premedication is given as for tonsillectomy.

Supine position on the operating table is used with the head extended.

Anesthesia

Since the injection of local anesthetic solution in inflammation (particularly cellulitis) carries the danger of spreading infection, intubation anesthesia is to be preferred. In an established abscess localized by a capsule, local anesthesia can be used, but the abscess must not be penetrated during the injection to prevent spread of organisms to the surrounding tissue. If the abscess cavity is entered, the injection needle should be changed.

Operative Technique

The operative technique is that of the customary tonsillectomy (see p. 365). Due to the danger of recurrence on the healthy side, both tonsils must be removed. The healthy tonsil is removed first in the usual way and the abscess tonsillectomy is then carried out. The latter part of the operation requires a suction apparatus.

Landmarks and Danger Points

Orientation is made more difficult because of edema of the entire peritonsillar area. The base of the uvula is an important landmark since the abscess usually occurs at this level. Medial displacement of the tonsil and edema of the faucial pillar make the medial edge more difficult to recognize. Careful pressure on the base of the tongue usually brings the triangular fold into view (provided the abscess is not intratonsillar); the triangular fold indicates the direction of the faucial pillar. Despite the edema, the capsule can usually be found relatively easily. The individual steps of the operation then proceed as for the usual tonsil enucleation.

- It is important to remember that a peritonsillar abscess arises from a crypt near the capsule; the capsule has usually been breached at this point and is granulating. The opposite side of the abscess membrane also demonstrates these granulations. They should not be removed during the enucleation since this can cause serious hemorrhage.

If dissection is not carried out accurately around the upper pole, damage to the supratonsillar artery can easily occur. This artery often tears because of previous erosion. Grasping the bleeding vessels in the granulation tissue is then difficult.

Rules, Hints and Typical Errors

- If a wide incision has been made previously in the anterior faucial pillar, it is advisable to insert 1 or 2 sutures through the site of the incision before spreading the edges of the wound since the faucial pillar can otherwise tear easily under light pressure. For this reason the operation must be carried out with particular care at this point.

- After releasing the upper pole, the incision along the posterior faucial pillar must be made with Cooper's scissors to avoid penetrating the muscles from the abscess cavity. Excessive retraction on the upper pole of the tonsil can tear the friable tonsillar tissue so that smooth dissection outside the tonsillar capsule is made more difficult.

- When the operation is carried out after an interval, firm scar tissue may have formed. This should be divided with the scissors since blunt dissection may tear the peritonsillar tissue.

- The lower pole is removed with the snare as for the usual tonsillectomy.

- If dissection is kept close to the tonsillar capsule, bleeding is not particularly heavy; a few ligatures usually suffice. If the abscess capsule is damaged, bleeding can be extremely severe and difficult to stop since the friable tissue tears easily when it is transfixed and the faucial pillars cannot be stitched together. The bleeding can then be stopped by suturing a tagged pack into the wound with the tape fixed to the cheek.

- Aftercare for abscess tonsillectomy is the same as for an ordinary tonsillectomy. Pain is usually less on the side of the abscess and secondary hemorrhage does not occur more frequently than after an ordinary tonsillectomy.

Important Modifications and Surgical Alternatives

Incision of the abscess

Indications. In an established paratonsillar or supratonsillar abscess with pronounced trismus or if the patient's general condition is poor, an immediate abscess tonsillectomy is contraindicated. In retrotonsillar and infratonsillar abscesses, the incision seldom releases the pus. In such cases abscess tonsillectomy is indicated as the first line of treatment.

Anesthesia for aspiration and incision. The mucosa around the upper pole is superficially infiltrated with 1% lidocaine (Xylocaine) with norepinephrine or epinephrine preceded by the application of pledgets soaked in 1% Pontocaine.

Technique of the Aspiration. A long, wide-bore cannula is used on a 10 ml syringe with a record needle. It is introduced immediately above the upper pole to a depth of about 2 to 3 cm. If pus is aspirated, the needle is left in situ and a wide incision is made along the cannula. The entry point of the needle should be in the middle of a line between the base of the uvula and the last molar tooth. The cannula must be introduced perpendicular and parallel to the midline to avoid damaging the lateral fascial spaces of the neck and their neurovascular contents.

Technique of the incision. The incision is made with a narrow, longhandled scalpel or with a lanceolate knife as wide as the required opening. The incision is made from above downward in the paramedian plane or, even better, in an oblique direction to achieve wide spreading of the incision (see Fig. 14.30). The edges of the wound are further opened with sinus forceps until the abscess has been emptied completely.

Postoperative Care. Since the edges of the wound tend to adhere to each other, the wound is opened daily with sinus forceps. This is done until only serous fluid appears or the cavity is completely dry.

Ice packs on the neck should be continued and high doses of antibiotics given if cellulitis is present.

Tonsillectomy should definitely be carried out if the course of the disease is prolonged or healing of the abscess is delayed.

Complications of incision of the abscess. Pronounced hemorrhage can occur from the supratonsillar artery. This can also happen due to the sudden release of pressure in the presence of previous erosion of the vessel. This requires immediate packing of the abscess cavity. Tonsillectomy then follows in which the bleeding vessel can be grasped and transfixed in the bed of the wound.

Opening of Parapharyngeal and Retropharyngeal Abscesses

Parapharyngeal and retropharyngeal abscesses usually arise from the tonsil and sometimes follow a tonsillectomy. In children the cause is often inflammation of the nasopharynx and the posterior part of the nose. Lymphadenitis in the retropharyngeal space develops which then undergoes liquefaction. The *treatment* is surgical opening and spreading of the wound for several days.

Anesthesia

After superficial anesthesia has been achieved by applying pledgets soaked in 1% Pontocaine solution with norepinephrine (levarterenol) or epinephrine to the mucosa over the abscess, the mucosa is infiltrated with 1% lidocaine (Xylocaine) solution. The patient should have received premedication.

Operative Technique

In *small children* the operation is carried out with the head lowered and a mouth gag in place. The tongue is depressed with a Hartmann's retractor and the abscess is suctioned thoroughly to prevent the danger of aspiration. A median or paramedian incision, depending on the side of the abscess, is then made from above downward (Fig. 14.31). The scalpel must not be directed outward in order to avoid damaging the great vessels of the neck.

In *older children* and occasionally in *adults*, the head must be bent forward immediately after the incision. This should be preceded by needle aspiration to avoid the danger of inhalation. Suction apparatus must be available.

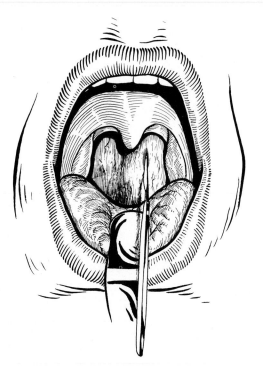

Fig. 14.31   Incision for opening of a parapharyngeal and retropharyngeal abscess.

Complications

● The principal complication is profuse immediate hemorrhage or a secondary hemorrhage. The palatine artery and the ascending pharyngeal artery are endangered the most; the internal jugular vein and the carotid artery are usually endangered only if the vessels are displaced. If it is not possible to grasp the bleeding vessel immediately with forceps and ligate it, the external carotid artery or the origin of the ascending pharyngeal artery and the ascending palatine artery must be exposed externally and ligated.

● If the abscess spreads into the parapharyngeal space, the spaces of the neck should be opened widely via an external incision. If a thrombosis has already developed, the affected vessel segment should be ligated and resected. It is also essential to open up the connective tissue spaces in the parapharyngeal and retropharyngeal spaces. Finally, a wide drain is introduced (see the next section).

Operations for Parapharyngeal Abscess of Tonsillar or Dental Origin and for Tonsillogenic Septicemia

Exposure of the Parapharyngeal Space

Parapharyngeal infection is rare today. It demands immediate attention because inadequate antibiotic therapy masks the course of the disease. Chills, septic pyrexia and even high fever may be absent. The cause is seldom an acute inflammation but rather a small abscess which remained following incomplete drainage of a peritonsillar abscess. This abscess develops over a long period and is very difficult to diagnose. This syndrome requires not only wide exposure externally but also tonsillectomy. Infection originating from a tooth should be dealt with in the same way.

Diagnosis

Sometimes the symptoms are fulminating, but usually there is less disturbance of the general condition and a moderate to high fever as well as a preceding tonsillar or peritonsillar inflammation. There is slight redness and possibly slight medial displacement of the tonsil, a degree of tenderness of the tonsil especially on palpation, enlargement of the jugulodigastric lymph node and sometimes a significant infiltration in the surrounding area. Leucocytosis is present.

Preparation for Surgery and Anesthetic

Premedication is given as usual. Intubation anesthesia is always used.

The **position** on the operating table is the same as for every external operation on the neck.

The **location of the surgical team** is the same as for operations on the external part of the neck.

Special Instruments

Only general surgical instruments are necessary.

Indications

The operation is indicated for the above-mentioned signs of parapharyngeal inflammation arising from the tonsil or the teeth, particularly the following:

● Chills during the course of but not at the beginning of a quinsy or after its apparent resolution;

● Septic pyrexia with disturbance of the general condition, and for a prolonged parapharyngeal inflammation with relatively mild systemic disturbance;

● Sensitivity to pressure which is seldom pronounced over the carotid sheath, the tonsillar parenchyma and in the tonsillar recess.

There are **no contraindications** since the operation is life saving.

Operative Technique

Figure 14.32 shows the topography of the fascial spaces of the neck.

A 6 to 8 cm long skin incision is made along the anterior border of the sternomastoid muscle from the angle of the jaw to the level of the cricoid cartilage; the fatty tissue, the platysma and the superficial fascia of the neck are divided. The anterior edge of the sternomastoid muscle is demonstrated and the carotid sheath is now exposed down to the omohyoid muscle using dissecting forceps or scissors. Dissection proceeds by carefully freeing the swollen lymph nodes adherent to the carotid sheath from below upward to the level of the carotid bifurcation where the larger lymph nodes are usually found. The nerves here, particularly the vagus nerve, the hypoglossal nerve with its descending branch and the accessory nerve, are carefully preserved.

The further course of the operation is dictated by the pathogenesis of the inflammation and by the principal pathological anomalies. Since inflammation usually spreads by a combination of hematogenous lymphatic and interstitial pathways, the operation is determined by the operative findings.

Sepsis arising from the tonsil or from the teeth, usually from an acute process, requires exposure of the carotid sheath in addition to tonsillectomy (see p. 365). If a thrombophlebitis is found, ligation of the internal jugular vein superior and inferior to the facial vein and of this vein itself (Fig. 14.33) is necessary.

The tonsillar vein should be traced back to the tonsillar bed and ligated at this point. The thrombus is removed and the affected segment of the vein resected.

In lymphatic extension of the disease, abscess formation in the region of the carotid bifurcation is usually present which ruptures into the internal jugular vein and leads to a thrombosis. Thrombophlebitis can be recognized by the discoloration of the vein wall, by absence of the venous pulse and often by a palpable thickening of the vein.

If thrombosis is present, the vein must be slit, the thrombus removed and the diseased wall of the vein resected. If the thrombosis extends far inferiorly, the omohyoid muscle is divided and, after extension of the skin incision to the sternoclavicular joint, the internal jugular vein is exposed as far as its termination in the brachiocephalic vein (Fig. 14.34). If necessary, it is resected. Under anesthesia with controlled respiration, a thrombus extending further inferiorly can be removed by suction or careful intravascular curettage.

If the sepsis stems from the teeth, the venous network over the facial vein is exposed and all thrombosed parts of the vessel are resected after the vessels have been ligated in a healthy segment.

Ligation of the jugular vein must not be carried out if thrombosis is not demonstrated. The facial vein and the posterior facial vein must, however, be ligated and slit. The thrombus is then sought. The posterior facial vein is ligated close to the tonsillar bed.

If in addition to lymphatic spread, spread by interstitial pathways is also present, it is particularly important to open up the fascial spaces of the neck toward the pharynx and drain them. Often small abscesses are found in the immediate neighborhood of the tonsil. They must be drained before healing can begin.

If the jugular vein has been ligated, the wound is usually closed in layers. In cellulitis the wound is left open, the fascial spaces are packed and the upper and lower corners of the incision are shortened with sutures. Drainage is best carried out with a rubber drain.

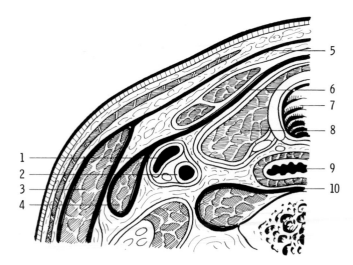

Fig. 14.32   Topography of the cervical fascial spaces:

1 = Internal jugular vein
2 = Common carotid artery and vagus nerve
3 = Sternomastoid muscle
4 = Omohyoid muscle
5 = Superficial fascia
6 = Pretracheal fascia
7 = Trachea
8 = Thyroid gland
9 = Esophagus
10 = Prevertebral fascia

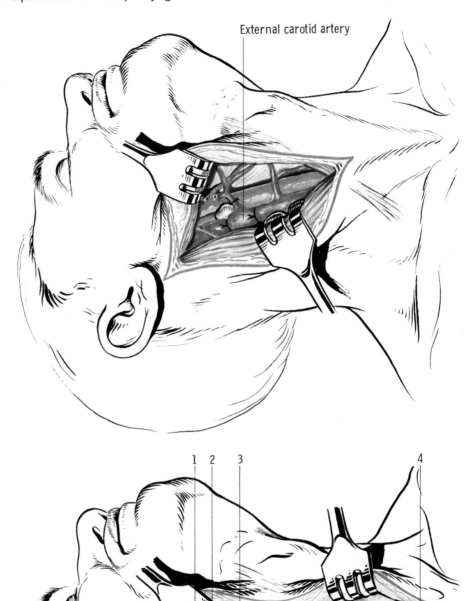

External carotid artery

Fig. 14.33

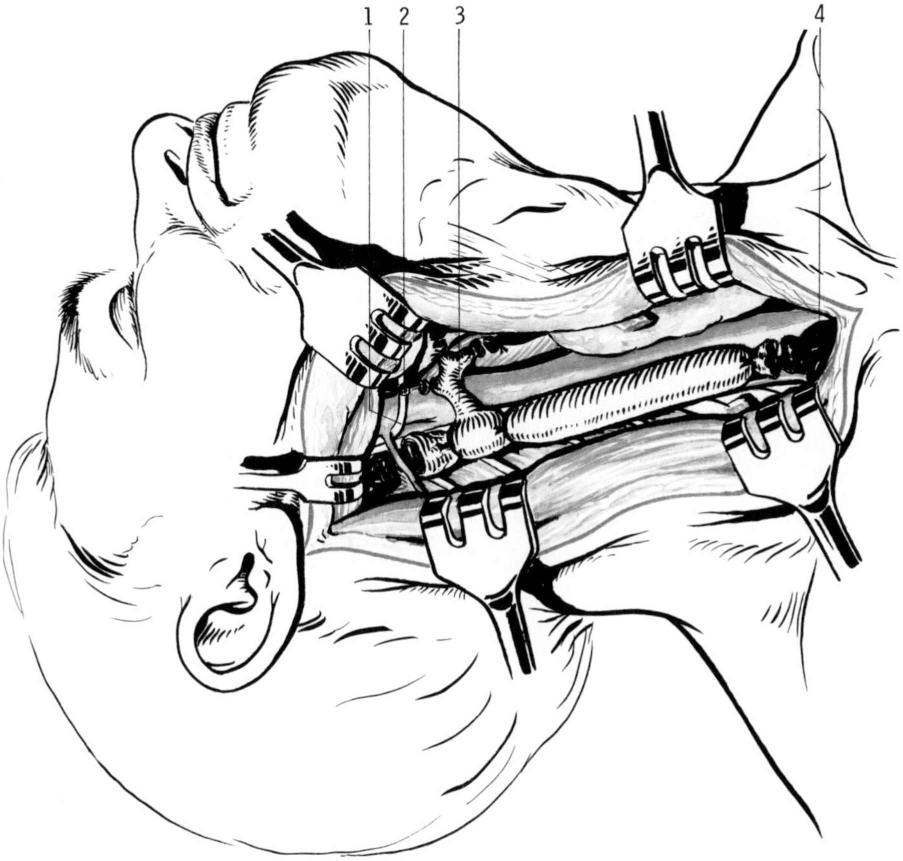

Fig. 14.34

1 = Hypoglossal nerve
2 = Posterior facial vein,
    ligated and divided
3 = Anterior facial vein
4 = Subclavian vein

Landmarks

These include the angle of the jaw and the anterior edge of the sternomastoid muscle. After dividing the cervical fascia, the superior belly of the omohyoid muscle is exposed. Directly under the muscle belly runs the carotid sheath.

Danger Points

● Damage to the internal jugular vein when inflamed lymph nodes are dissected from it. Dissection of the tissue surrounding the internal jugular vein should, therefore, always be carried out in a longitudinal direction in order to prevent damage.

● A tape should be passed around the lower end of the jugular vein; if there is danger of an air embolus, it can be prevented by traction on this tape. Positive pressure respiration can be used as an alternative.

● The vagus may also be damaged when the carotid sheath is opened; the nerve should be exposed to prevent this.

Complications

● Damage to the internal jugular vein when exposing the carotid sheath. Small bleeding points can be controlled by packing, suturing or carefully suturing a small muscle flap to the vessel. But ligation of the vessel may be necessary after complete exposure.

● Extension of the thrombus superiorly into the sigmoid sinus requires operative exposure via a mastoidectomy; the sinus should be packed superiorly and the thrombus removed from the bulb of the jugular vein.

● Septic metastases require general surgical management.

Postoperative Care

High doses of antibiotics are given using either penicillin or broad-spectrum antibiotics. The packing is changed after 2 to 3 days and a rubber drain is reinserted.

Surgery of Tumors of the Mesopharynx

Sites: The tonsil, the base of the tongue (see Chap. 13) and the lateral and posterior pharyngeal walls between the uvula and the epiglottis.

The prognosis for these tumors is extremely poor except for those confined to the tonsil and the anterior faucial pillar or small exophytic tumors on the posterior or lateral pharyngeal wall. Involvement of the posterior part of the linguoalveolar sulcus is also very unfavorable. From here a tumor can easily involve the periosteum of the mandible and extend along the medial pterygoid muscle toward the pterygopalatine fossa and into the parapharyngeal space.

Depending on the localization of the tumor, its extent and its depth, several routes of access are available which are not exclusively applicable to only one tumor site.

The following different routes are available:

1. The transoral route (Fig. 14.35 A),

2. The transmandibular route (Fig. 14.35 B),

3. The submandibular cervical route (Fig. 14.35 C 1–3),

4. The lateral route (Fig. 14.35 D).

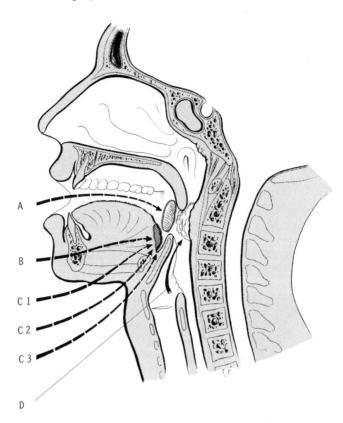

Fig. 14.35 Routes of access
for removal of mesopharyngeal tumors:

A = Transoral
B = Transmandibular
C_1 = Suprahyoid
C_2 = Transhyoid
C_3 = Infrahyoid
D = Lateral access

Principal Indications for the Different Routes of Access

The **transoral route** is indicated for all benign tumors and for malignant oropharyngeal tumors if they are exophytic, small and localized to the posterior pharyngeal wall, the tonsil or the anterior faucial pillar. The tumor must also be fully mobile, the medial pterygoid muscle must not be involved and no palpable lymph nodes should be present.

This route of access is not satisfactory if the posterior part of the linguoalveolar sulcus, the ascending ramus of the mandible, the base of the tongue, the alveolus, the pterygopalatine fossa as well as the lateral or posterior walls of the pharynx are involved. For this reason, it is seldom used today.

The **submandibular cervical route** of access may be either by a median or a lateral pharyngotomy.

Median pharyngotomy is used for small circumscribed tumors of the base of the tongue (see also

Chap. 13) and of the posterior wall of the pharynx. There are several modifications: Subhyoid, suprahyoid, transhyoid, infrahyoid and translaryngeal pharyngotomies, but these only serve as guidelines since the surgical procedure depends on the findings. The view of the operative field of the oropharynx is good in a transhyoid pharyngotomy if it is combined with a resection of the entire hyoid (Pietrantoni 1951) or a temporary resection of this structure (Rethi 1959). This operation, however, is seldom indicated.

Lateral pharyngotomy, which basically preserves the muscles for swallowing and allows exposure and clearance of the lymphatic areas, has more and more replaced median pharyngotomy. It, however, permits only a relatively narrow view into the pharynx; access is through either the digastric or carotid triangles. It is, therefore, only to be used for removing small tumors on the posterior pharyngeal wall or a small recurrence. A *lateral* tumor of the oropharynx should *not* be handled by this route since the pharynx is opened in the immediate neighborhood of the tumor, if not actually through the tumor itself.

The **transmandibular route** is either median (paramedian) through the mandible which is temporarily divided as well as through the horizontal plane of the ascending ramus of the mandible or the angle of the jaw which are permanently resected. This guarantees a wider view of the entire tumor area.

The seldom used median access with temporary division of the mandible is based on Conley 's procedure (1970). Here a tumor on the posterior wall of the pharynx is removed after a temporary median split of the mandible and the base of the tongue. According to Conley, this operation is indicated for primary tumors of the pharynx which are radioresistant, limited to the posterior pharyngeal wall and free of metastasis.

While temporary median division of the mandible is very limited, lateral division with simultaneous partial or complete resection of one-half of the mandible is frequently used in the monoblock operation. This operation is indicated for extensive tumors of the oropharynx and tonsil, particularly if the tumor extends to the posterior part of the linguoalveolar sulcus, the alveolus, the mandible, the floor of the mouth and the pterygopalatine fossa.

Operation by the Transoral Route

Tumor Tonsillectomy

Diagnostic Preoperative Measures

After a biopsy has been conducted direct inspection with a mirror is carried out; the mobility and extent of the tumor are ascertained. Radiographs of the mandible are taken to exclude the possibility of extension to the bone. A general physical examination is performed including chest radiographs, etc.

Principles of the Operation

The tonsil with the neighboring tissue including the faucial pillars, the neighboring part of the base of the tongue and the lateral wall of the pharynx are removed.

Preparation for Surgery

General physical examination and premedication.

Special Instruments

The same instruments are used as for a tonsillectomy.

Anesthesia

The operation can be carried out under local anesthetic (an extended tonsillectomy anesthetic including the base of the tongue and the lateral and posterior wall of the pharynx). It can also be carried out under general anesthesia, particularly after preliminary ligation of the vessels. In this case the entire operative area should be infiltrated with a vasoconstrictor solution to reduce the danger of hemorrhage.

Operative Technique

If general anesthesia is used, the operation is carried out with the head extended on the operating table. The operating table is tilted slightly with the head downward (see p. 360).

If brisk hemorrhage is expected, it is advisable to place a suture around the external carotid artery and to ligate the lingual artery when the carotid sheath is exposed during the neck dissection (Fig. 14.36).

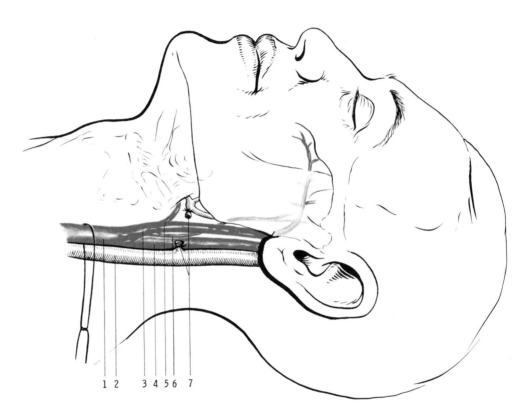

Fig. 14.36 Anatomical sites for arterial ligature after double ligature and division of the facial vein:

1 = Common carotid artery
2 = Internal jugular vein
3 = External carotid artery
4 = Internal carotid artery
5 = Lingual artery
6 = Ascending pharyngeal artery
7 = Common facial vein, doubly ligated and divided

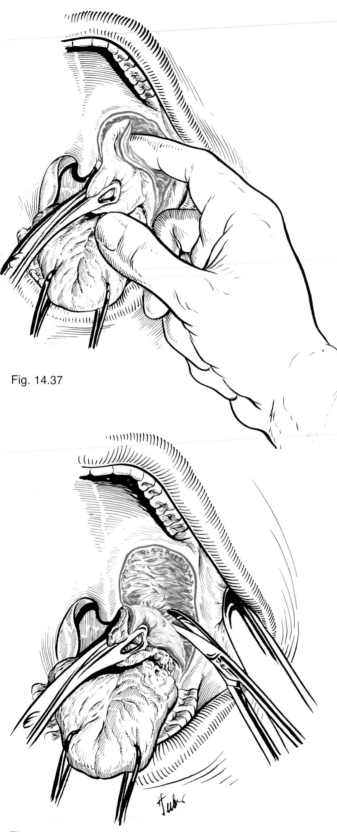

Fig. 14.37

Fig. 14.38

The operation is basically the same as for an ordinary tonsillectomy (see p. 365), except that after the mouth gag or the anesthetic mouth gag has been inserted, the anterior faucial pillar is incised laterally in order to remove the tumor with a healthy margin. The incision must lie far enough laterally to allow the Henke's tonsil elevator to be introduced directly into the paratonsillar space. The enucleation is thus carried out outside the capsule. The forefinger should preferably be used after extension and deepening of the incision because differentiation between the tumor and normal tissue is more certain (Fig. 14.37).

After the tissues have been divided above the upper pole of the tonsil, the tonsil is divided posteriorly with the scissors (Fig. 14.38). Often the faucial pillar must be sacrificed. At the lower pole, the tonsil should only be removed with a snare if the tumor is confined to the upper and middle portions of the tonsil and has not reached the lower pole.

If the tumor extends toward the base of the tongue, 1.5 cm of healthy tissue must be removed at this site, preferably with cutting diathermy. It should be removed in one block with the tonsil. The tongue is held with 1 or 2 sutures in its anterior portion and pulled forward, thereby allowing the tumor to be removed easily and under direct vision.

A preliminary neck dissection (a functional neck dissection) and, if necessary, ligation of the vessels (see. Fig. 14.36) is also necessary if the procedure is extended to the base of the tongue or if the tumor extends to the soft palate.

Surgical Alternatives

Extensive tumors of the tonsil involving not only the lateral and posterior walls of the pharynx but also the base of the tongue, the floor of the mouth and the mandible require a neck dissection in addition to wide external exposure with a hemimandibulectomy (see p. 408 and Vol. 1, Chap. 6).

Landmarks and Danger Points

- During endoral tumor tonsillectomy, attention must be paid to the neighboring large vessels, particularly the external carotid artery and the ascending pharyngeal artery. If they are exposed, they must be covered with mucosal flaps from the surrounding area (the posterior pharyngeal wall).

- To prevent damage to the vessels, a tonsillar tumor is best removed with the finger.

Postoperative Care and Complications

These are the same as following the usual tonsillectomy (see p. 376). The cervical wound caused by ligating the vessels and by the neck dissection is closed primarily. The rubber or suction drain is removed on the second day.

Disturbances in swallowing may occur following surgery on the lateral and posterior walls of the pharynx, but they usually resolve rapidly.

Disturbances in taste are possible following extensive resection of the neighboring portion of the tongue, but they are usually unilateral.

Transoral Access for Small Tumors of the Posterior Wall of the Pharynx

Diagnostic Preoperative Measures

These are described on page 386.

Indications

This operation should only be considered for very small, benign or malignant tumors of the posterior pharyngeal wall where there is no extension to the prevertebral fascia and no metastases.

Principle of the Operation

The tumor is excised with a healthy margin without any particular method of access.

Preparation for Surgery

The patient is positioned on the operative table half sitting or lying. The mouth gag is inserted.

Location of the surgical team is as for tumor tonsillectomy.

Special Instruments

Diathermy with spherical attachments and a long handle.

Anesthesia

Local infiltration anesthesia is satisfactory, but intubation anesthesia may be necessary.

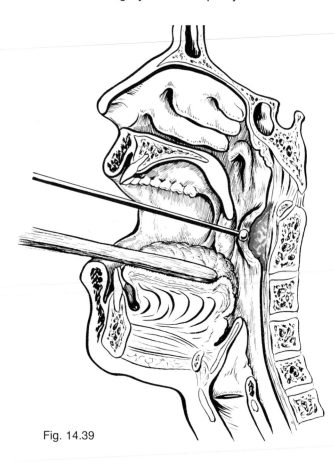

Fig. 14.39

Operative Technique

After introduction of a wood or plastic tongue blade (not metal), the tumor is completely diathermised with the ball electrode and peeled off in layers (Fig. 14.39). If necessary, the soft palate must be retracted from the operative field with a rubber catheter introduced through the nose.

Landmarks and Danger Points

● The prevertebral fascia should not be included in the slough since this can easily lead to necrosis of the vertebral column.

● If bleeding occurs, it is controlled by long forceps and diathermy as for a tonsillectomy.

Modification

If the excision is carried out with a knife, coagulation is necessary.

Submandibular Cervical Access

Median Pharyngotomy

Diagnostic Preoperative Measures

The nasopharynx, oropharynx, hypopharynx and the larynx are examined with the mirror. Frontal and lateral radiographs of the cervical spine should be made to assess the cervical vertebra and the prevertebral soft tissues (the prevertebral soft tissues are widened if tumor infiltration and destruction of the cervical vertebra is present).

Indications

These include: benign and localized malignant tumors of the posterior pharyngeal wall and of the base of the tongue (lingual thyroid and benign and malignant tumors which have not extended beyond the apex of the angle of the circumvallate papillae; tumors of the base of the tongue tend particularly to infiltrate inferiorly toward the epiglottis via the lymphatic pathway). The view with this method extends over the base of the tongue and the posterior pharyngeal wall down to the laryngeal inlet and the piriform sinus.

Contraindications

These include: tumors situated in the lateral part of the pharynx or extending to the lateral wall of the pharynx, the tonsil, the faucial pillars and the prevertebral fascia. Extension of the tumor or its lymph node metastases to the internal or common carotid artery, distant metastases and serious general disorders are absolute contraindications.

Note

Depending on the findings, the procedure described above can be extended or modified at any time; the typical procedure described should serve only as a guideline. If the tumor extends to the epiglottis, the median pharyngotomy can be extended by a perpendicular T-incision (Fig. 14.40) for simultaneous frontal resection of the involved part of the larynx.

Principles of the Operation

Access is gained to the oropharynx with a good view over the base of the tongue and the posterior pharyngeal wall so that localized benign and malignant tumors can be removed radically.

Preparation for Surgery

The **position** of the patient on the operating table is as for external operations on the neck.

Anesthesia

Intubation anesthesia is used, preceded if necessary by a tracheostomy.

If *local anesthesia* is to be used, it is injected subcutaneously in a horizontal direction over the hyoid bone. If the base of the tongue is involved, injection is done with a long cannula radiating from a point just above the hyoid bone into the base of the tongue. The cannula should be guided with a finger introduced within the mouth. The superior laryngeal nerve is blocked on both sides. The thyrohyoid membrane is always infiltrated.

We prefer tracheal intubation anesthesia.

Special Instruments

Special instruments are not necessary for this operation except for electrocautery equipment and suitable attachments.

Operative Technique

Removing a malignant tumor of the oropharynx from an incision along the anterior border of the sternomastoid muscle must always be preceded by neck dissection on the side most involved (the other side is dealt with 3 weeks later).

A curved skin incision is then made over the hyoid bone from one sternomastoid muscle to the other (Fig. 14.40). The subcutaneous tissue and the platysma are divided at the same time (Fig. 14.41).

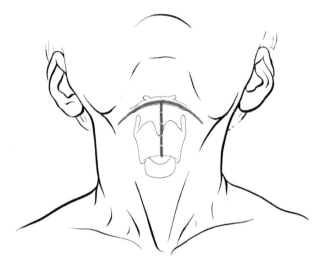

Fig. 14.40   Transverse skin incision for median pharyngotomy: The broken line shows an extension of the skin incision to provide a better view and for simultaneous frontal resection of the larynx if necessary.

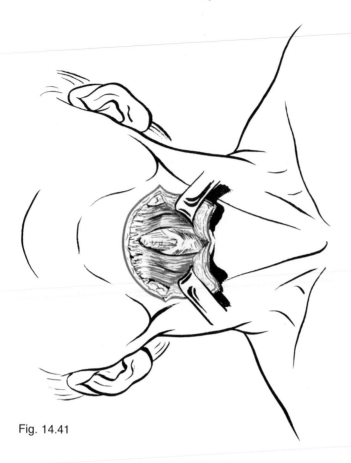

Fig. 14.41

The superficial veins of the neck are ligated and divided. The cervical fascia is divided. The strap muscles are divided immediately inferior to the hyoid bone in order to preserve the superior laryngeal nerve and the accompanying vessels (Fig. 14.42).

The muscular insertions superior to the hyoid bone are similarly divided with cutting diathermy (Fig. 14.43).

The body of the hyoid bone is freed by dividing the fascia lying posterior to it from above and below by resection of the central part of the hyoid bone. Cutting diathermy stops most of the bleeding at this point.

The median thyrohyoid ligament and the neighboring thyrohyoid membrane are divided transversely. The incision must not be carried too far laterally in order to preserve the vessels and the superior laryngeal nerve. The pre-epiglottic fat pad is resected if the tumor is malignant. The pharyngeal mucosa bulges forward, after this.

The mucosa is incised carefully and then the pharynx is opened widely to provide a good

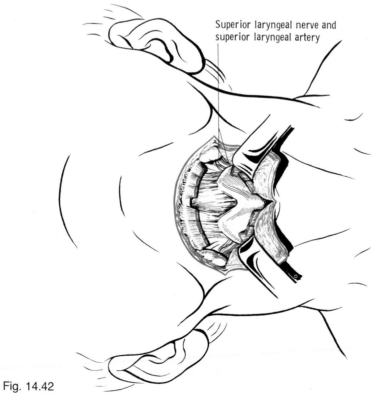

Superior laryngeal nerve and superior laryngeal artery

Fig. 14.42

view of the neighboring base of the tongue. A stay suture is placed in the epiglottis; it should be pulled anteriorly and inferiorly (Fig. 14.44).

The tumor of the base of the tongue or the posterior pharyngeal wall is now resected with cutting diathermy. The borders of the tumor can be easily palpated at this time.

Hemostasis after removal of a tumor of the base of the tongue is achieved by unilateral ligation of the lingual artery during the preceding neck dissection. Bilateral ligation carries the danger of necrosis of the entire tongue.

The resulting defect is closed with deep sutures. If the tumor is on the posterior pharyngeal wall, a split or full-thickness skin graft can be introduced if it is not possible to achieve direct closure after undermining the neighboring tissues in a benign tumor.

The wound is now closed. Closure is easy following resection of the hyoid bone, particularly if relaxation is achieved by elevating the head and bringing the chin downward.

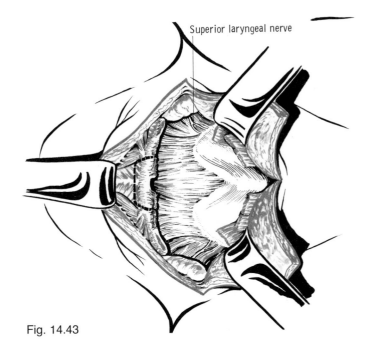

Fig. 14.43

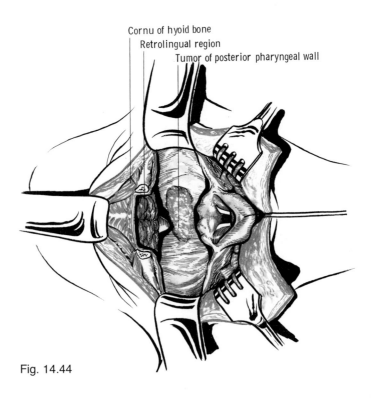

Fig. 14.44

Important Modifications and Surgical Alternatives

A similar wide exposure of the oropharynx is achieved with the next method, but the temporarily divided body of the hyoid bone is preserved.

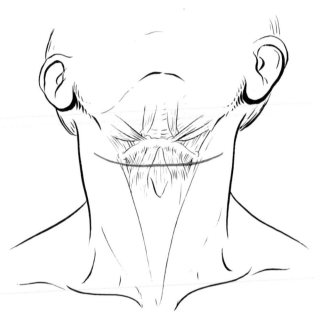

Fig. 14.45

Transverse Transhyoid Pharyngotomy (Réthi's Method)

The indications are identical to those for the method just described. Also, this method provides an equally wide exposure. This operation is also employed by Réthi (1959) for excising a solid or membraneous stenosis of the oropharynx and hypopharynx using suitable flaps. The operative prerequisites, therefore, are the same.

Technique: A 10–12 cm long transverse incision is made at the level of the hyoid bone (Fig. 14.45). The superficial veins are doubly ligated, and divided; the superficial fascia is incised.

The body of the hyoid bone and the lateral cornua (Fig. 14.46) are exposed.

The body of the hyoid bone is undermined with a slightly curved elevator on both sides obliquely from inferoexternal to superointernal. A Gigli saw is introduced or the bone is divided with a Stryker saw (Fig. 14.47). Before the bone is divided, burr holes are drilled in the hyoid bone for the sutures.

The muscles inserted into the *lower edge* of the *body of the hyoid bone* are then divided. The superior tendinous insertion of the stylohyoid and digastric muscle and the insertion of the hyoglossus muscle are divided in the region of the *hyoid cornu*. The suprahyoid musculature remains attached to the body of the hyoid bone and the infrahyoid muscles remain attached to the hyoid cornu.

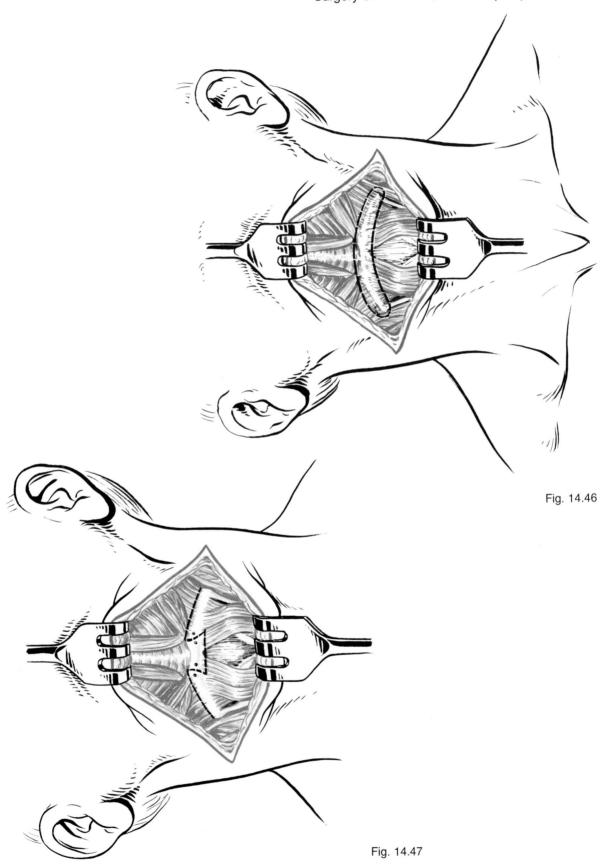

Fig. 14.46

Fig. 14.47

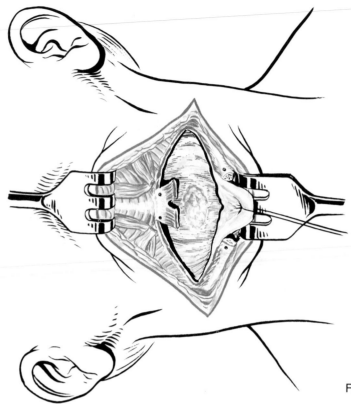

After separating the pre-epiglottic fat pad, the pharynx is opened with a transverse incision at the level of the vallecula. An excellent view of the entire oropharynx is then obtained by retracting the wound edges superiorly and inferiorly (Fig. 14.48).

When the wound is closed, the body of the hyoid bone is fixed to the cornua using the previously made burr holes and wire ligatures; the wound is then closed in layers in the usual way (Fig. 14.49).

Fig. 14.48

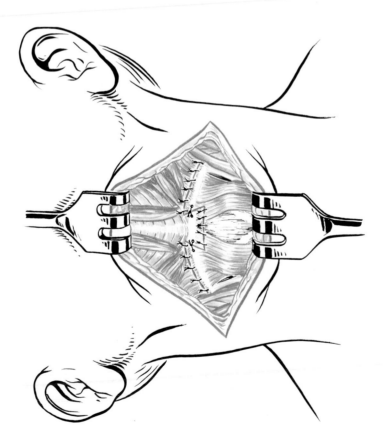

Fig. 14.49

Pietrantoni's Transhyoid Pharyngotomy

Without doubt this method permits the widest access to the oropharynx since the view of the base of the tongue, the epiglottis and vallecula is excellent and the entire area including the preepiglottic space down to the petiolus of the epiglottis can be resected en bloc. The subsequent disturbance of swallowing can be partially compensated by ensuring that the resection does not include the apex of the circumvallate line.

Technique: A preliminary tracheostomy is always necessary.

A wide transverse incision is made immediately inferior to the hyoid bone through the skin and platysma from one sternomastoid muscle to the other.

The superficial veins are ligated and the superficial fascia is divided.

The muscles are divided superiorly and inferiorly, not only from the body but also from the cornua.

The entire hyoid bone is resected including the cornua.

The thyrohyoid membrane is divided horizontally superior and lateral to the superior laryngeal nerve. The incision runs inferiorly to the superior edge of the thyroid cartilage and passes posterior to it so that the petiolus can be freed and divided (Fig. 14.50).

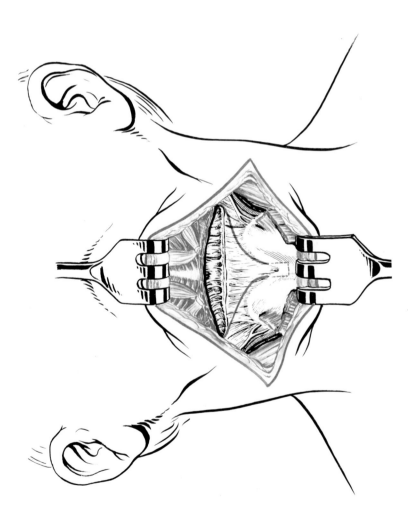

Fig. 14.50

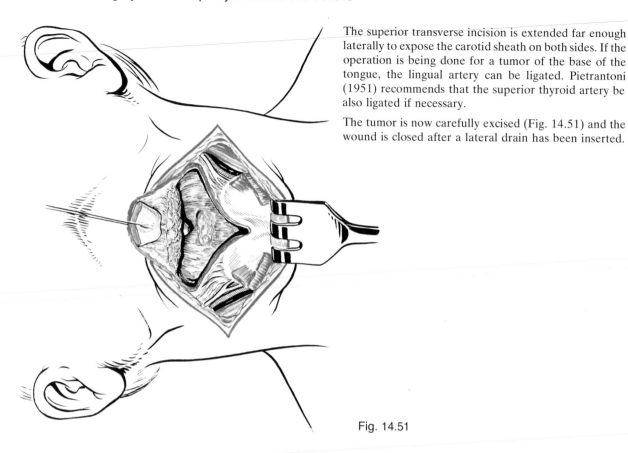

The superior transverse incision is extended far enough laterally to expose the carotid sheath on both sides. If the operation is being done for a tumor of the base of the tongue, the lingual artery can be ligated. Pietrantoni (1951) recommends that the superior thyroid artery be also ligated if necessary.

The tumor is now carefully excised (Fig. 14.51) and the wound is closed after a lateral drain has been inserted.

Fig. 14.51

Transmandibular Access

Transmandibular access is a worthwhile procedure for tumors of the posterior pharyngeal wall.

Conley's Transmandibular Pharyngotomy

Indications

This operation is restricted to radioresistant, circumscribed tumors of the posterior pharyngeal wall or the center of the base of the tongue (see Chap. 13) without regional metastases.

Principles of the Operation

Access is gained through the center of the lower lip, the mandible and the tongue. This provides an excellent view of the operative field. The advantage of the method is that sensory or motor symptoms do not occur. In addition the external incision in the lower lip is not disfiguring.

Anesthesia

Endotracheal intubation anesthesia is used.

Operative Technique

A median incision is made through the lower lip, curved around the chin (see Fig. 14.55) and then continued to the thyroid notch. Small vessels are coagulated and larger ones are ligated. The mandible is split in the midline by a step incision (see Fig. 14.54). The incision in the bone is made with a Gigli or Stryker saw after the external and internal periosteum has been elevated. Corresponding small burr holes must first be made on both sides (see Fig. 14.54).

Next the tongue is split back to its base in the midline, and the resulting wound in the mandible, tongue and base of the tongue is widely retracted with hooks. This provides a satisfactory view of the oropharynx (Fig. 14.52). The tumor can now be freed from the prevertebral fascia and removed with an adequate margin. The prevertebral fascia must be preserved as far as possible. The resulting large defect is covered with a split-skin graft from the upper thigh (Fig. 14.53).

(Application of this operation for tumors of the base of the tongue is described in Chapter 13).

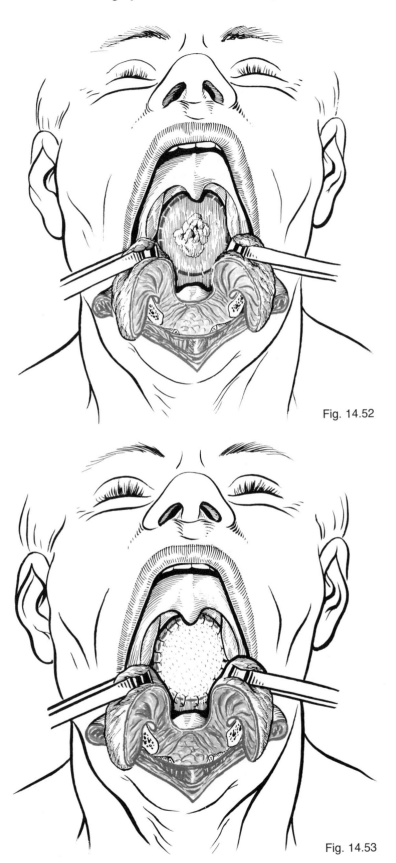

Fig. 14.52

Fig. 14.53

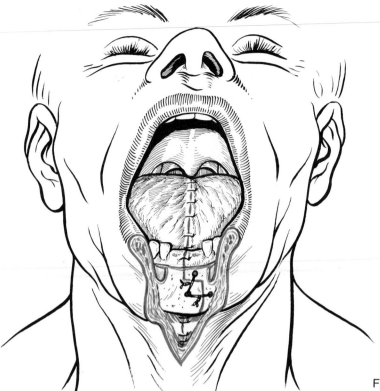

Inverting mucosal sutures are now introduced into the tongue, deep chromic catgut sutures are used for the muscles, and the floor of the mouth is sutured. The mandible is reunited with wire sutures (Fig. 14.54) and the lower lip is sutured (Fig. 14.55) using monofilament nylon. The mandible is fixed to the upper jaw for 4 to 6 weeks by intermaxillary fixation to guarantee immobilization and to prevent pseudoarthrosis. A plaster of Paris impression as well as plates for the upper and lower jaw must be prepared before the operation.

Fig. 14.54

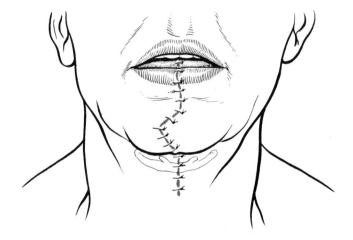

Fig. 14.55

Lateral Pharyngotomy

Indications

- Tumors of the lateral part of the base of the tongue with extension to the lateral wall of the pharynx and the piriform fossa. Tumors of the posterior pharyngeal wall.

Principle of the Operation

The principle of the operation is to create access for resecting a tumor which has spread superiorly and deeply into the oropharynx.

Anesthesia

Local anesthesia is induced by infiltration of the entire operative field. Intubation anesthesia after a preliminary tracheostomy is preferable. A tracheostomy is only essential when an oral intubation tube will get in the way because the tumor is extensive.

Landmarks and Danger Points

Damage to important nerves (hypoglossal and lingual nerve) and to the large vessels (lingual artery) are the main dangers.

Operative Technique

A slightly curved, convex skin incision is made from the angle of the jaw to the center of the hyoid bone or to a point just inferior to the center of the chin (Ward et al. 1959). A neck dissection or a functional neck dissection is always recommended and can be done by extending the incision from the lower border of the curve along the sternomastoid muscle down to the point where the omohyoid muscle crosses the carotid sheath (Fig. 14.56). Extensions of this incision are shown in broken lines in Figure 14.56.

The subcutaneous tissue and platysma are divided, and the external jugular vein is doubly ligated and divided. The flap, skin and platsyma are elevated superiorly as far as the inferior border of the mandible.

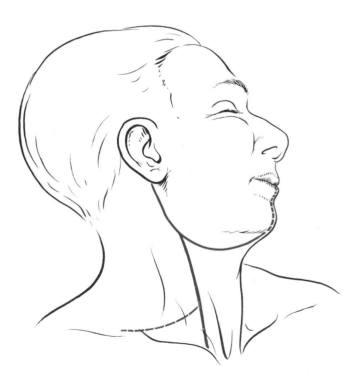

Fig. 14.56

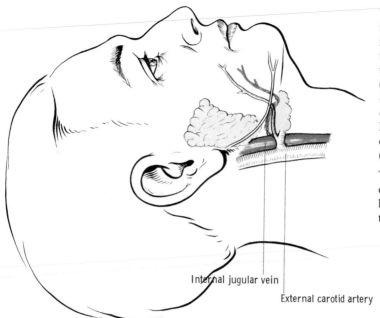

The inferior division of the facial nerve runs in the area of the submandibular triangle immediately medial to the fascia and maintains a constant relationship to the facial artery and vein where they cross the mandible (Fig. 14.57). Both vessels are doubly ligated immediately superior to the submandibular gland and then divided and elevated. In this way the nerve is removed from the operative area and damage is prevented (Legler 1961) (Fig. 14.58).

The fascia is divided along the inferior edge of the gland, immediately superior to the hyoid bone (Fig. 14.58) and turned up over the edge of the mandible (Fig. 14.59).

Internal jugular vein

External carotid artery   Fig. 14.57

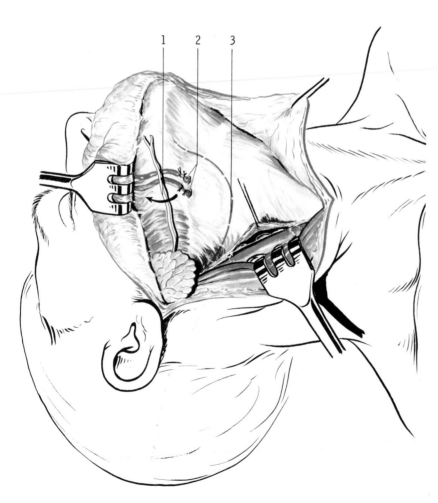

Fig. 14.58

1 = Marginal mandibular
    branch of the facial nerve
2 = Facial artery and vein,
    ligated
3 = Incision in the fascia along
    the inferior edge of the
    submandibular gland

The submandibular gland is removed together with the lymph nodes of the submandibular space. The gland is dissected bluntly with forceps or scissors. The facial artery, its branches and accompanying veins are freed and ligated at its posterior edge. The submandibular duct is also ligated. The gland including the lymph nodes can now be removed cleanly (Fig. 14.60). The hypoglossal nerve is elevated from the field; the mylohyoid muscle is opened to expose the lingual artery, which is now isolated, ligated and divided (Fig. 14.60).

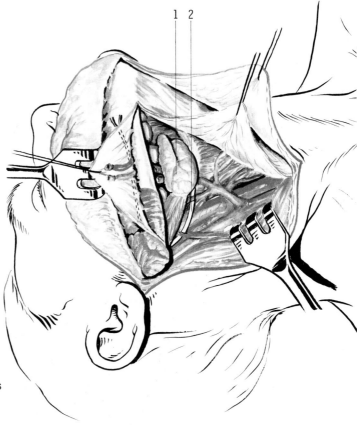

Fig. 14.59
1 = Submandibular gland, dissected from its bed
2 = Hypoglossal nerve

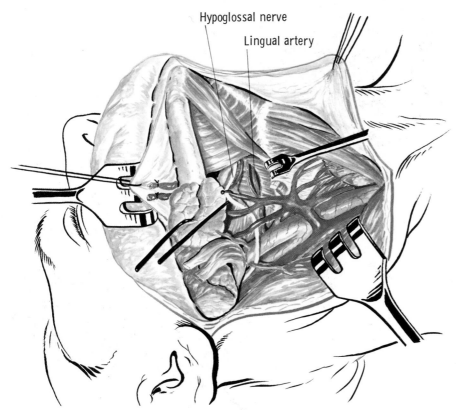

Hypoglossal nerve
Lingual artery

Fig. 14.60

The tendinous insertion of the posterior belly of the digastric muscle and the stylohyoid muscle are divided from the cornu of the hyoid bone, exposing the lateral pharyngeal wall widely (Fig. 14.61). The vessels crossing this space are divided.

The lateral pharyngeal wall is opened in the same direction as the skin incision (Fig. 14.61, black broken line), and retractors are introduced to provide access to the oropharynx (Fig. 14.62). The tumor can now be excised with a wide margin. The pharyngeal wall is sutured carefully. This can usually be carried out easily after the posterior pharyngeal wall has been mobilized. The wound is closed in layers and a suction drain left in place (Fig. 14.63).

Rarely, it is necessary to make a pharyngostoma when direct suture of the pharynx is not possible due to the size of the defect. This pharyngostoma is later closed by a secondary plastic procedure after healing has occurred.

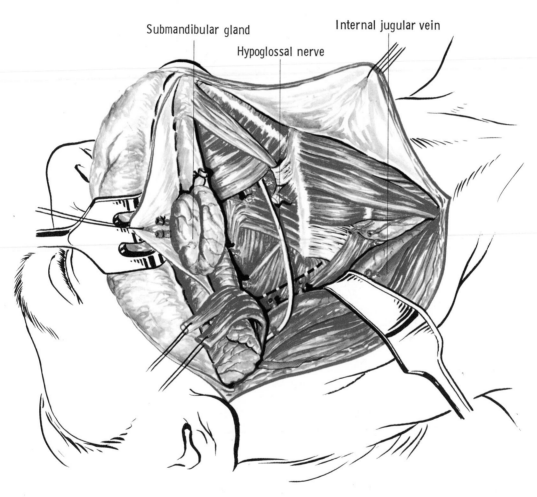

Submandibular gland   Hypoglossal nerve   Internal jugular vein

Fig. 14.61

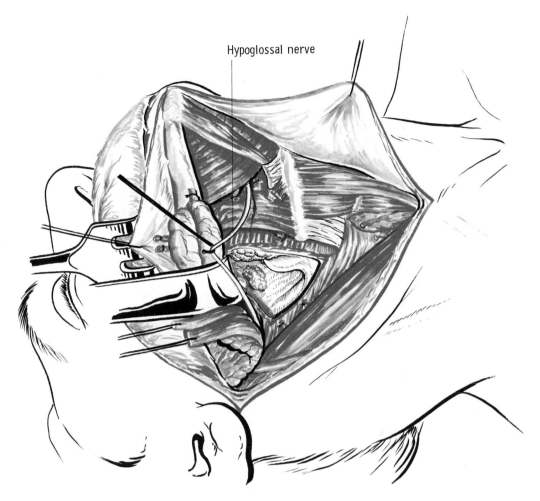

Hypoglossal nerve

Fig. 14.62

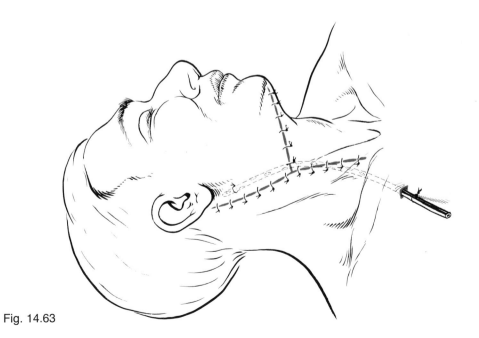

Fig. 14.63

Important Modifications and Surgical Alternatives

Pietrantoni's Lateral Pharyngotomy

The *principle of this operation* is to use both the digastric and carotid triangles as routes of access at the same time in order to improve the view of the oropharynx considerably. A neck dissection can be incorporated in the operation.

Anesthesia. Endotracheal anesthesia is used after a previous tracheotomy.

Technique. A curved skin incision is made from the angle of the jaw to the center of the chin and from the hyoid bone in the midline, proceeding inferiorly to the inferior edge of the thyroid cartilage. Here the incision curves externally toward the sternomastoid muscle and is continued to the sternal notch (Fig. 14.64). This provides good access and avoids having the layers of sutures directly over each other. A neck dissection is carried out in conjunction with clearance of the submandibular space (see p. 403).

The posterior belly of the digastric and the stylohyoid muscle are divided from the hyoid bone (Fig. 14.65).

The superior laryngeal, lingual and facial arteries crossing this space are ligated.

Next, an incision is made in the middle and inferior constrictor muscles from the angle of the jaw to the level of the cricoid cartilage; the pharyngeal mucosa is opened in the same direction. From the upper end, an incision is made in an anterosuperior direction through the hyoglossus and mylohyoid muscles (Fig. 14.65).

An incision is now made in the mucosa of the tonsillolingual sulcus. It is extended anteriorly in the floor of the mouth as necessary.

Wide access to the entire base of the tongue and the lateral and posterior walls of the pharynx is obtained by retracting with sharp hooks. This wide incision also permits a view of the vallecula and the epiglottis.

The tumor is excised with cutting diathermy; the wound is closed carefully in layers with monofilament nylon after a suction drain has been introduced.

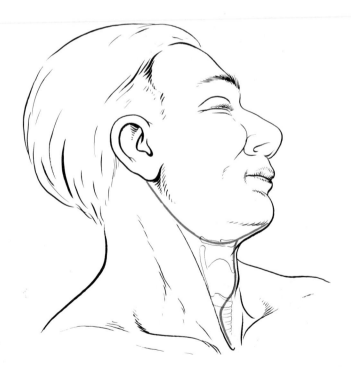

Fig. 14.64

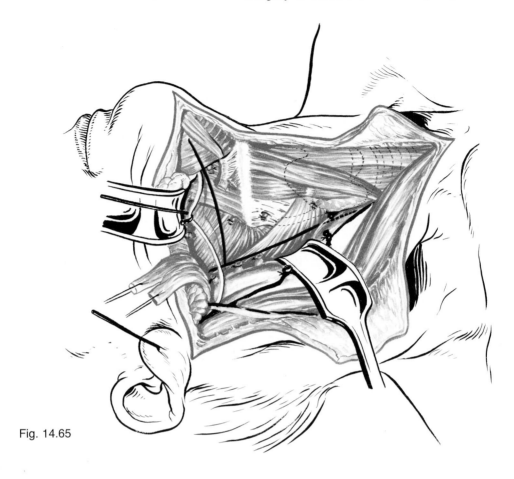

Fig. 14.65

Postoperative Care

Treatment with high doses of antibiotics is indicated after all forms of pharyngotomy because of the danger of infection. The suction drain is removed on the second or third day. If there is difficulty with swallowing, a nasogastric tube is introduced.

Postoperative Complications

Wound infection is the principal complication. It is treated with high doses of antibiotics and requires external drainage.

Hemorrhage is treated by exposing and ligating the bleeding vessel.

Functional Sequelae

The principal functional disturbance results from damage to the superior laryngeal nerve. This is particularly serious if the nerve is damaged on both sides. Obviously, a nasogastric tube should be introduced immediately; Pietrantoni (1951) even advises a gastrostomy. Swallowing disturbances seldom occur following conservative types of median pharyngotomy.

Monoblock Operation for Malignant Mesopharyngeal Tumors

These operations can be carried out either with or without splitting the mandible, after its partial removal or after a hemimandibulectomy. Extensive tumors of the lateral and posterior walls of the pharynx or of the tonsil, particularly if they involve the base of the tongue and the retromolar portion of the mandible or the pterygopalatine fossa, are best approached by a partial mandibulectomy or hemimandibulectomy combined with a neck dissection.

Indications

Indications for the major monoblock operation with resection of the mandible are as follows:

● Malignant tumors of the tonsil, particularly with involvement of the retromolar mucosa, the floor of the mouth and the bone of the mandible itself.

● Tumors of the lateral and posterior walls of the ortopharynx with extensive involvement of the base of the tongue.

The tumor must be unilateral, but if a tonsillar carcinoma extends over the tonsilloglossal sulcus deep into the base of the tongue, the line of resection must cross the midline.

Principles of the Operation

The principle of the operation is *to remove the primary tumor with its lymphatic drainage en bloc via a neck dissection.* To ensure conformity to the principle of radicality, the resected part of the mandible must be included on the specimen. A hemimandibulectomy is preferable to a partial resection of the horizontal or ascending ramus or of the angle of the jaw. This procedure considerably improves the access, provides an excellent view of the entire operative area and facilitates apposition of the wound edges when the large pharyngeal defect is closed. If necessary, this may be supplemented by a reconstructive procedure.

Preparation for Surgery

The **position** of the patient on the operating table is the usual one for external operations on the neck; the head is turned to the healthy side.

The **location** of the surgical team is the same as for external operations on the neck.

Special Instruments

In addition to the usual instruments for soft tissue and bone surgery, a Gigli and a Stryker saw are necessary.

Anesthesia

General intubation anesthesia is definitely required.

Since a *tracheostomy* is *always* necessary to prevent aspiration pneumonia, the intubation is via this route. The tendency to bleed can be reduced by additionally infiltrating the soft tissues with a vasoconstrictor solution.

Operative Technique

A modified Kocher's incision (Fig. 14.66) or a double Y-incision (Fig. 14.67) are used. Kocher's incision is modified by extending the inferior end over the origin of the sternomastoid muscle and then horizontally over the clavicle (see Fig. 14.66). If necessary, the incision is extended superiorly from the chin through the lower lip in the midline so that the entire lower part of the cheek can be turned backward. Rankow's incision is also useful (see Chap. 13).

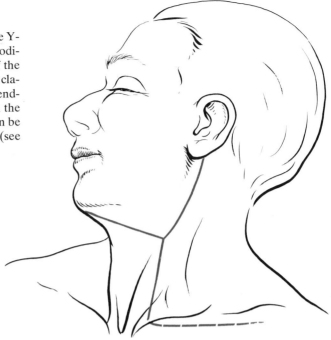

Fig. 14.66 Kocher's modified skin incision for the monoblock operation.

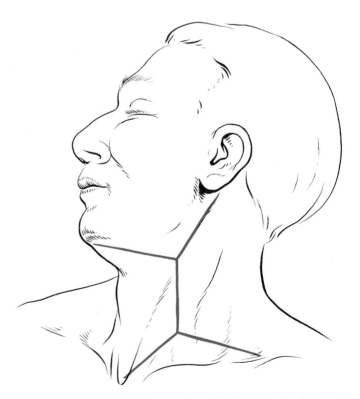

Fig. 14.67 Double Y-incision for the monoblock operation.

The operation begins inferiorly, just above the clavicle, with a neck dissection carried out in the usual manner.

The hypoglossal nerve is preserved as long as tumor extension to the entire half of the tongue and the floor of the mouth does not make this a waste of time.

Anesthesia of the carotid bifurcation abolishes the carotid sinus reflex.

The external carotid artery, which is recognized by its branches, is ligated superior to the superior thyroid artery. The individual branches (lingual artery, ascending pharyngeal artery and facial artery) should also be ligated individually.

Although the internal jugular vein is usually ligated and divided where it passes under the belly of the digastric muscle, in this case it is followed to the base of the skull after the posterior belly of the digastric muscle and the stylohyoid and styloglossus muscles have been divided (Fig. 14.68). It is ligated and divided at this point.

The submental and submandibular spaces with the enclosed lymph nodes are included in the block.

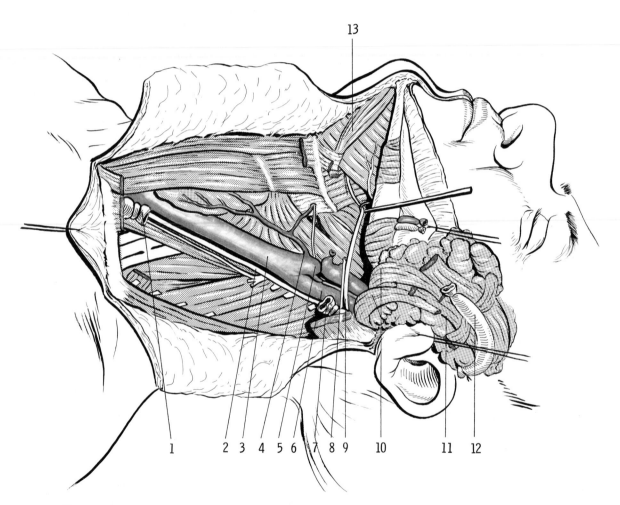

Fig. 14.68   Anatomical relationships during neck dissection:

1 = Lower end of the internal jugular vein
2 = Vagus nerve
3 = Common carotid artery
4 = Superior thyroid artery
5 = External carotid artery
6 = Internal carotid artery
7 = Superior end of the internal jugular vein
8 = Facial artery, ligated
9 = Hypoglossal nerve
10 = Posterior belly of the digastric muscle and the stylohyoid muscle
11 = Sternomastoid muscle
12 = Jugular vein on the block
13 = Anterior belly of the digastric muscle

Before dividing the fascia covering the submandibular gland immediately superior to the hyoid bone, the facial vein and the posterior facial vein are doubly ligated immediately superior to the gland and are turned up so that the lowest division of the facial nerve running over the venous bifurcation is preserved (see Figs. 14.57, 14.58).

In order to reduce the danger of infection of the vascular spaces due to opening of the oral and pharyngeal cavities, the entire supraclavicular area is closed off by stitching the skin flap to the cervical muscles at the level of the hyoid bone. Drainage of wound secretions is assured by a suction drain. The drain is introduced through the skin and brought out below the clavicle (see Fig. 14.63).

Hemimandibulectomy now follows (see Chap. 13). We almost always split the lower lip, as described by Kocher, because this not only facilitates removal of the mandible but also permits a better view of the surgical field. Splitting or partial resection of the mandible follows the principles laid down in Chapter 13 (Fig. 14.69).

Resection of the *anterior* belly of the digastric and of the geniohyoid and hyoglossus muscles is only required during a radical operation for an oropharyngeal tumor if the disease has extended to the floor of the mouth.

After incising the oral mucosa at least 1.5 to 2 cm from the edge of the tumor, a view of the entire oropharyngeal area is obtained. The tongue is retracted to the healthy side and the soft tissue incision is extended posteriorly and inferiorly until the entire area lies free.

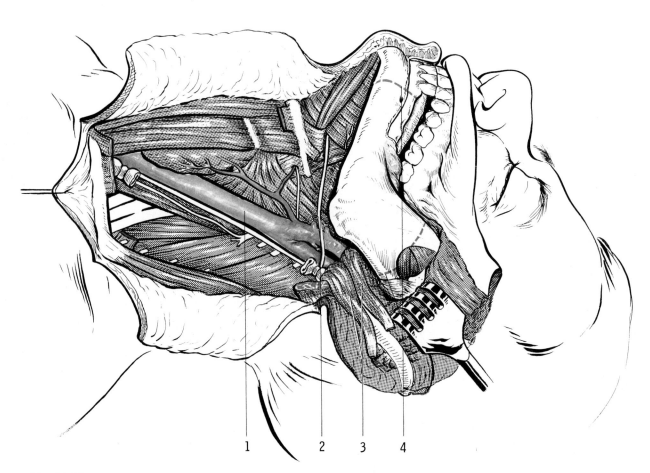

Fig. 14.69

1 = Common carotid artery
2 = Hypoglossal nerve
3 = Digastric muscle (posterior belly) and the stylohyoid muscle included on the block
4 = Anterior and posterior limits of resection

Depending on the extent of the tumor in the tonsillar and parapharyngeal areas, the medial pterygoid and lateral pterygoid and stylopharyngeus muscles must be included in the block (Fig. 14.70).

Frozen section is indicated during the operation if extension of the tumor into the surrounding tissue, particularly into the pterygopalatine fossa, is suspected. In this way the infratemporal fossa can be cleared with cutting diathermy if necessary.

Involvement of the lateral and particularly the posterior pharyngeal walls by the tumor necessitates exposure of the prevertebral fascia, occasionally beyond the midline.

If possible, the prevertebral fascia should be preserved. Dissection of the tumor then is carried out only in the lateral part of the pharyngeal wall which is lined by muscles in order to prevent damaging the prevertebral fascia, which can lead to necrosis of the cervical spine.

The retropharyngeal lymph nodes are often involved and must always be removed in continuity with the block. After cutting around the tumor area along the posterior and lateral pharyngeal wall about 1.5 cm from the tumor, the block is divided from the surrounding tissue and removed together with the neck dissection (Fig. 14.71). The size of the defect of the lateral and posterior pharyngeal walls and of the base of the tongue is determined by the extent of the tumor.

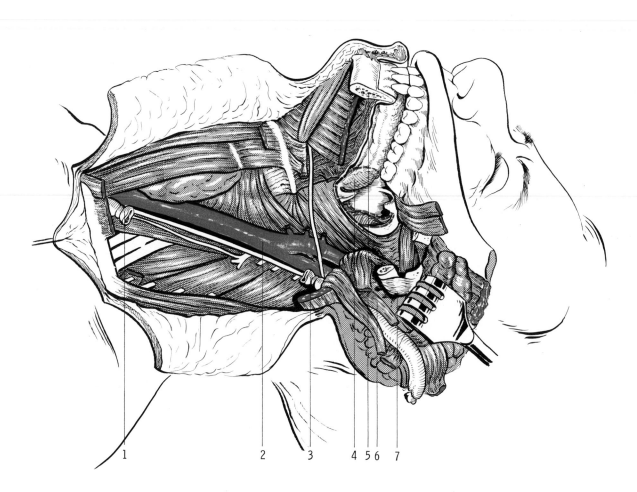

Fig. 14.70

1 = Inferior end of the internal jugular vein
2 = Common carotid artery
3 = Superior end of the internal jugular vein
4 = Wound resulting from excision of a tumor on the posterior pharyngeal wall and the base of the tongue

5 = Anterior saw cut through the mandible
6 = Posterior belly of the digastric muscle and the stylohyoid muscle, reflected posteriorly
7 = Neck dissection specimen

Closure of the wound by undermining the surrounding mucosal edges and direct suture is only possible with small tumors. Resection of the pharyngeal soft tissues including the lymphatic drainage area in the monoblock operation produces a defect so large that reconstructive procedures are necessary to restore the ability to swallow. This is particularly true if the tumor has extended across the midline of the base of the tongue and involved the hypoglossal nerve deep within the body of the tongue.

Such a plastic closure should always be attempted if possible. It is certainly preferable to the creation of a pharyngeal stoma, which should only be necessary in certain cases. The principle of the necessary reconstructive operations is not only closure of the large defect by local or distant flaps (e.g., forehead flap, see Chap. 13) but also more or less complete restoration of the function of the pharynx plus the possibility of velar occlusion. Sometimes such a defect can be closed by rotation flaps from the neighboring mucosa (mucosal-muscle flaps), if necessary from the soft palate. Flaps from the lateral part of the tongue and the dorsum of the tongue are very useful also. The edges of the defect can be undermined and sutured together exactly. The edge of the incision of the tongue is then stitched carefully to the lateral edge of the defect. This method of closure is limited by the size of the remaining tongue stump. At least half of the tongue should be preserved (Conley 1970). This method sufficiently compensates the oropharyngeal defect and swal-

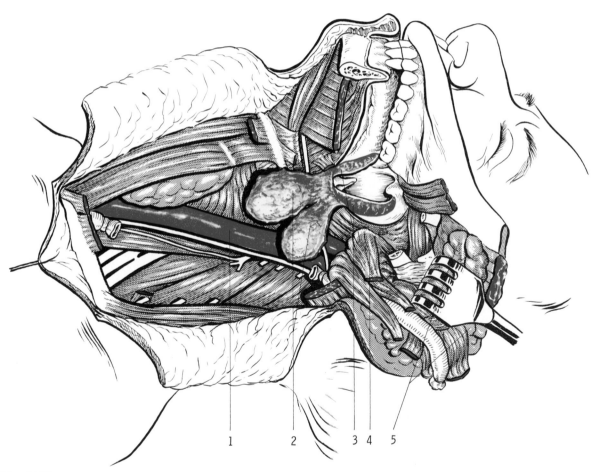

Fig. 14.71

1 = Common carotid artery

2 = Tumor specimen from the posterior pharyngeal wall and the base of the tongue

3 = Wound surfaces on the posterior pharyngeal wall and the base of the tongue

4 = Pterygoid, digastric and stylohyoid muscles, reflected posteriorly

5 = Neck dissection specimen

lowing is only temporarily disturbed. Larger defects of the tonsillar area may be covered by mucosal flaps from the cheek or the floor of the mouth. After this, the resulting defect of the buccal mucosa is easily closed by direct suture. If the defect extends into the soft palate, the buccal soft tissues are elevated, displaced medially and sutured to the edge of the wound of the soft palate.

In large tumors extending into the infratemporal fossa, it is recommended that the soft tissues of the cheek be displaced as far as the inferior surface of the opening of the eustachian tube (Zehn). The results in regard to speech and swallowing are reputed to be good.

Since malignant tumors of the tonsil often extend into the floor of the mouth, this area must be removed en bloc, thereby causing an extensive defect of the floor of the mouth. After the standard resection of the horizontal ramus of the mandible or hemimandibulectomy, the edge of the tongue can be easily sutured to the buccal mucosa. This may be supplemented if necessary by an external pressure bandage. Zehn recommends vertical buried sutures for this. Many authors prefer the introduction of a split-skin graft to improve function (Conley 1970, Mündnich 1960, Rankow and others).

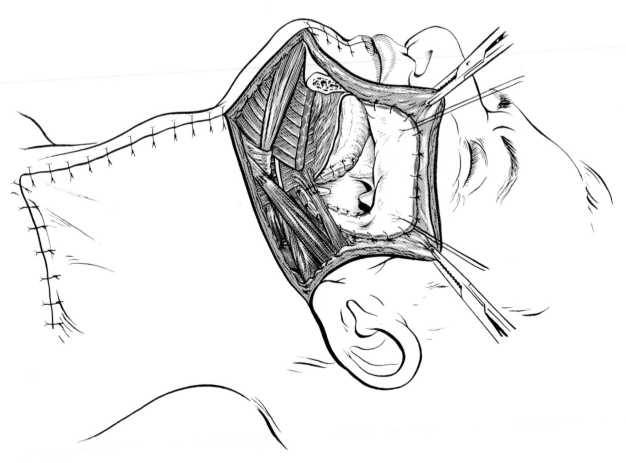

Fig. 14.72

The graft for reconstructing the floor of the mouth is fixed by a muslin pledget; the silk sutures are knotted over it. Conley uses a metal plate padded with foam rubber and fixed with wire. The author has used silicone foam cut to size and fixed with percutaneous wire. The operation described by Dargent (1954) appears to be particularly useful. At the conclusion of the operation, the platysma is freed from the skin flap which is turned upward.

A split-skin graft the size of the pharyngeal defect is attached to the inner surface of the flap and fixed by accurately placed sutures (Fig. 14.72). The edges of the split-skin graft can then be easily sutured into the defect of the pharynx and the floor of the mouth (Fig. 14.73). It is obvious that a previous resection of the mandible is required. The remaining soft tissues of the floor of the mouth, the pharynx and the skin are closed in layers.

Prosthetic management of the stumps of the mandible following partial resection must always be planned with the orthodontist before the operation and should be carried out in cooperation with the prosthetist. The procedures necessary (wire sutures and plastic mandibular splints) for resection of the body of the mandible are described in Chapter 13.

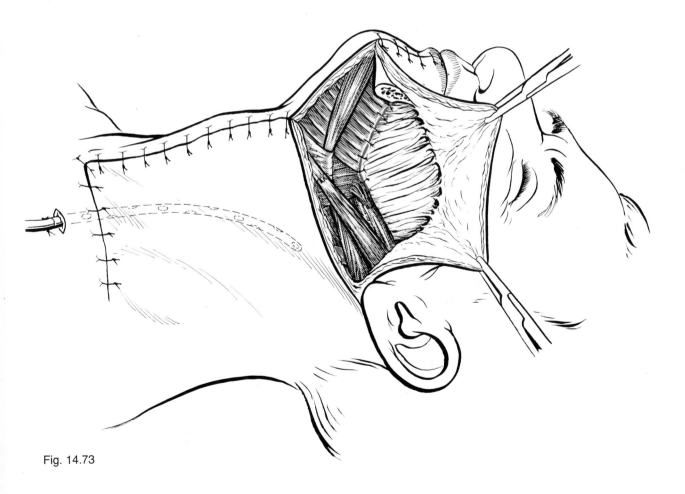

Fig. 14.73

Landmarks and Danger Points

Extreme care should be exercised when using cutting diathermy because of the proximity of the carotid sheath to tumors of the lateral pharyngeal wall and the tonsil. Extreme care is also required when removing tumors of the posterior pharyngeal wall in order to preserve the prevertebral fascia as much as possible. Damage to this structure can cause necrosis of the vertebral bodies.

Rules, Hints and Typical Errors

● The branches of the external carotid artery as well as the artery itself must be ligated with silk. The external carotid artery should always be doubly ligated. Catgut ligatures can easily slip and serious reactionary hemorrhage can result.

● When the mucosal incision is made through the floor of the mouth along the mandible (if the mandible is to be preserved), a 5–6 mm strip of mucosa should be retained along the mandible to facilitate suturing the floor of the mouth later.

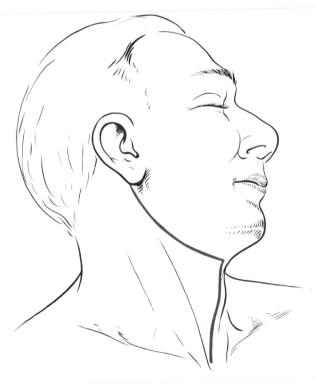

Fig. 14.74 Incision for a monoblock operation without division of the mandible.

● Due to the danger of hematoma or seroma, suction drainage should always be introduced at the end of the operation.

Important Modifications and Surgical Alternatives

Monoblock operations for malignant pharyngeal tumors can also be carried out through a special incision without dividing the mandible (Fig. 14.74) (Raven 1959) or after temporary division of the mandible (Kremen 1951 and Ward et al. 1959). The "pull-through" method is described in Chapter 13. A prerequisite for these operations is that the tumor does not extend into the immediate neighborhood of the bone or involve it. In the latter case, a wide resection of the mandible is required, if possible a hemimandibulectomy. Management of the defect after an extensive resection including part of the floor of the mouth and the base of the tongue is considerably more difficult than after resection of the horizontal and ascending ramus of the mandible, the angle of the jaw or after hemimandibulectomy.

Postoperative Care and Complications

● Obviously the operation must be carried out under massive antibiotic cover for 8 to 10 days.

● Blood should always be available for transfusion in case of serious blood loss.

● The suction drain is removed on the second or third day.

● A nasogastric tube is introduced during the operation.

● If aspiration of secretions occurs during the use of a nasogastric tube, even with a previously created tracheostomy, it is advisable to introduce the tube by means of a cervical esophagotomy. Rügheimer's tracheal cannula provides good protection because it can be blocked off and left in place for several days. Care must be taken, however, to prevent tracheal stenosis.

● The most important postoperative complications are hemorrhage and wound dehiscence with infection of the wound bed.

- Reactionary hemorrhage can easily occur from arteries which were not carefully ligated (see above) or from secondary infection of the wound bed which can lead to a fatal hemorrhage from the carotid vessels. To avoid this problem, the carotid sheath must be protected during the operation itself and before the oral cavity is opened; furthermore the suturing of the pharynx and the floor of the mouth must be carried out exactly. The levator scapulae muscle is recommended for protection of the carotid artery (see Chap. 13).

- The tracheostomy tube should be removed only after swallowing has resumed and after the edema has resolved.

- If movement of the tongue is restricted, it should be mobilized 3 to 4 months later by introducing a split-skin graft.

Functional Sequelae

The most important functional disturbances after surgery on the oropharynx are those affecting speaking, swallowing and chewing. The speaking and swallowing defects caused by extensive operations on the tongue are dealt with in Chapter 13. Defects or fixation of the soft palate by scar tissue lead to rhinolalia aperta. A pharyngoveloplasty with Schönborn-Rosenthal's method is seldom indicated. Removal of a tonsillar carcinoma extending to the base of the tongue and the floor of the mouth produces a large defect. Fixation of the remaining part of the tongue by suturing it to the cheek or the pharyngeal wall as well as closure of the resulting defect considerably affects the mobility of the tongue and leads to further speech disturbances. The vocal function after extensive resection of the tongue is otherwise generally good if the muscles of the floor of the mouth are preserved so that they can partially take over the function of the tongue.

Considerable disturbance of masticatory function is also produced by fixation of the tongue, particularly if the musculature of the floor of the mouth is extensively removed.

Hemimandibulectomy does not cause severe defects of masticatory function if prosthetic treatment of the remaining part of the mandible is begun immediately.

According to Mündnich (1953) the base of the tongue should not be resected if unilateral vocal cord paralysis is present, to prevent disturbances in swallowing. This is recommended because the recurrent laryngeal nerve must be intact if the superior laryngeal nerve is deficient to prevent difficulties in swallowing.

Similar disturbances of swallowing are less apt to occur after resection of *half* the base of the tongue since the larynx is drawn over to the side of the remaining base of the tongue (Taillens 1953). According to Pietrantoni (1951), resection of a tumor of the tongue with simultaneous removal of the hyoid bone should not extend past the circumvallate line since compensation then requires a long time. Cricopharyngeal myotomy can sometimes considerably improve swallowing if it is disturbed, although a serious functional disturbance may resolve spontaneously over a long period of time. The extent of the operation is however limited, particularly in elderly patients where the will to cooperate in function-restoring therapy is often lacking. Furthermore, it should not be forgotten that surgical mortality for an extensive monoblock operation is still quite high.

Operative Procedures for Neurogenic Dysphagia

Etiology

These lesions are caused by paralysis of the glosso-pharyngeal, vagus or hypoglossal nerves due to surgical trauma or tumors, particularly a neurilemmoma. They can also be caused by a fracture of the base of the skull (jugular foramen syndrome) and by operations for cerebellopontine angle tumors.

Principles of the Operation

That portion of the swallowing musculature which is no longer innervated is excised in order to reduce the diameter of the pharynx (to almost half its diameter). After closing the wound, the noninnervated half of the esophageal lumen is put out of use and the new lumen is slowly reinnervated from the healthy side.

Operative Technique

A skin incision is made along the anterior edge of the sternomastoid muscle. The subcutaneous tissue, platysma and superficial cervical fascia are divided. The incision is extended by blunt dissection between the carotid sheath and the thyroid gland or the lateral wall of the hypopharynx toward the prevertebral fascia.

The lateral pharyngeal wall is exposed between the lower pole of the tonsil and the upper end of the esophagus.

The paralyzed part of the hypopharynx is now excised. The section to be excised can be recognized by the atrophic muscle fibers, particularly when the patient swallows if the operation is carried out under local anesthetic (the operation can be carried out as early as 3 to 4 weeks after removal of a tumor).

A cricopharyngeal myotomy is done in the same way as in the operation for a pharyngeal pouch.

The pharynx is closed with an inverting 3×0 catgut suture through all layers. The skin is sutured; suction drainage is applied. A feeding tube is left in for several days.

Postoperative Complications

These are only to be expected if wound dehiscence is present. In such cases the skin wound should be reopened and drainage applied.

Bibliography

Conley, J. J.: Concepts in Head and Neck Surgery. Thieme, Stuttgart 1970

Dargent, M.: La pharyngectomie latérale transmaxillaire avec pharyngoplastie immediate. J. Chir. (Paris) 70: 810, 1954

Dargent, M.: Le cancer de la langue. Bull. Soc. Int. Chir. 16: 523, 1957

Denecke, H. J.: Die oto-rhino-laryngologischen Operationen. In: Allgemeine und spezielle chirurgische Operationslehre, ed. by N. Guleke, R. Zenker. Springer, Berlin 1953

Denecke, H. J.: Korrektur des Schluckaktes bei einseitiger Pharynx- und Larynxlähmung. H. N. O. 14: 351, 1961

Falk, P.: Entwicklungsgeschichte, Anatomie, Mißbildungen, Physiologie und Pathophysiologie des Rachens (einschließlich Tonsillen). In: Hals-Nasen-Ohren-Heilkunde, Vol. II/1, ed. by J. Berendes, R. Link, F. Zöllner. Thieme, Stuttgart 1963

Falk, P., H. Maurer: Die entzündlichen Erkrankungen des Rachens. In: Hals-Nasen-Ohren-Heilkunde, Vol. II/1, ed. by J. Berendes, R. Link, F. Zöllner. Thieme, Stuttgart 1963 (p. 71)

Herrmann, A.: Gefahren bei Operationen an Hals, Ohr und Gesicht und die Korrektur fehlerhafter Eingriffe. Springer, Berlin 1968

Kremen, A. J.: Cancer of the tongue. – A surgical technique for a primary combined en bloc resection of the tongue, floor of the mouth and cervical lymphatics. Surgery 30: 227, 1951

Krönlein: Über Pharynxcarcinom und Pharynxexstirpation. Beitr. Chir. 19: 61, 1897

Legler, U.: Die Verletzung des Ramus marginalis mandibulae des N. facialis, ihre Verhütung und Behandlung. Z. Laryng. Rhinol. 40: 399, 1961

Menzel, H., R. Maurer: Insufflation oder Intubation bei Adeno-tonsillektomie. Z. Laryng. Rhinol. 5ß: 412, 1971

Miehlke, A.: Über den heutigen Stand der Chirurgie des Zungenkarzinoms. Z. Laryng. Rhinol. 38: 525, 1959

Mündnich, K.: Neue Wege bei der Radikaloperation des Zungenkrebses. Arch. Ohren-, Nasen-, Kehlkopfheilk. 163: 379, 1953

Mündnich, K.: Die malignen Tumoren des Mesopharynx. Arch. Ohren-, Nasen-, Kehlkopfheilk. 176: 237, 1960

Mündnich, K.: Die Geschwülste des Mesopharynx. In: Hals-Nasen-Ohren-Heilkunde, Vol. II/1, ed. by J. Berendes, R. Link, F. Zöllner. Thieme, Stuttgart 1963 (p. 32)

Naumann, H. H.: Die Lymphknotenmetastasen beim Krebs der Mundhöhle und der oberen Luftwege. Dtsch. Med. Wochenschr. 82 (1957) 1263

Pernkopf, E.: Topographische Anatomie des Menschen, Vol. III. Urban & Schwarzenberg, Vienna 1952

Pietrantoni, L.: La chirurgia dei tumori della base della lingua. Arch. Ital. Otol. 62: 477, 1951

Portmann, G.: Voie d'abord de la base de la langue. 45e Congrès Franç. d'O. R. L., 1947

Portmann, G.: L'ablation du cancer de la base de la langue par voie latérale. Rev. Laryng. (Bordeaux) 76: 1, 1955

Portmann, G.: Traité de Technique Operatoire oto-rhino-laryngologique, Vol. II. Masson, Paris 1962

Raven, R. W.: Carcinoma of the pharynx. In: Operative Surgery, ed. by Ch. Rob, R. Smith. Butterworth, London 1959

Réthi, A.: Chirurgie der Verengerungen der oberen Luftwege. Thieme, Stuttgart 1959

Ritter, R.: Gesicht, Gesichtsschädel, Kiefer. In: Allgemeine und spezielle chirurgische Operationslehre, ed. by N. Guleke, R. Zenker. Springer, Berlin 1956

Schwab, W.: Die Operationen an Nase, Mund und Hals, 5th edn., Vol. II. Barth, Leipzig 1964

Seifert, A.: Die Operationen an Nase, Mund und Hals, 3rd edn. Kabitzsch, Leipzig 1936

Stierlen, G.: Zur Tonsillektomie in Lokalanästhesie und Narkose (ein neuer Mundsperrer). Z. Laryngol. Rhinol. 36: 605, 1957

Stierlen, G.: Über Durchführung, Vorteile und Gefahren der Narkose-Tonsillektomie. H. N. O. 9: 241, 1961

Taillens, J. P.: Les limites de la chirurgie fonctionelle en cancérologie pharyngée. Pract. Oto-rhino-laryng. (Basel) 15: 180, 1953

Theissing, G.: Kurze HNO-Operationslehre, Vol. I. Thieme, Stuttgart 1971

Ward, G. E., et al.: Cancer of the oral cavity and pharynx and results of treatment by means of the composite operation. Ann. Surg. 150: 202, 1959

Ward, G. E., J. W. Hendrick: Tumors of the Head and Neck. Williams & Wilkins, Baltimore 1950

Zange, J.: Die Mandeln als Quelle von Herdinfektionen. Arch. Ohren-, Nasen-, Kehlkopfheilk. 156: 333, 1949

Zange, J.: Diagnostische und therapeutische Probleme bei bösartigen Geschwülsten des Mundrachens. Z. Laryng. Rhinol. 39: 266, 1960

Zehm, S., W. Prott: Die funktionelle Rehabilitation des Schlundes bei Tumoroperationen. Z. Laryng. Rhinol. 50: 776, 1971

15 Surgery of the Salivary Glands and the Extratemporal Portion of the Facial Nerve

By A. Miehlke

Diagnostic Preoperative Procedures

Regardless of the history, the findings on mirror examination and on general examination, the following must be done:

- *Exclusion of systemic diseases* involving the salivary glands by appropriate clinical and laboratory investigation.

- Suitable *radiographs* to exclude cysts of the ascending ramus of the mandible, which can occasionally present as a parotid swelling.

- *Palpation* to determine whether the tumor is mobile or fixed in the retromandibular fossa and whether it is a dumbbell tumor. The latter is determined by palpation posterior to the tonsillar bed. Obviously the neck must be examined for lymph node involvement.

- The *Wasserman reaction* to exclude a syphilitic parotid swelling.

- *Examination of the function of all branches of the facial nerve* to determine invasion of the nerve by the tumor. Invasion accompanied by pain indicates malignancy.

- *Sialography* is not necessary for all parotid tumors and need not be carried out if palpation demonstrates the presence of a tumor beyond any doubt. The true extent and type of the tumor are clarified by the operative findings and histological examination by frozen section during the operation if malignancy is suspected.

In certain cases sialography is definitely indicated, particularly if an inflammatory parotid swelling cannot be excluded with certainty by a clinical examination. In such cases sialography is particularly valuable since it demonstrates the characteristic changes (constriction, stenosis and peripheral ectasia) of chronic parotitis which usually can be clearly differentiated from tumorous processes. It should be stated that there are other swellings of the parotid gland which are not caused by tumors, and these have to be considered in differential diagnosis. Viral sialadenitis, allergic sialadenitis, myoepithelial sialadenitis (Sjögren's syndrome), sialadenoses in endocrine disorders, neurogenic sialadenoses, and finally sialadenoses during antihypertensive treatment. More information on this subject can be found in the literature. (In particular, a report by Haubrich 1976).

Indications

Approximately 70% of all tumors of the parotid gland are benign (fibromas, lymphangiomas, Warthin's tumor or cystic adenolymphomas, true adenomas, etc.). The remaining 30% are malignant. Depending on the size and histological character, 10 to 15% of these tumors can be operated on in such a way that the facial nerve is preserved. The remaining 15 to 20% require partial or complete resection of the facial nerve with all its attendant consequences. If the histological examination, the size and the clinical behavior of the tumor necessitate such a serious decision, any attempt to avoid this procedure will have lethal consequences for the patient. Although the operation may be successful from a medical point of view, the patient may not regard it as quite so gratifying since he must put up with a severe facial deformity. The following pages, therefore, not only illustrate parotidectomy with maintenance of the facial nerve but also show the possibilities for reconstructing lost facial expression.

Parotidectomy with Maintenance of Continuity of the Facial Nerve

Surgical Anatomy

The facial nerve and its branches lie loosely between the lobes of the parotid gland. All branches of the facial nerve run in a plane parallel to the medial surface of the superficial lobe of the parotid gland (Fig. 15.1). Bailey's remark (1941) that "the facial nerve should be looked upon as the meat within a parotid sandwich" humorously and appropriately illustrates the anatomical situation. It makes clear that the parotid gland can be divided into two lobes by the plane of the facial nerve. These lobes can be separated into the so-called superficial lobe and the deep lobe which are joined by an isthmus anterior to the bifurcation of the facial nerve. However, there is no actual separation by *connective tissue* between these two layers!

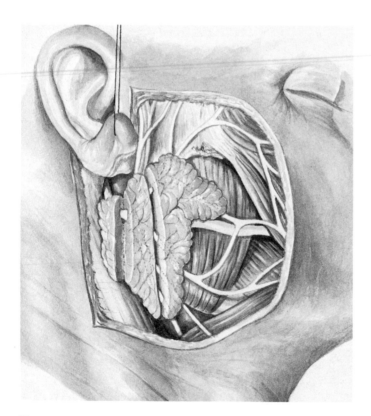

Fig. 15.1 a)   Course of the facial nerve in the parotid gland.

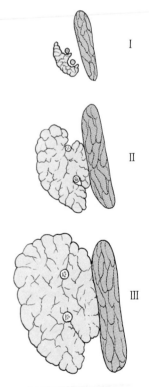

Fig. 15.1 b)   Stages of progressive envelopment (I–III) of the facial nerve by the parotid gland during development (according to McWorther, Martin, Cody).

Principles of the Operation

In contrast to many authors, especially in the Latin countries, we feel that identification of the facial nerve trunk is an important prerequisite for a successful and safe parotidectomy.

After demonstration of the trunk of the facial nerve in the retromandibular fossa, the bifurcation of the nerve is exposed. The entire parotid plexus is then exposed by piecemeal division of the superficial lobe of the parotid gland. The branches of the facial nerve are used as guidelines through the tissue of the parotid gland.

Preparation for Surgery

Premedication. In addition to the usual premedication before the operation, an optimal bloodless field is obtained by infiltrating the area with anesthetic solution.

Positioning of the patient. The head of the patient is raised slightly by tilting the operating table down-ward; the head is turned toward the healthy side. The area is covered with drapes which may cover the face but must leave the region anterior and posterior to the ear widely exposed. The drapes are stitched with nylon sutures to the facial and cervical skin as well as to the skin behind the mastoid process.

Special Instruments

All the instruments necessary for a parotidectomy are included in the following collection:

- Muck's periosteal knife (Fig. 15.2 a).
- Jansen's 14 mm wide elevator (Fig. 15.2 b).
- Freer's straight double elevator, both sides blunt, for protection of the facial nerve during parotid surgery (Fig. 15.2 c).
- Freer's curved double elevator, both sides blunt and extra narrow (2 or 2.5 mm wide), for protection of the facial nerve in its bony canal during drilling (Fig. 15.2 d).

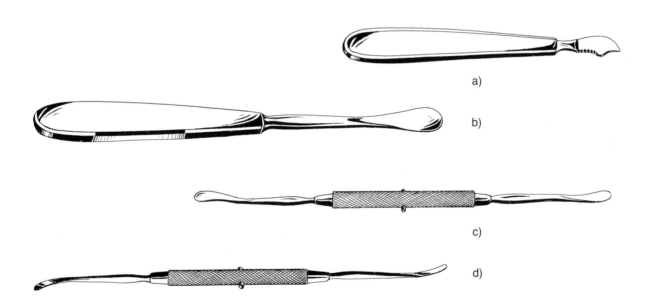

a)

b)

c)

d)

Fig. 15.2   Instruments for parotidectomy
a) Muck's periosteal knife
b) Jansen's raspatory
c) Straight Freer's double elevator
d) Curved Freer's double elevator

- Freer's raspatory, curved anteriorly (Fig. 15.2 e).
- Schönborn's thyroid hooks, angled posteriorly for traction on the parotid (Fig. 15.2 f).
- Curved scissors 14.5 cm long, blunt/sharp points (Fig. 15.2 g).
- Metzenbaum-Lahey's dissecting scissors; extra narrow, curved, 14 cm long, blunt (Fig. 15.2 h).

- Reynold's dissecting scissors; extra narrow, slightly curved (blunt/blunt), 15 cm long for deep dissection (Fig. 15.2 i).
- Joseph's plastic surgery scissors; straight, 14 cm long, sharp/sharp points (Fig. 15.2 j).
- Vanna's dissecting scissors; curved, 8 cm, for dissecting the nerve and for nerve grafts.
- Lempert's excavator right and left for splitting the wall of the facial canal.

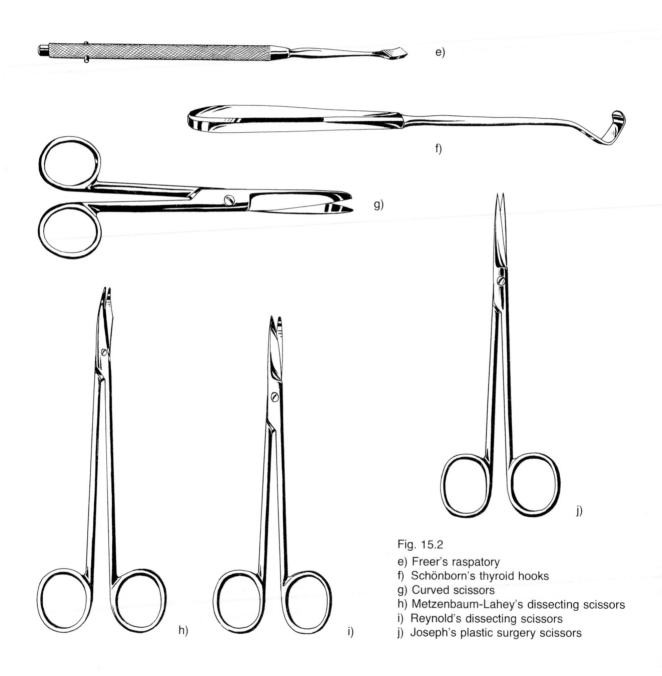

e)

f)

g)

h)

i)

j)

Fig. 15.2
e) Freer's raspatory
f) Schönborn's thyroid hooks
g) Curved scissors
h) Metzenbaum-Lahey's dissecting scissors
i) Reynold's dissecting scissors
j) Joseph's plastic surgery scissors

- Malis' coagulation forceps; bipolar, curved anteriorly, blunt, 15 cm long.
- Malis' coagulation forceps; bipolar, curved anteriorly, sharp, 15 cm long.
- Dissecting forceps without teeth; 13 cm long, fine.
- Dissecting forceps without teeth; very fine, 10 cm long.
- Dissecting forceps without teeth; fine, 10 cm long.
- Narrow dissecting forceps without teeth, 7 cm long.
- Dissecting forceps with teeth; fine, 1:2 teeth, 10 cm long.
- Special needle holder for work in the cerebellopontine angle (Fig. 15.2 k).
- Needle holder with hardened jaws and gold plated handles, 13 cm long (Fig. 15.2 l).
- Battery driven disposable electroprobe (Fig. 15.2 m).
- The following attachments for coagulation forceps:

  microcoagulator, adjustable supply of special current for bipolar coagulation, antistatic foot pedal; lead with special coupling for bipolar forceps.

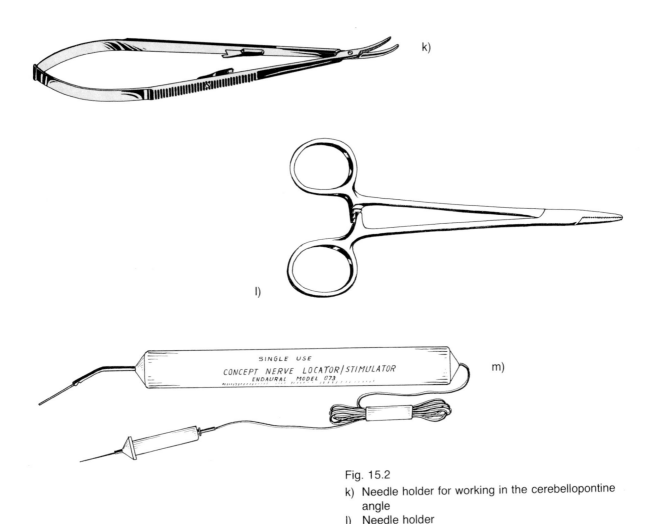

Fig. 15.2
k) Needle holder for working in the cerebellopontine angle
l) Needle holder
m) Disposable stimulator

Operative Technique

Removal of the Superficial Lobe of the Parotid Gland

A Y-shaped incision is made around the ear and toward the angle of the jaw, utilizing one of the skin creases. The size of the incision depends on the size of the tumor. This Y-incision is extended by a 2–3 cm long subsidiary incision which runs anterior to the tragus, just inferior to the hairline and toward the orbit. This incision provides optimal access. The preauricular incision is only partly anterior to the ear. At the level of the external auditory canal, the incision runs inside the canal 2–3 mm posterior to the tragus so that the scar is later invisible. The lobe of the ear is retracted with a nylon stay suture (Fig. 15.3).

The retroauricular incision is carried down to the bone with a periosteal knife as for a mastoidectomy. The cutaneous posterior wall of the external auditory canal is pushed forward with Freer's elevator and Lahey's swabs until the suprameatal spine can be seen posterosuperiorly (Fig. 15.4).

The parotid gland anterior and inferior to the ear is exposed by sharp dissection of the subcutaneous tissue until the anterior edge of the gland can be seen. The knife is tilted slightly away from the gland into the subcutaneous tissues. Since the branches of the facial nerve at the anterior edge of the parotid gland lie very superficially in the fascia over the masseter muscle, elevation of the skin should not be continued this far at this stage. The resulting skin flap is fixed to the drapes with 2 silk stay sutures.

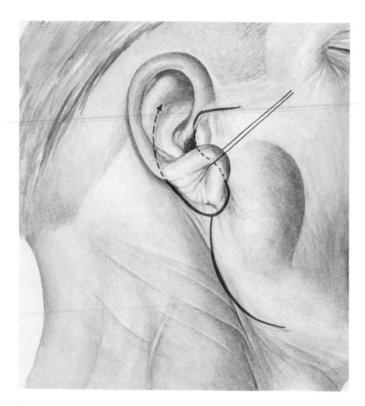

Fig. 15.3   Y-incision for parotidectomy.

The lobe of the ear is now retracted anteriorly using the nylon stay suture, and the incision running toward the angle of the jaw is deepened. At the same time, the posterior edge of the parotid gland is freed without opening its capsule, and is pushed anteriorly with an elevator. During this maneuver the great auricular nerve is often encountered and should always be marked with a black silk suture. This nerve is now divided so that the posteroinferior quadrant of the parotid gland can be mobilized. Sharp dissection is continued along the an-terior edge of the sternomastoid muscle with simultaneous anterior retraction of the posterior part of the parotid gland and slight posterior retraction of the sternomastoid muscle and the posterior belly of the digastric muscle, using both index fingers for this maneuver. The decisive part of the operation follows, i. e., the search for the trunk of the facial nerve in the retromandibular fossa. A surgical maneuver first described by Hogg and Kratz (1958) is used to ensure the success of this part of the operation.

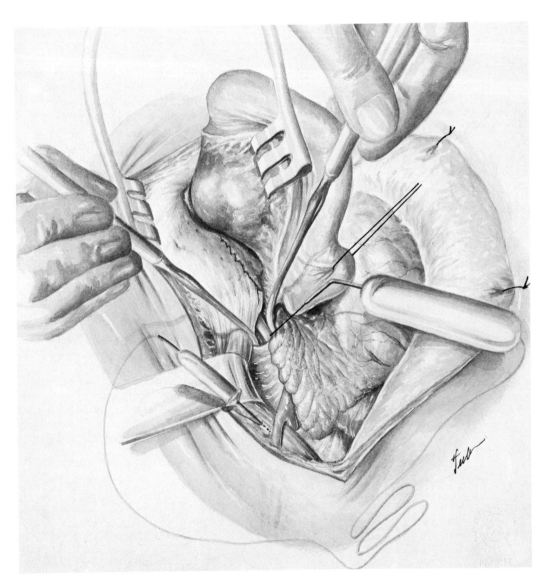

Fig. 15.4

These authors pointed out that the tympanomastoid fissure is an excellent guide for *directly* finding the trunk of the facial nerve anterior to the stylomastoid foramen. *The facial nerve always lies 6–8 mm medial to the end of the tympanomastoid fissure.*

The membranous external auditory canal is now carefully freed deeply from the wall of the meatus until the tympanomastoid fissure has been found running from the suprameatal spine and the end of this fissure. If the parotid conceals the retromandibular fossa, 10 ml of hyaluronidase solution is injected into the posterior part of the parotid to shrink the tissues. Meanwhile, the surgeon is fitted with magnifying glasses ($\times 2.5$). Two Freer's elevators are then introduced deeply into the retromandibular fossa at the end of the tympanomastoid fissure, while the capsule of the posterior part of the parotid gland is retracted anteriorly with a wide elevator or a Schönborn hook. The trunk of the facial nerve is found enclosed in fatty tissue at a depth of 6–8 mm (see above). It runs diagonally through the retromandibular fossa like a silvery white cord; it is approximately as thick as a knitting needle.

Figure 15.4 shows the search for the trunk of the facial nerve with an electric stimulator.

The trunk of the nerve can be expected to be found at the above-mentioned depth from the end of the tympanomastoid fissure; the stylomastoid foramen lies 1 cm medial to this point. Since the trunk of the nerve turns laterally (i.e., toward the operator) immediately after leaving the stylomastoid foramen, it appears to be somewhat more superficial. Often the facial nerve is concealed by one or two branches of the posterior facial vein as it rises out of the depth of the retromandibular fossa. This vessel is coagulated with Malis' bipolar coagulation forceps and divided (current strength: 3–4 milliamps).

Sometimes the trunk of the nerve is not found at the first attempt, but this should be no cause for alarm. A pledget, soaked in epinephrine solution and then wrung out is introduced into the operative defect after consultation with the anesthetist. The surgeon should then wait and relax for 2 to 3 minutes.

During this time of resting, one thing should be kept in mind: It seems highly questionable and probably dangerous to use the styloid process as a guide for finding the trunk of the facial nerve as several authors have suggested. Research by Davis et al. (1956) on 350 specimens showed that the styloid process was absent in one-third of all cases; in many other cases, it was not palpable clinically. Since the facial nerve runs lateral to the styloid process, attempts to find it carry the dissection medial to the nerve, which can be damaged by this approach.

An electro-stimulator may be useful for identifying the facial nerve, particularly in dumbbell tumors which displace the trunk of the nerve laterally from its course and thin it out so that it occasionally looks like a band of connective tissue. Usually the trunk of the nerve can be found without the electroprobe, but this apparatus is still extremely valuable when operating for a recurrence. The stimulator is indispensable for accurately determining the innervation area of individual branches of the nerve when dissecting out the periphery of the nerve. This will be dealt with again later.

After waiting 2 to 3 minutes for the surgeon to rest his eyes, the operation proceeds again exactly as described above. Both elevators are introduced into the surgical field, which can be extended by having the assistant retract the mandible anteriorly. Often the course of the nerve can be estimated or felt before the nerve itself is seen. This phase of the operation is best carried out using magnifying glasses rather than the operating microscope, which does not permit simultaneous assessment of a wide enough area around the course of the nerve. As soon as the shining trunk of the nerve is exposed running diagonally across the retromandibular fossa, a rubber sling (cut from a surgeon's glove) is placed around it.

The next step follows immediately: The dissection toward the periphery by elevating the tissues of the superficial lobe of the parotid gland with the raspatory or Schönborn hooks until the bifurcation of the nerve can be clearly seen. Another short pause can be taken only after this has been done. During this pause a gauze swab soaked in epinephrine is laid in the wound. If halothane anesthesia is used, this practice is not advisable.

Dissection of the branches of the facial nerve follows until the parotid plexus is completely exposed. Depending on the tumor site, the temporofacial or cervicofacial branch is followed. The branch furthest from the tumor should be chosen first. Since most benign tumors of the parotid gland lie in the inferior part of the superficial lobe, the main temporofacial branch is usually exposed first.

We have developed the socalled tunneling technique for this operation. The principle of this operation is segmental division of the superficial lobe of the parotid gland by introducing a Freer's elevator in a peripheral direction directly over the branches of the facial nerve (Fig. 15.5). With the elevator resting on the nerve, the blade of a pair of narrow scissors is introduced into the tunnel over the instrument, and the parotid tissue lying over it is divided

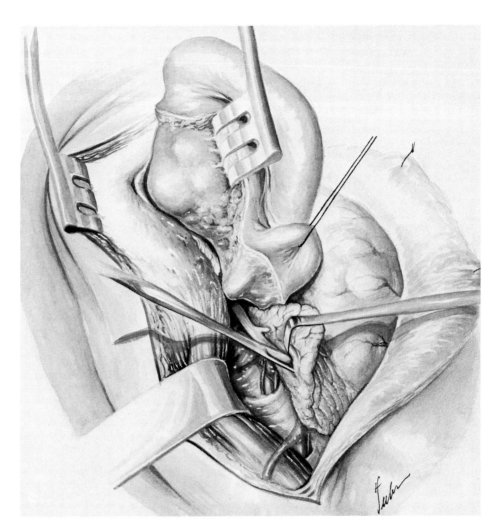

Fig. 15.5

(Fig. 15.6). The operation progresses step by step toward the periphery of the nerve branches so that the mass of the superficial lobe of the parotid gland becomes thinner. Finally, the exposed peripheral branches of the facial nerve turn deeply to reach the muscles of expression. The dissection ends here. By demonstrating the individual branches of the facial nerve in the manner described, the superficial lobe of the parotid gland is divided into several sectors (Fig. 15.7). Since the surgeon always works with the nerve in view, the individual segments of the gland can be removed without danger of damaging the nerve.

Dissection of the tumor-bearing part of the parotid gland is continued by the tunneling technique around the tumor. The intention is to remove the tumor intact together with its surrounding tissue. This is usually successful be-cause the nerve is pushed aside by the tumor. Other techniques are available for malignant tumors (see p. 440).

The parotid duct is inevitably exposed during dissection of the buccal branch. Often several buccal branches running parallel to the duct are present which must be divided in order to remove the gland completely (Fig. 15.8). The peripheral stump of the duct is ligated with chromic catgut to prevent undesirable reflux of saliva from the mouth into the surgical field. Small blood vessels are either ligated or coagulated with Malis' bipolar coagulation forceps. In chronic parotitis the vessels are ligated with chromic catgut; in noninfected tumor cases, with silk or chromic catgut. Figure 15.9 illustrates sharp dissection of the remaining posteroinferior quadrant; Figure 15.10 shows removal of the remaining posterosuperior quadrant of the parotid gland.

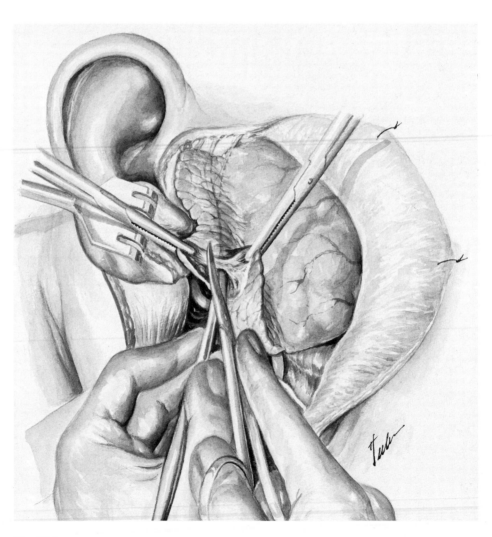

Fig. 15.6

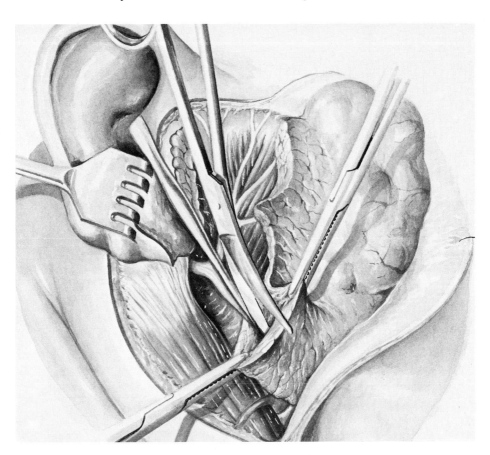

Fig. 15.7

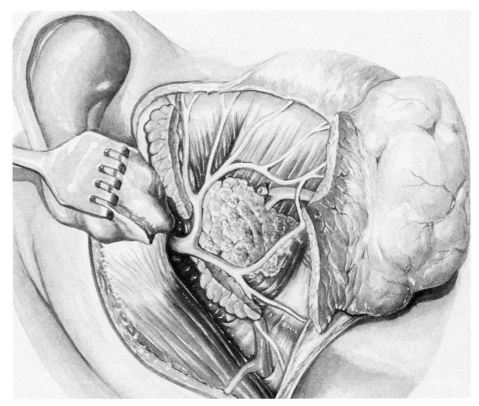

Fig. 15.8

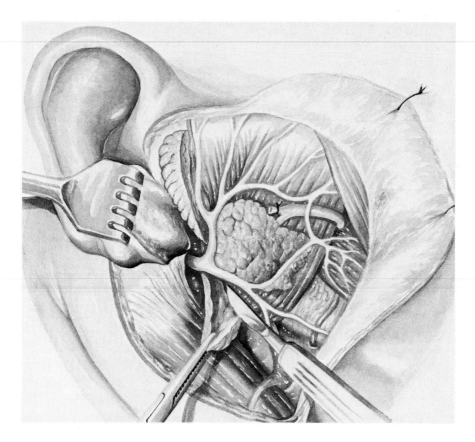

Fig. 15.9

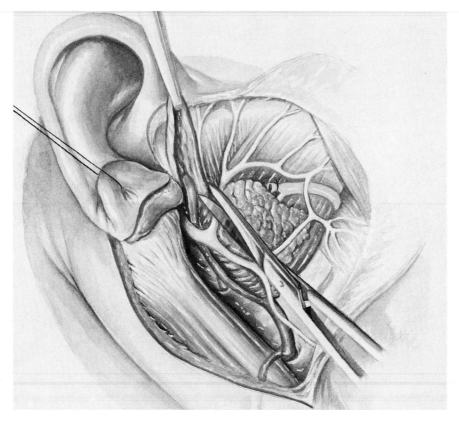

Fig. 15.10

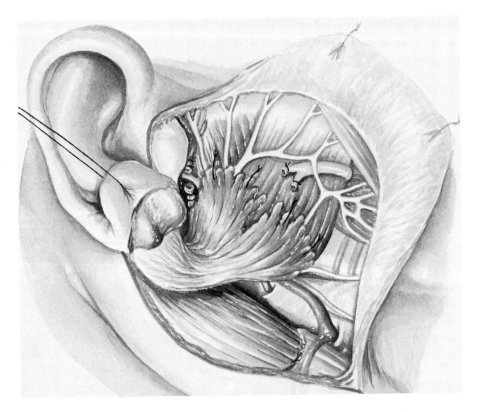

Fig. 15.11

Where desirable, a frozen section is done. If the tumor is benign and embedded in normal parotid tissue, the operation is now finished. The surgeon has thus carried out a superficial parotidectomy. For cosmetic reasons, the deep operative defect behind the ascending ramus of the mandible, created during the course of the parotidectomy, is filled out by a muscle flap from the sternomastoid muscle. The flap is fanned out over both main branches of the facial nerve and fixed in place with catgut (Fig. 15.11).

According to French studies, transposition of muscle tissue over the branches of the facial nerve prevents the development of the auriculotemporal syndrome, the cause of which is still unclear.

A comparative study of 35 patients with and without this muscle flap has indicated that use of this flap in no way prevents the appearance of Frey's syndrome (Kornblut, Westphal and Miehlke, 1974).

After the muscle graft has been fixed, a suction drain (Redon's drain) is introduced and the wound is closed in layers with subcutaneous and skin sutures (Fig. 15.12).

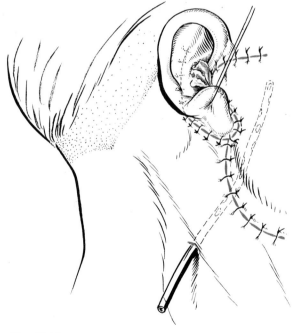

Fig. 15.12

Total Parotidectomy with Preservation of the Facial Nerve

If the benign tumor lies in the isthmus or the deep lobe or if it is a recurrent tumor, total parotidectomy with preservation of the facial nerve is indicated. The facial nerve must be carefully elevated from the deep lobe before the latter is removed. Small rubber bands are carefully placed around its individual branches, and the medial surface of the nerve is carefully dissected free from the deep lobe with fine, curved scissors. Each branch of the nerve not being worked on is covered during the intervening period with small compresses moistened in Ringer's solution.

The deep lobe is now isolated; sometimes it is adherent to the temporomandibular joint, the mandible or the muscles of this region (stylohyoid, styloglossus, digastric). This part of the lobe lies immediately on the external carotid artery and maxillary artery. Double ligation of the external carotid artery is often indicated. Finally, the deep lobe is carefully retracted between the branches of the facial nerve which are gently separated and then removed (Fig. 15.13).

Facial paralysis sometimes occurs following this type of total parotidectomy. Since the lesion is a neuropraxia or an axonotmesis at most, the mild paralysis resolves spontaneously.

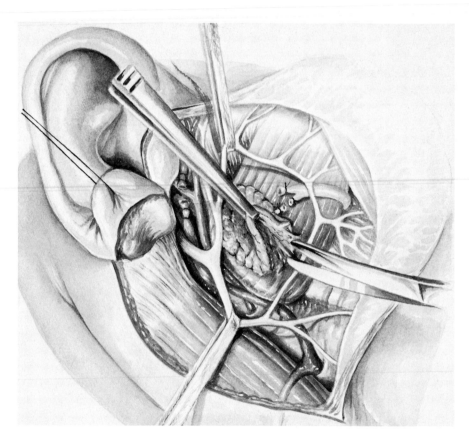

Fig. 15.13

Removal of a Deep Lobe Tumor

Removing a tumor of the retromandibular section or of the pharyngeal prolongation of the parotid gland is more difficult (Fig. 15.14a). Many of these socalled dumbbell tumors are recognized late because of their concealed location. For this reason, the characteristic tenderness in front of the mastoid process (Denecke 1958) should be noted. Often these tumors become apparent only after the pharyngeal wall or the tonsillar region has been displaced (Fig. 15.14b). Removal is made difficult because of the extent of the dumbbell constriction around the styloid process and the stylomandibular ligament.

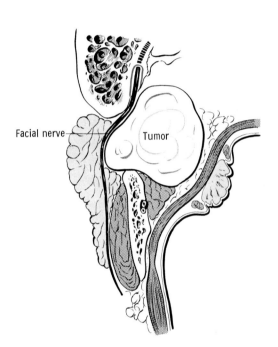

Fig. 15.14 a)   Dumbbell tumor of the parotid in horizontal section.

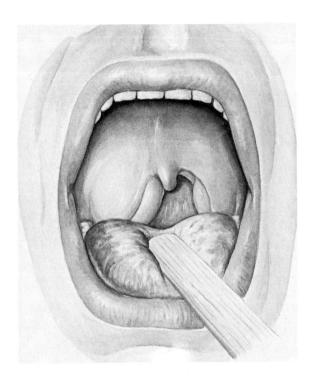

Fig. 15.14 b)   Dumbbell tumor presenting as a swelling behind the tonsillar region.

Technique. In these cases the stylomandibular ligament is divided in order to open up the surgical field. The ascending ramus of the mandible is subluxated anteriorly as far as possible with a hook. It is advantageous to ligate the external carotid artery or the maxillary artery as well as the superficial temporal artery and their corresponding veins. The trunk of the facial nerve is exposed first as described above and the superficial lobe is removed. Extra space is achieved by removing the tip of the mastoid process and the posterior part of the ascending ramus with the chisel or drill. Sometimes the styloid process is also removed. Occasionally, temporary division of the ascending ramus of the mandible is indicated. In such cases the bone is fixed by intraosseous wires after removal of the tumor; (osteosynthesis); the fragments are carefully adapted (see Fig. 11.19).

The tumor is then mobilized by blunt dissection with an elevator. If the trunk of the facial nerve is in danger of being overstretched during luxation of the dumbbell tumor from the depths of the retromandibular fossa, the fallopian canal should be opened and the mastoidal segment of the facial nerve should be widely lifted out of the canal. Figure 15.15 shows exposure of the nerve in the fallopian canal and the surface of the dumbbell tumor medial to the nerve.

Once the tumor has been mobilized from inferior or superior, it is relatively easy to retract the trunk of the facial nerve superiorly or inferiorly over the tumor and then to remove the tumor without further damaging the nerve. Following removal of a dumbbell tumor, a muscle graft is always introduced to reduce the size of the operative cavity (see p. 433). A suction drain is introduced and the wound is closed in layers.

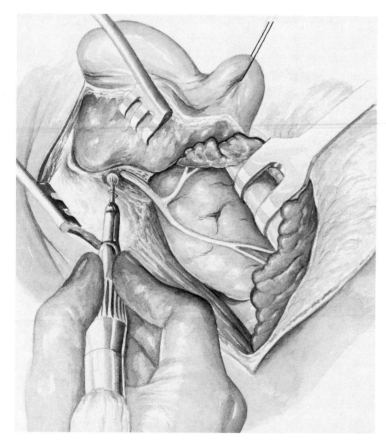

Fig. 15.15

Surgical Alternatives for Parotidectomy

Exposure of the facial nerve within the parotid gland is absolutely necessary first, not only for a subtotal but also for a total parotidectomy. There are different views on how the nerve might best be found. Direct access to the trunk of the nerve as used by the author is one possibility. An alternative is to find the branches peripherally and dissect posteriorly over the bifurcation to the trunk of the facial nerve.

If the parotid gland is regarded schematically as a triangle standing on its apex, access to the nerve can be found from any side or from the apex of the triangle. Several authors first seek the marginal mandibular branch of the nerve at the inferior pole of the gland and use it to guide them to the trunk of the nerve. Bailey (1941) began the dissection at the anterior edge of the parotid gland, and State searched for the parotid duct as a landmark. From here it is easy to find the parallel buccal branch or branches. When the buccal branch has been demonstrated, dissection is carried posteriorly to the bifurcation and over it to the trunk of the nerve. Finally the temporal branches can be sought at the superior edge of the parotid gland halfway between the outer canthus and the tragus; dissection is then continued backward along it (Trueblood and Moser's operation).

Although the author generally finds the procedures beginning at the periphery to be less advantageous and more difficult, the surgeon who carries out parotid surgery should be familiar with these routes of access since he will occasionally find them indispensable, e.g., for operations for a recurrence when scar tissue makes it dangerous to look for the trunk of the facial nerve in the retromandibular fossa.

Surgical alternatives are also available for access to the trunk of the facial nerve at its exit from the base of the skull anterior to the stylomastoid foramen. The first method can be carried out quickly at the end of a neck dissection.

The following method can be used to find the trunk of the nerve. After exposing the tip of the mastoid and its anterior edge, the volar surface of the index finger is introduced along the posterior belly of the digastric as far as its origin (Fig. 15.16). At this point the trunk of the facial nerve lies directly on the finger nail. After pushing the posterior part of the parotid gland forward, the trunk of the facial nerve is easily found immediately before it enters the gland.

The access preferred by Conley (1951) using the "pointer" as a guideline also deserves mention. The "pointer" is the pointed prolongation of the cartilaginous external auditory meatus. Access using this "pointer" as a guide requires deepening of the preauricular incision lying directly anterior to the tragus. Dissection then proceeds obliquely around the cartilaginous external meatus; anteroinferiorly, a pointed prolongation of the cartilage, the "pointer", is found (see Fig. 15.5). A point halfway between the "pointer" and the tip of the mastoid process is now visualized; dissection deeply at this point demonstrates the trunk of the facial nerve lying in loose fatty tissue.

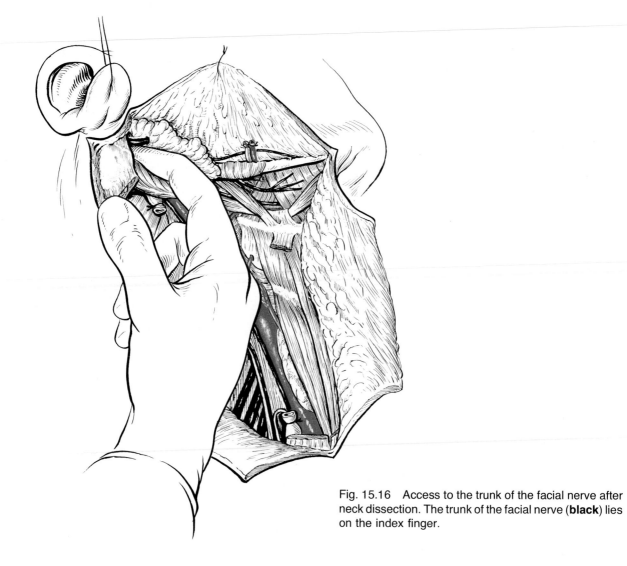

Fig. 15.16   Access to the trunk of the facial nerve after neck dissection. The trunk of the facial nerve (**black**) lies on the index finger.

Rules, Hints and Typical Errors

● Hogg and Kratz's procedure (1958) for finding the trunk of the facial nerve should always be followed as closely as possible:

a) The suprameatal spine is used as a landmark.

b) The tympanomastoid fissure and its end are sought.

c) Dissection is carried out 6–8 mm deep at this point followed by palpation with Freer's elevator and retraction of the fatty tissue to demonstrate the somewhat thicker tissue of the trunk of the facial nerve which runs obliquely through the retromandibular fossa.

- As soon as the trunk of the nerve is exposed, it should be followed *immediately* to the bifurcation. This is done by spreading the tissue lying over it with Freer's elevators.

- Bleeding from one of the tributaries of the posterior facial vein crossing the nerve should be dealt with immediately by ligature or coagulation with Malis' bipolar coagulation forceps before the fatty tissue in the depth of the retromandibular fossa around the presumed course of the nerve becomes impregnated with blood.

- Use of the styloid process as a landmark for finding the trunk of the facial nerve is not advocated, even though several authors recommend it. In such a procedure, the nerve can be damaged in attempts to find the styloid process in the depth of the wound.

- In all situations where the anatomy is not clear, the stimulator should be used to identify the trunk of the facial nerve and its peripheral branches.

- Becker (1958) has provided impressive evidence that all the peripheral branches of the facial nerve *always lie in a plane* parallel to the medial surface of the superficial lobe of the parotid gland. If this is kept in mind, all structures which look like nervous tissue, but which lie external to this plane, can be divided. In practice such structures are usually fine blood vessels put under tension during dissection. They are, therefore, empty of blood due to the tension and look like nerves. This knowledge allows dissection of the peripheral branches of the nerve to be carried out with certainty, speed and surgical elegance.

- All branches of the facial nerve which are not being worked on should be covered with swabs soaked in Ringer's solution to prevent these fine branches of the nerve from drying out. Saline solution should not be used (Shambaugh 1967) since this can damage the nerve.

Postoperative Care

As described above, a suction drain is introduced into the operative cavity. All preauricular stitches are made with the finest Mersilene on atraumatic needles to keep the stitch holes very small. A moderate-sized headband is applied for 3 to 4 days. The suction drain is removed at the end of this period as well as some of the sutures. The remaining sutures are removed on the sixth day.

Occasionally, facial paralysis occurs after parotidectomy. It is the author's experience that this paralysis can never be predicted, and the surgeon can only partly control its occurrence. Sometimes it is necessary to stretch and retract the nerve, and one is then convinced that a postoperative facial paralysis will result. Such patients, however, sometimes recover from the anesthetic without the slightest functional disturbance of the facial musculature. On the other hand, there are patients where the facial nerve has barely been disturbed during the operation and one is almost certain that postoperative paresis will not occur, and yet it does. The author has made it a practice, therefore, to warn the patient before the operation of the possibility of a temporary facial paresis due to a neuropraxia. It resolves after a few days or weeks.

A *seroma* occasionally occurs after the first 2 weeks but resolves spontaneously. Opening the wound with a blunt probe is sometimes indicated. A *salivary fistula* is a rare, but possible, complication. The fistula usually closes spontaneously within several days. If it does not close spontaneously, the salivary secretion can be dried up with a dose of radiation between 1,000 and 1,200 rad administered over a period of 8 to 10 days.

The region around the ear is insensitive for 2 to 3 months. The patient should be warned before the operation of this feeling of numbness "as if his ear did not belong to him". Sometimes about a year after the operation, the socalled gustatory sweating (Frey's syndrome) occurs. This is not the place to discuss the incompletely explained cause of this phenomenon. The circumscribed reddening and sweating over the operated area is occasionally a little disturbing for the patient; it should be explained to him, but the condition requires no specific management. The author himself suffers from Frey's syndrome following a parotidectomy but consoles himself with the knowledge that gustatory sweating disappears, or at least decreases, with increasing age.

Total Parotidectomy with Sacrifice of the Facial Nerve, Reconstruction of the Facial Nerve by a Free Autogenous Nerve Graft

If histological examination of the parotid tumor demands the most radical form of parotid surgery, a total parotidectomy is carried out with deliberate sacrifice of the facial nerve, often if not always accompanied by a simultaneous partial mandibulectomy and neck dissection en bloc. The decision as to whether reconstruction of the facial nerve is justifiable or indicated must be made in each individual case. If so, it should be decided which of the surgical possibilities should be used to reconstruct the facial nerve. Basically, there are three methods available:

1. Direct anastomosis,
2. Indirect anastomosis,
3. Autogenous nerve grafts.

The necessary surgical steps in each individual case will be discussed later.

In all cases where a malignant tumor is suspected because of rapid growth, pain, partial or complete facial paralysis and, sometimes, palpable lymph node metastases in the neck, a specimen is taken for frozen section immediately after making the incision. Special care should be taken so that tumor tissue is not carelessly spread from the biopsy wound.

A slightly curved double incision for the neck dissection is added to the Y-incision for the parotidectomy. After the end-branches of the facial nerve at the anterior border of the parotid gland have been identified, a total parotidectomy is carried out. A reliable method for identifying these end branches is described on page 437. The peripheral branches of the facial nerve are marked with colored silk. The tip of the mastoid process is removed down to the digastric fossa, and the fallopian canal is opened widely within the mastoid process so that the facial nerve can be divided just inferior to the origin of the chorda tympani nerve and at a safe distance from the tumor in healthy tissues.

The resulting gutter of the facial canal provides an excellent base for the nerve graft if reconstruction of the nerve is carried out later. The superficial temporal artery is ligated superiorly, the maxillary artery medially and the external carotid artery at a suitable point, usually just above the origin of the superior thyroid artery. The vessels are doubly ligated and divided. The corresponding veins are dealt with similarly. The parotid duct is ligated. The posterior portion of the masseter muscle is resected. Depending on the site of the tumor, a partial mandibulectomy is carried out, but this is not obligatory. Whether or not not the condyle should be preserved must be decided in each individual case.

The Stryker saw is an outstanding instrument for working quickly. The posterior belly of the digastric muscle and the stylohyoid as well as the styloglossus muscle are divided at a distance from the tumor-bearing parotid tissue. The superior constrictor muscle of the pharynx can now be seen. The histopathology of the tumor forms the basis for deciding whether reconstruction of the facial nerve should be undertaken (see Table 15.1). Of the three possibilities of rehabilitation mentioned above, direct anastomosis is not possible because of the extent of the defect. However, for didactic reasons the technique will be described because the principles of anastomosis formation constitute the basis for all reconstructive methods.

Table 15.1   When dealing with the fairly common metastases to the intraglandular and paraglandular lymph nodes of the parotid gland, where the primary tumor may be unknown, the surgeon must be flexible with regard to preservation or resection of the facial nerve. This applies also to the question of a possible reconstruction of the nerve (in group 3 or 4 or both groups combined). (After Haubrich and Miehlke, 1978)

Group 1	Group 2	Group 3	Group 4
Superficial or total parotidectomy with preservation of the facial nerve	Superficial or even total parotidectomy with preservation of the facial nerve, or partial resection with reconstruction by direct or indirect anastomosis (Conley's "big-little" operation)	Total parotidectomy with preservation of the facial nerve or partial resection and reconstruction by direct or indirect anastomosis	Total parotidectomy, neck dissection and resection of the mandible if necessary with sacrifice of the facial nerve without nerve reconstruction (Conley's "big-big" operation
No irradiation	No irradiation	Irradiation	Irradiation
Monomorphic adenoma (oncocytoma, basal-cell adenoma)	Mucoepidermoid tumor ("low grade type")	Recurrent acinic-cell tumor	Secondary malignant mixed tumor at an advanced stage
Pleomorphic adenoma (mixed tumor)	Acinic-cell tumor	Secondary malignant mixed tumor (carcinoma within a pleomorphic adenoma)	Mucoepidermoid tumor ("high grade type" at an advanced stage)
Cystadenolymphoma (Warthin's tumor)		Mucoepidermoid tumor ("high grade type")	Adenoidcystic carcinoma (cylindroma)
Lymphangioma			Adenocarcinoma
Schwannoma of the facial nerve is included here, because the surgical approach is similar. It is only occasionally possible to preserve the facial nerve which must therefore be reconstructed if necessary			Undifferentiated carcinoma
			In principle all tumors causing preoperative facial paresis

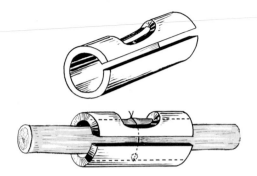

Fig. 15.17 Formation of the anastomosis at the periphery using a split silicone or collagen tube.

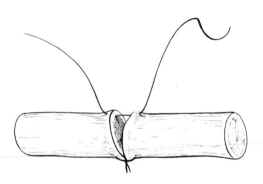

Fig. 15.18 Nerve suture. Individual atraumatic monofilament sutures passed through the epineurium.

Operative Technique of Nerve Anastomosis

To obtain good results in *nerve suture*, all tension must be avoided on the suture site when making the anastomosis of the divided nerve. Tension on the anastomosis produces a fairly severe connective tissue reaction at the anastomotic site which hinders the growth of the axons. According to Millesi et al. (1972), it is even possible that axons which have already reached the distal stump can be damaged by the contraction process of the scar tissue. If direct anastomosis of the nerve stumps is possible, it is carried out using an individual 10×0 monofilament suture through the substance of the nerve or the perineurium (Fig. 15.17).

Figure 15.18 shows the introduction of several individual epineural sutures.

The site of the anastomosis is protected by a silicone or collagen cylinder which, at the same time, also prevents the formation of undesirable scar tissue around the sutures. A drop of autogenous plasma is introduced through a window in the cylinder (Fig. 15.19). This helps stabilize the nerve and forms a bridge for the new growth of Schwann cells. A drop of the tissue glue Histoacryl is introduced with a pipette at each end of the tube (Fig. 15.19).

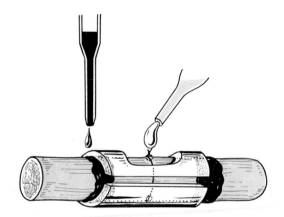

Fig. 15.19 Stabilization of the nerve and the suture by a tube, plasma (**center**) and tissue glue (**side**).

Extremely careful adaptation of the nerve stumps is a prerequisite if successful results are to be achieved.

This is done with fine silver probes introduced through the hole in the silicone cylinder; they are used to manipulate the stumps of the nerve until exact apposition is achieved (Fig. 15.20). The procedure is carried out very carefully under the operating microscope and is an essential prerequisite for the success of the operation. Until recently, this technique of anastomosis has generally been used with good results by surgeons (notably Conley) who have concentrated on surgery of the extratemporal part of the facial nerve. We have also used this technique with equally good results. The author has recently, however, been influenced by Millesi et al. (1972) to change over to the socalled fascicular suture for surgery of the facial nerve also. In this technique the epineurium of the nerve stump is first resected (Fig. 15.21) in order to remove the principal source of connective tissue proliferation. The fascicles of the facial nerve, which can be easily recognized under the microscope, are now sutured with 10×0 monofilament as for a perineural suture. If this is not possible, a suture is introduced through the fascicle itself so that the proximal and distal stumps of the facial nerve are exactly apposed (Fig. 15.21).

While Millesi does not use any covering for this suture in surgery of the extremities, the author does not wish to give up the additional protection for the fine anastomosis used in surgery of the facial nerve. For this reason the nerve suture is protected with a tube of collagen or silicone. At present one material does not appear to have an advantage over the other. The tube is fashioned as illustrated in Figure 15.17 and placed around the anastomosis. A drop of autologous plasma is introduced with a pipette through the hole in the tube. A drop of Histoacryl is introduced at both ends of the tube to anchor the reunited nerve in position.

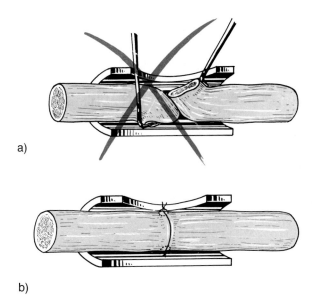

a)

b)

Fig. 15.20   Exact approximation of the nerve stumps in the silicone cylinder.
a) Incorrect,
b) Correct.

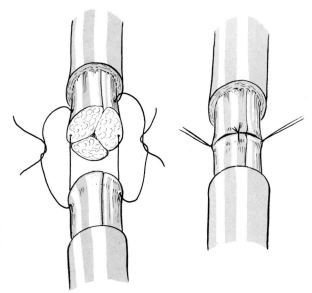

Fig. 15.21   Millesi's fascicular suture.

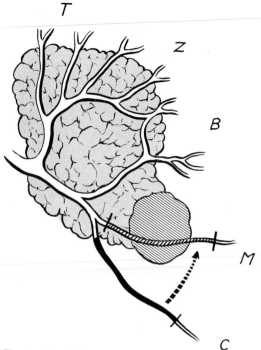

Fig. 15.22   Indirect anastomosis

T = Temporal branches
Z = Zygomatic branches
B = Buccal branches
M = Marginal mandibular branch
C = Cervical branch

It is conceivable that, when the tumor is widely resected, one of the important end-branches had to be sacrificed while one of the other less important branches could be preserved. The remaining longer segment of the latter nerve may then be anastomosed to a more important branch, i.e., the so-called *indirect anastomosis* (Fig. 15.22).

If the trunk of the facial nerve must be sacrificed and if several peripheral branches must be resected, the methods discussed up to this point are no longer practicable and a *free autogenous nerve graft* must be used. The author prefers to use the great auricular nerve or branches of the cervical plexus as the donor nerve. The donor nerve is removed from the contralateral side of the neck due to the danger of lymph node metastases on the homolateral side.

In order to *find the great auricular nerve*, a perpendicular line is visualized from the external auditory canal to the first skin crease of the neck. An incision in the skin crease at this point exposes the donor nerve just dorsal to the external jugular vein running in the subcutaneous tissue (Fig. 15.23). A segment of the donor nerve corresponding to the defect is now taken. If reconstruction of the entire parotid plexus is needed, further segments should be taken from the cervical plexus which are found spreading out from the primary ramus in the depths of the wound.

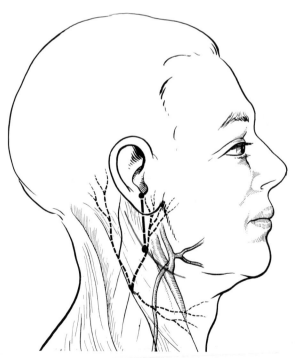

Fig. 15.23   Incision for taking a free autogenous nerve graft.

It has been the author's practice recently to replace the site of the anastomosis in the gutter of the facial canal after having introduced the sutures into the trunk of the facial nerve. It does not seem to be significant whether the autogenous nerve is a little too long or too short. Exact apposition of the axons and fixing them in the optimal position is much more important. The open gutter of the facial canal provides the best conditions. Figure 15.24 shows the anastomosis with the trunk of the nerve lying in the gutter at the mastoid end as well as reconstruction of the trunk and branches of the facial nerve.

The trunk of the facial nerve is divided just distal to the origin of the chorda tympani unless there is a reason for dividing it higher. A small scalpel or a piece of razor blade is used. The nerve is divided transversely with one cut. The distal stump is then dissected from the canal. The transverse connective tissue adhesions across the stylomastoid foramen are divided parallel to the course of the nerve and spread apart so that the distal part of the nerve can be easily removed. Anastomosis of the nerve trunk with the graft trunk now follows. The anastomosis is covered with collagen or silicone foil and the graft is secured with Histoacryl.

In the periphery, the fine branches of the nerve are sutured to the branches of the donor nerve with a fascicular suture and secured with a silicone or col-

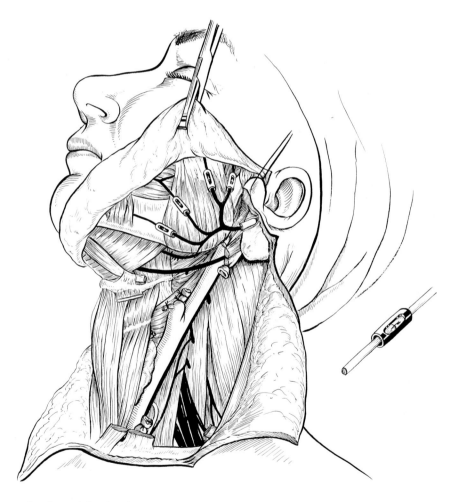

Fig. 15.24 Situation after reconstruction of the trunk and branches of the facial nerve (from Conley, J.: Concepts in Head and Neck Surgery. Thieme, Stuttgart 1970).

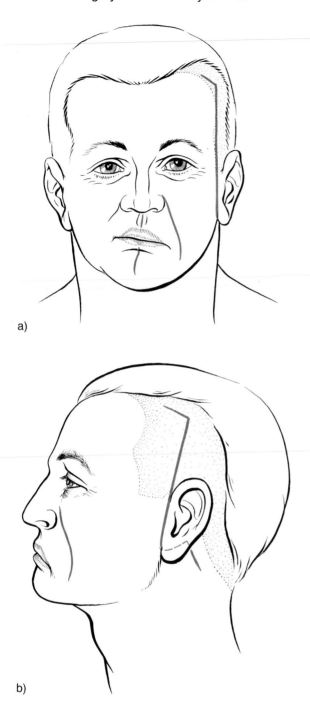

a)

b)

Fig. 15.25 a), b)   Incision for insertion of plastic mesh.

lagen tube. The relative position of the fascicles is checked through the hole in the cylinder and corrected with the operating microscope if necessary.

Drops of plasma are infused in the anastomosis itself and the whole is secured with drops of Histoacryl at both ends of the collagen or silicone cylinder.

If the extent of the resection in the region of the masseter muscle permits, the anterior part of this muscle is occasionally freed from its insertion and stitched with silk sutures to the orbicularis oris muscle medial to the reconstructed facial nerve. This is done for cosmetic reasons to provide partial suspension of the face during the interval required for reinnervation of the muscles of expression.

Finally the wound is closed in layers. A suction drain is introduced at a distance from the anastomotic site. For those cases where the type and extent of the tumor does not permit reconstruction of the facial nerve, other considerations supervene.

If the external auditory meatus or the ascending ramus of the mandible appear to be endangered by the extent of the tumor, these structures are included in the specimen according to the principles described in other chapters of this book. If reconstruction of the facial nerve is not possible, the paralyzed side of the face is suspended after removal of the tumor using one of the muscle-fascia techniques described by Lexer (1931), Rosenthal (1930), Ragnell (1958) and McLaughlin (1953). The author prefers Mennig's (1964) technique for suspension of the face using a nylon net (Figs. 15.25–15.27), particularly where postoperative radiotherapy will not be used (e.g., after resection of an adenoidcystic carcinoma [formerly cylindroma]). The advantage of this method compared to the myofascioplasty is that wide implantation of a bifurcate plastic net within the subcutaneous tissues not only elevates the face but also stabilizes the cheek which improves vocalization of the labial "p" which is otherwise difficult with a facial paralysis. If postoperative radiotherapy is to be carried out, the plastic net should not be introduced before radiotherapy since it can lead to prolonged inflammation with partial or complete rejection of the net. In this case either a myofascioplasty should be carried out at the same time as the operation or a nylon net should be implanted at a later date. A plastic net should be used only if the patient has been free of recurrence for a long period of time and if additional radiotherapy is not planned.

Plastic Procedures for Irreparable Facial Paralysis

Fitting of a Bifurcate Plastic Net

Mennig's operation (1964) mentioned above proceeds as follows: The incision is made as in Figure 15.25. The facial skin is undermined widely to reach an incision in the nasolabial fold. Further tunneling of the skin of the upper and lower lip is carried a little beyond the midline incision to the intact side of the face. An individually shaped piece of plastic mesh (Fig. 15.26) is now introduced subcutaneously via the incision. It is fastened with mattress sutures of chromic catgut and silk. Both ends of the net are deliberately pulled slightly over to the healthy side and attached (Fig. 15.27). With the mesh protruding from the incision in the nasolabial fold the end is pulled slightly posterosuperiorly so that the mouth is brought into a horizontal position. The ends of the mesh are fixed in this position by several mattress sutures. Next, the wide part of the plastic mesh is retracted posterosuperiorly via the posterior incision in order to overcorrect the anterior part of the face on the paralyzed side. The mesh is now fixed in this position with multiple mattress sutures to the underlying tissue, the zygoma, the masseter and occasionally the periosteum of the ascending ramus of the mandible. If the released facial skin is stretched posterosuperiorly after the incision in the nasolabial fold has been sutured, the amount of facial skin to be resected is the same as for the usual face lift (see Vol. 1, Chap. 3).

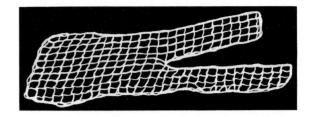

Fig. 15.26   Plastic mesh.

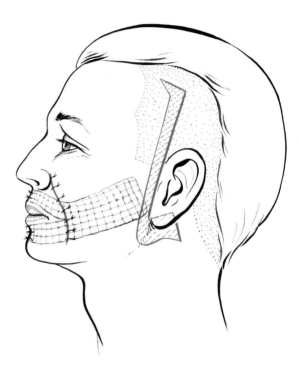

Fig. 15.27   Site of implanted plastic mesh.

"Muscular Neurotization" and Myofascioplasty

Rosenthal (1916) developed a muscular neurotization operation for re-innervation of the paralyzed muscle of facial expression. On the basis of the research of the orthopedic surgeon Erlacher (1914), he assumed that nerve fibers could grow from healthy tissue into the paralyzed muscle which then recovered tone and a certain amount of voluntary movement. The prerequisite for such a myoneurotization was a wide connection of the donor muscles to the paralyzed musculature.

According to Lexer (1931) and Gohrbandt (1950), parts of the masseter and temporalis muscle innervated by the motor division of the trigeminal nerve are used for the transplant. The procedure is only applicable if the trigeminal nerve is intact, which is not always the case (e.g., facial paralysis after operation for tumors of the cerebellopontine angle).

Figure 15.28 shows the principles of the operation: The interrupted red lines show the position of the skin incision.

Taking the course of the trigeminal nerve into account (Fig. 15.28), segments are split off from the above muscles and transposed by tunneling to the orbicularis oris and orbicularis oculi muscles. Rosenthal's operation is based on the purely mechanical procedure of muscle rotation plasty worked out by Lexer. Today it is known as the Lexer-Rosenthal procedure.

Rosenthal's attractive theoretical supposition has not remained undisputed. Recently Felix (1961) raised significant objections based on animal experiments conducted by his collaborator deWeese. These objections were confirmed in 8 patients who had been operated on by the Rosenthal-Lexer-Gohrbandt method. He concluded that "the sup-

posed myoneurotization does not occur. The only facial structures which move after this plastic operation are the temporalis or masseter muscles which are innervated by the motor root of the trigeminal nerve." This is supported by the electromyographic findings of Struppler and Scheininger (1961) on patients who had undergone the Lexer-Rosenthal operation. A re-innervation of the muscles of expression from the motor branches of the trigeminal nerve could be ruled out by taking simultaneous recordings from the synergistic muscles supplied by the facial and trigeminal nerves.

It should be emphasized that the slight movement achieved by the masseter or temporalis muscle and a certain tone of the face together with improved masticatory and speech functions is of great importance for the patient.

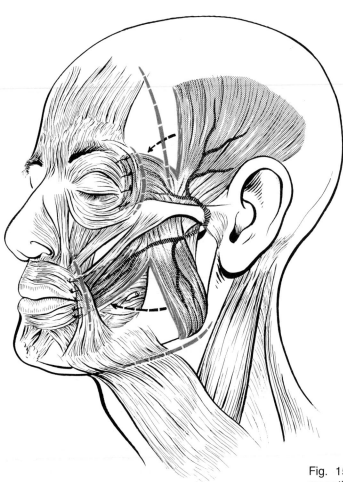

Fig. 15.28   Incision for and diagram of "muscular neurotization".

The muscle transposition described should be tried in young patients who are prepared to undertake the tiresome self-training required for transferring the action of the masseter and temporalis muscles to the paralyzed facial muscles. A simple *fascioplasty* with suspension of the paralyzed muscles by a wire sling should be used to produce simple improvement at rest in older patients.

There are several varied modifications of fascioplasty, the standardization of which is associated with the name Blair (1926). As first described by Stein (1913), the donor site is the fascia lata of the thigh. Transplanted fascia is nourished at the receptor site by ingrowing blood vessels; retraction is maintained by wound contraction. The principle of the operation is to enclose the sphincter muscles of the mouth with a subcutaneously introduced fascial sling suspended from the anterior part of the zygomatic arch. Gillies (1934) used an additional narrow fascial strip drawn in a figure of eight around the paralyzed side of the mouth to improve suspension of the angle of the mouth.

Finally, musculoplasty and fascioplasty can be combined as in the method described by McLaughlin (1953). This procedure serves as a model for the similar operations used by Aschan (1956) and Ragnell (1958) (Fig. 15.29). The movement of the temporalis muscle is transmitted to the paralyzed half of the mouth by interposition of a strip of fascia lata.

The interrupted red lines in Figure 15.29 mark the site of the necessary skin incision. The tendon of the temporalis muscle together with the coronoid process is divided from the mandible and is united by a short, narrow fascial strip with an additional fascial sling drawn in a figure of eight around the paralyzed muscles of the mouth.

The author usually combines this type of operation with a face lift (see Vol. 1, Chap. 3) via a correspondingly extended skin incision.

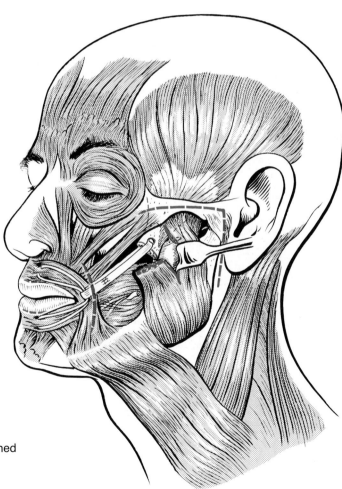

Fig. 15.29 Incision for and diagram of combined musculoplasty and fascioplasty.

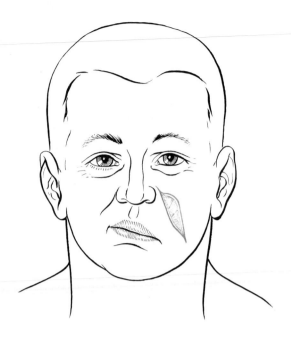

Fig. 15.30   Incision for correction of a drooping corner of the mouth.

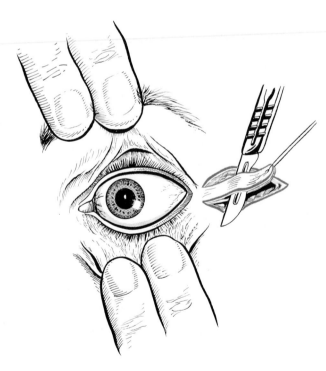

Fig. 15.31   Incision for elimination of an ectropion.

Suppression of the Function of the Antagonists

Increased muscle tone on the contralateral side is often observed in a facial paralysis. It can considerably accentuate the already pronounced asymmetry. The situation can be improved by suppressing the increased muscle tone of the opposite side. Approximately 1 cm of tissue is excised from the hypertonic muscles, particularly the zygomatic muscles and the levator labii superioris, via an incision in the nasolabial fold. The fibers of the depressor labii inferioris and depressor anguli oris are divided via an oral mucosal incision.

Corrective Operations on the Soft Tissues of the Face

Plication of the facial skin as described by Joseph, Lexer and others is only to be regarded as a palliative operation. According to Schuchardt (1954) the undermining of the skin of the cheek should be carried as far as the nasolabial fold to allow ingrowth of scar tissue over as wide an area as possible. This prevents a recurrence of the skin laxity.

Plication of the facial skin alone is seldom adequate. The *dependent corner of the mouth*, in particular, and the philtrum which is drawn to the healthy side are often not satisfactorily managed. An S-shaped excision of skin of the cheek from the nasolabial fold, therefore, is required at a second operation in order to add some animation to an otherwise smooth and lifeless cheek (Fig. 15.30).

In the *presence of an ectropion*, the lacrimal punctum is no longer bathed in tears; the physiological drainage of the tears is disturbed and epiphora develops. After careful consideration of the pros and cons, the ophthalmologist is occasionally prepared to reduce the secretion of tears artificially by removing the palpebral part of the lacrimal gland. The orbital part of the gland should always be preserved "since an excess of tears has never yet damaged an eye, but too little has sometimes led to damaged vision due to corneal desiccation" (Sautter 1956). Physiologically, it is undoubtedly better to try to deal with the ectropion. The author has had good results with Edgerton and Wolfort's procedure (1969) (dermal-flap canthal lift). A 2.5 × 0.5 cm

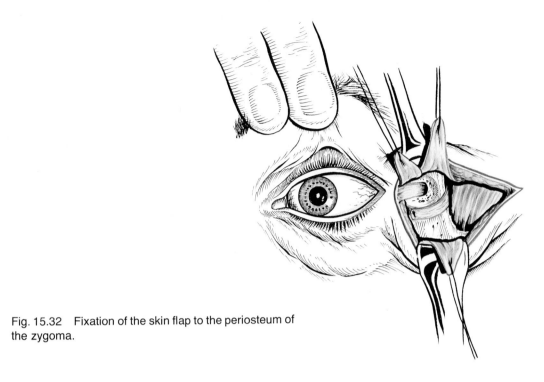

Fig. 15.32   Fixation of the skin flap to the periosteum of the zygoma.

skin flap is formed at the lateral canthus as shown in Figure 15.31; an epidermal shave is carried out at the appropriate point. At the medial end of the origin of the zygoma, an elliptical groove is formed and a tunnel is drilled with a medium-sized burr from this groove to the posterior surface of the zygoma. The skin flap is now drawn through this tunnel and fixed to the periosteum of the zygoma with a slight overcorrection (Fig. 15.32). Up to now this method has succeeded in eliminating the ectropion and a satisfactory cosmetic result has been produced. The often ugly result of a tarsorrhaphy can thus be avoided.

Mühlbauer (1973) has developed a simple and elegant procedure for narrowing the palpebral cleft in patients with paralysis. Magnets shaped in the form of the eyelids are implanted in the upper and lower lids on the cartilage of the tarsal plate; their mutual attraction facilitates closure of the lids.

Rules, Hints and Typical Errors

In reconstructing the extratemporal section of the facial nerve (e.g., after lacerations), the following should be observed particularly:

● Care must be taken to ensure that there is no tension on the anastomosis site, and that the operative trauma to the nerve is minimized while preparing the stumps for suture. Recent research by Millesi et al. (1972) has shown that the neighboring connective tissue can grow into the anastomosis if given an opportunity because of sloppy technique or tension on the sutures. As few sutures as possible should be introduced.

● In surgery of the extratemporal part of the facial nerve, the author has made it a rule always to place the proximal anastomosis in the gutter of the fallopian canal in doubtful cases. The advantages of this procedure are that:

a) the anastomosis is protected to a certain extent by the fallopian canal,

b) suturing can be avoided.

● Anastomosis directly at the bifurcation of the nerve is unfavorable since the junction of two donor nerves on the trunk of the nerve increases the danger of connective tissue ingrowth between the anastomosis.

● Due to the very extensive anastomosis formation in the parotid plexus, reconstruction of the peripheral branches of the second order is not recommended. Experience has shown that, even after loss of either the main superior or the inferior branches with preservation of the other main branches, only about a 15% deficit occurs (Conley 1961). Nevertheless, reconstruction of *these* main branches is always necessary in an attempt to achieve optimal results.

● The marginal mandibular branch is an exception; it anastomoses to the remaining part of the plexus in only 5 to 12% of the patients. Since it divides peripherally into two branches much more often than was previously thought, reconstruction of the marginal mandibular branch is only advisable if a defect is present in the proximal portion in the area of the origin of the cervicofacial branch. The fact that the marginal mandibular branch often divides peripherally explains why the occasional paralysis of the lower lip following operations in the upper part of the neck often resolves spontaneously.

● Lesions of the facial nerve in deep wounds of the face deserve special mention. Good results are achieved with primary restitution of continuity of the facial nerve. If the primary suture is not possible for any reason, equally good results can be achieved with the socalled early secondary suture. The doctor who first sees the patient at the site of the accident should mark the stumps of the nerve with a preliminary stay suture (colored silk, if possible) and, at the same time, prevent their retraction by fixing them to the underlying tissue. In this way the damaged branches of the nerve can be found relatively easily 3 weeks later and dealt with.

● There is no reason for resignation in patients where neither a primary nor an early secondary suture has been undertaken. Recent experience has shown that reconstructive surgery can be successful as long as the muscles of expression are prepared for re-innervation. The chances for rehabilitation are good within the first month. After 5 months, the chances decrease rapidly, and after 1 year, the prospects for resumption of function from a reconstruction of the nerve are usually very slight but not altogether hopeless. In these patients the author bases his decision on the results of galvanic stimulation, EMG, and Nessel's (1970) succinyl tests.

Removal of the Submandibular Gland

Indication

Excision of the submandibular gland is advised in many patients because of *chronic inflammation*, with or without *stone formation*. The stone generally occurs in the duct of the gland. The symptoms are well known: Severe pain with swelling of the gland during eating, thick purulent secretion from Wharton's duct or complete absence of secretions. The radiopaque calculus can often, if not always, be demonstrated by radiographs. The calculus can often be felt in the duct and palpated with a probe. In the latter case, the duct should first of all be split on the probe as a therapeutic trial so as to be able to get away with as minimal surgery as necessary.

All *neoplasms* constitute a further indication for removing the submandibular gland. The relatively frequent adenoidcystic carcinoma (cylindroma) with its extremely gloomy prognosis should be noted in particular.

Loss of the gland has no functional consequences, particularly in cases of chronic inflammation and neoplasms where the function of the gland has usually already been lost.

Surgical Anatomy

The submandibular gland lies on the hyoglossus muscle in the triangle between the anterior and posterior bellies of the digastric muscle. A branch of the gland lies along the mylohyoid muscle; the remaining part of the body of the gland lies on the hyoglossus muscle. Superiorly, the gland extends just inferior to the edge of the mandible; large and possibly congested glands often overlap the posterior belly of the digastric muscle inferiorly.

Through a gap between the posterior edge of the mylohyoid muscle and the anterior edge of the hyoglossus muscle, the submandibular gland comes into direct contact with the sublingual gland which sits in the floor of the mouth superior to the mylohyoid muscle. The duct of the submandibular gland (Wharton's duct) passes through the above-mentioned cleft in the muscles toward the floor of the mouth and then toward its orifice on the superior surface of the floor of the mouth on the medial side of the sublingual gland.

Critical Structures

1. The marginal mandibular branch of the facial nerve crossing the facial artery and vein at the inferior edge of the mandible.

2. The hypoglossal and lingual nerves and the submandibular ganglion between the medial side of the body of the gland and the course of the lingual artery.

Special Instruments

These include soft tissue instruments and Malis' bipolar coagulation forceps; the stimulator may be useful for the beginner to identify the marginal mandibular nerve (see Fig. 15.34).

Position

The head of the patient is slightly extended by tilting the operating table downward; the head is turned to the healthy side. Drapes are applied and stitched in place or secured with towel clips.

Operative Technique

A 5 cm long sickle-shaped skin incision (convexity inferiorly) is made one fingerbreadth inferior to the angle of the mandible, beginning just anterior to the lateral cornu of the hyoid bone (Fig. 15.33). (The following figures are based on Rankow 1968).

The platysma is divided and the facial artery and vein are sought at the inferior edge of the mandible. These vessels are found on the external surface of the mandible and the anterior edge of the masseter muscle. The following trick can be used to ensure preservation of the marginal mandibular branch: the above-mentioned vessels are ligated 1 cm inferior to the edge of the mandible and divided. They are then displaced superiorly and fixed to the slightly retracted soft tissues of the cheek with a catgut suture (Fig. 15.34).

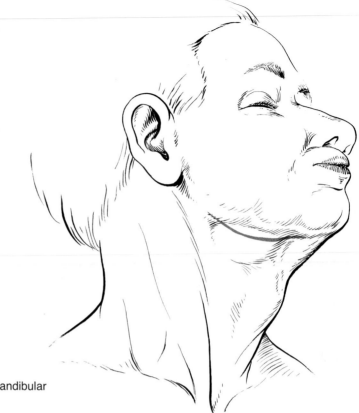

Fig. 15.33   Incision for removal of the submandibular gland.

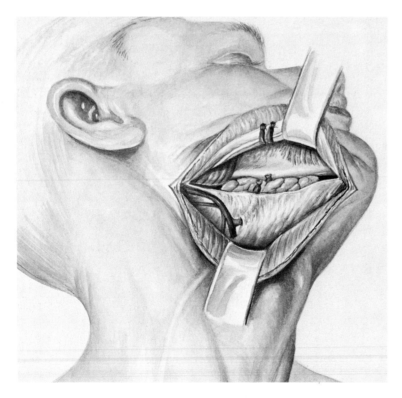

Fig. 15.34

Since the facial artery and vein are crossed by the marginal mandibular branch, this branch is caught up by retracting the vessels superiorly and thus protected from damage. The marginal mandibular branch only anastomoses with the other end-branches of the facial nerve in 5 to 12% of the patients. It is, therefore, very important to preserve this branch since its division promptly leads to a noticeable paralysis of the lower lip (see also p. 452.

Unlike the facial artery, the facial vein does not run deeply in the digastric triangle but over the belly of the submandibular gland. It should, therefore, be doubly ligated and divided at the inferior border of the gland. Only then can the submandibular gland be elevated. The anterior belly of the digastric muscle comes into view; posterior retraction of the body of the gland demonstrates the posterior edge of the mylohyoid muscle.

The mylohyoid muscle serves as a guide for finding the hypoglossal and lingual nerves as well as Wharton's duct. This muscle is forcibly retracted anteriorly with a double hook which opens up the anterior part of the digastric triangle far enough to demonstrate Wharton's duct in the center of this region, the lingual nerve superior to it and the hypoglossal nerve running anterosuperiorly inferior to it. Finally the submandibular ganglion lying just inferior to the lingual nerve is demonstrated by blunt separation of the capsule of the gland from the underlying tissues (Fig. 15.35). The gland is further freed from the space by double ligation and division of Wharton's duct (Fig. 15.36). Holding the stump of the duct with forceps, the body of the gland is now turned posteriorly so that the posterior surface with the facial artery attached can be seen (Fig. 15.36).

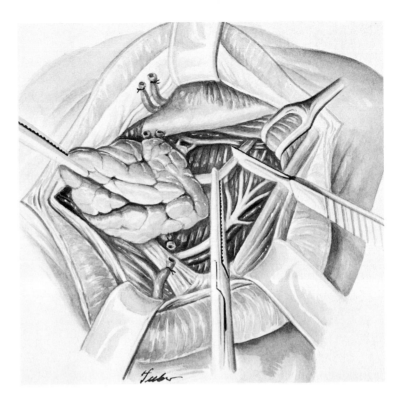

Fig. 15.35

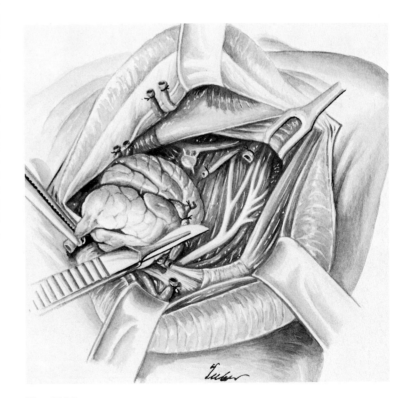

Fig. 15.36

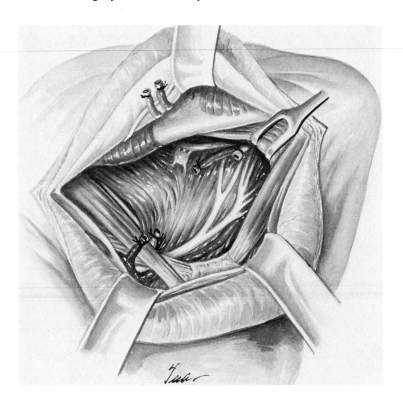

This vessel is again doubly ligated and divided. The submandibular gland is then removed from the wound bed. Figure 15.37 shows the resulting situation.

After careful hemostasis using Malis' bipolar coagulation forceps if possible, a Penrose drain is introduced and the wound is closed in layers (Fig. 15.38).

Fig. 15.37

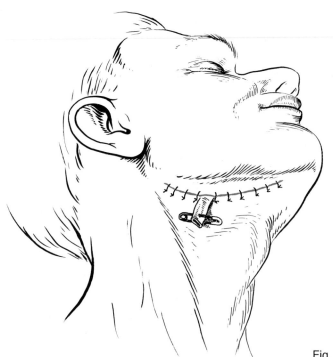

Fig. 15.38

Excision of the Sublingual Gland

The sublingual gland is about one-third the size of the submandibular gland and lies beneath the mucosa of the floor of the mouth between the tongue and the mandible on the mylohyoid muscle. This gland has several ducts one or more of which occasionally open directly into Wharton's duct. The best known and most frequent disorder of the sublingual gland is a *ranula*, a cystic submucosal swelling caused by blockage of one or more of the ducts (Fig. 15.39).

Malignant tumors of the sublingual gland occur but are very rare. If they occur, they are dealt with surgically by a procedure identical to that for carcinoma of the floor of the mouth. An en bloc removal is done by a partial glossectomy combined with resection of the floor of the mouth, partial mandibulectomy and neck dissection (for details see Chap. 13). The removal of a ranula will now be illustrated.

Special Instruments

These include small soft-tissue instruments and Malis' coagulation forceps.

Operative Technique

A thin silver probe is introduced into Wharton's duct and an elliptical incision is then made over the curve of the cystic swelling in the floor of the mouth (Fig. 15.39). The mucosal flaps are grasped with mosquito forceps and retracted during exposure of the ranula.

Figure 15.40 shows the mucosal flaps already dissected from the cyst lining; a plastic tube has been introduced into Wharton's duct. Figure 15.41 shows the situation from the side.

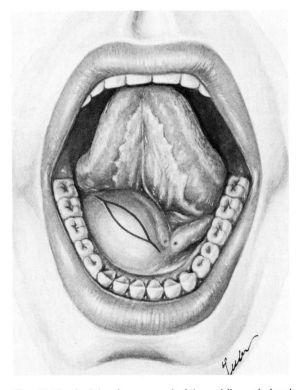

Fig. 15.39 Incision for removal of the sublingual gland.

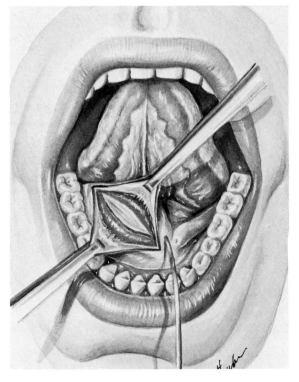

Fig. 15.40

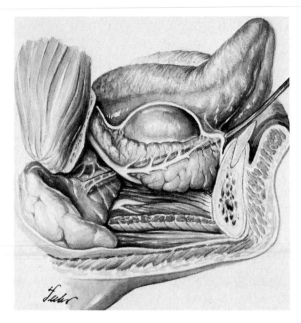

Fig. 15.41

The incision is extended anteriorly and posteriorly. The mucosal flaps over the cyst are carefully freed from the ranula, partly by blunt and partly by sharp dissection, with careful scissor strokes. The ranula thus becomes more and more mobile in the direction of the surgeon (Fig. 15.42).

The cystic swelling is now grasped with serrated forceps and freed from Wharton's duct by blunt dissection.

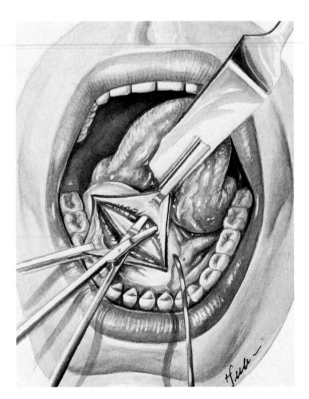

Fig. 15.42

The cyst is now free from the connective tissue and from its connections with the underlying mylohyoid muscle (Fig. 15.43). All small vessels in the field are dealt with by bipolar coagulation forceps. After removing the ranula together with the sublingual gland, the undamaged lingual nerve can be seen lying in the floor of the mouth next to Wharton's duct (Fig. 15.44).

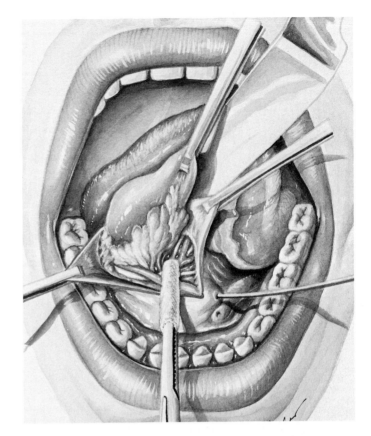

Fig. 15.43

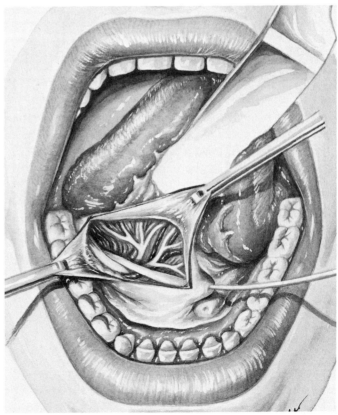

Fig. 15.44

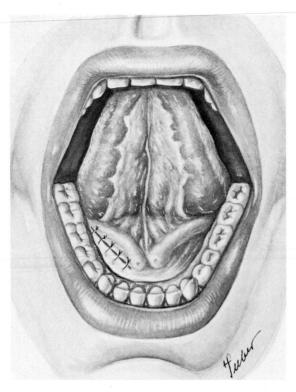

Fig. 15.45

The mucosa is now closed with 2 or 3 catgut sutures (Fig. 15.45).

Postoperative Care

A fluid diet and later a puréed diet is ordered for the first few days. Careful mouthwashes are useful.

Operations for Hemifacial Spasm

The term "hemifacial spasm" refers to uncoordinated, paroxysmal, involuntary movements of a clonic or fibrillary character in the muscles of facial expression supplied by the facial nerve.

The disease is usually unilateral (hemifacial spasm) and begins around the eye. Later it spreads inferiorly so that the lower part of the face and occasionally even the platysma are involved. Although the patient feels no actual pain during an attack, he finds these attacks disturbing, particularly in regard to his social life since facial spasm causes a severe deformity.

Facial spasm should be divided into primary and secondary types. The etiology and pathology of the first type have not yet been explained; the second is an undesirable residual condition arising from a previous facial paralysis.

Indications for the Operation

The cause of primary hemifacial spasm is unknown, but the patient expects relief from the physician. At the present time, surgical procedures must be used which suppress the symptoms, particularly the spasms of the muscles of expression.

In the last few years, two operations have emerged out of a whole series of different operations. Both of these operations attempt to eliminate excessive impulses in the peripheral neuron by attacking the extratemporal course of the facial nerve. These are the operations described by Scoville (1955), Miehlke (1959) and by Fisch (1972). Since this treatment only suppresses the symptoms but not the cause of the facial spasms, recurrence must be expected. This was certainly confirmed by a long-term follow-up of 30 patients. It is not yet known which operation yields the best results. It is to be hoped that these surgical methods will become superfluous when the etiology of the spasms has been discovered and a causal therapy can be developed. Both of the above-mentioned procedures will be described in brief.

Instruments

These are exactly the same as for a simple parotidectomy; the use of a stimulator (electroprobe), however, is obligatory. Fine neurectomy scissors from the set for surgery of the internal auditory meatus and Malis' coagulation forceps are useful.

Operative Technique

Scoville-Miehlke's Technique

A partial resection of the extratemporal course of the facial nerve is done as shown in Figure 15.46. Scoville carries out this partial resection on the trunk of the nerve in the retromandibular fossa. The author has modified this technique in an attempt to carry out a partial resection only on those branches of the facial nerve with the most severe spasm, leaving alone those branches which are not involved or are only minimally involved in the facial spasm. The purpose of this modification is to ensure that facial symmetry is not too noticeably affected after the operation. The branches of the facial nerve most affected by the spasm are sought in their course through the parotid gland *distal to the bifurcation*; the area of the facial musculature which they supply is checked with the stimulator. The branch intended for partial resection is isolated with a rubber band, elevated slightly from its bed and divided halfway through with a razor blade (Fig. 15.46).

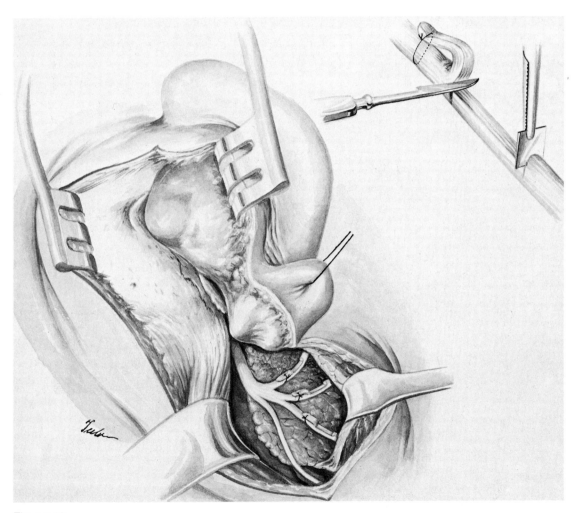

Fig. 15.46

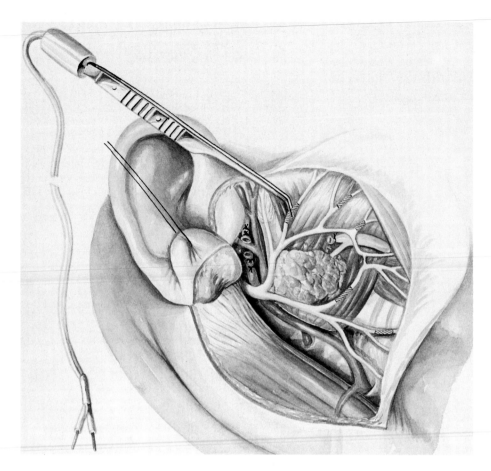

Fig. 15.47

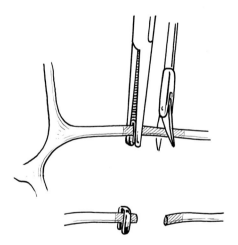

Fig. 15.48

The divided axon of the nerve is now turned back for 5 mm with fine neurectomy scissors and sutured to the epineurium in the direction of the facial nerve bifurcation. This prevents the new growth of axons into the periphery.

Fisch's Operation

The *most affected branches are completely divided and avulsed* further peripherally near the anterior edge of the parotid gland. This requires a superficial parotidectomy first.

The branches of the nerve to be divided are selected with the help of a stimulator. After identifying the area of distribution of the facial nerve branches, they are coagulated with Malis' coagulation forceps and divided (Fig. 15.47). The peripheral stumps are avulsed and a fine silver clip is placed on the central stump of the branch of the nerve to prevent peripheral growth of the axons (Fig. 15.48). In this way 75 to 80% of the peripheral branches of the facial nerve are eliminated. Only those few branches remain which were previously selected with the stimulator. These nerves maintain the symmetry of the face at rest (figures based on those of Fisch).

Postoperative Care and Functional Sequelae

A suction drain is left in for 2 to 3 days after the operation; the wound is closed in layers.

In both operations the tone and minimal function of the muscles of expression are retained. The patient must be emphatically warned about this before the operation. The author never fails to explain to the patient that he must expect a reduction in facial expression for a certain period of time after the operation (8 to 10 weeks) and a certain degree of facial paralysis. Electrotherapy and exercises for the movement of the muscles of expression are strictly forbidden during the postoperative phase even though they may seem to be appropriate because of the mild postoperative paralysis.

Bibliography

Aschan, P. E.: Muskel- und Sehnentransplantation bei Fazialis-parese. Fortschr. Kiefer- u. Gesichtschir. 2: 143, 1956

Bailey, H.: Treatment of tumours of parotid gland with special reference to total parotidectomy. Br. J. Surg. 28: 337, 1941

Bailey, H.: Parotidectomy; indications and results. Br. Med. J. 1: 404, 1947

Becker, W.: Die Klinik der Erkrankung der großen Kopfspeicheldrüsen. Z. Laryng. Rhinol. 37: 205, 1958

Blair, V. P.: Notes on the operative correction of the facial palsy. S. Afr. Med. J. 19: 116, 1926

Conley, J. J.: Tumors of the parotid gland. Surg. Clin. North Am. 51 (1951) 5

Davis, R. A., Anson, B. J., Büdinger, J. M., Kurth, L. E.: Surgical anatomy of the facial nerve and parotid gland based upon a study of 350 cervicofacial halves. Surg. Gynec. Obstet. 102: 384, 1956

Denecke, H. J.: Zur Chirurgie der Parotiserkrankungen unter Berücksichtigung des N. facialis. Z. Laryng. Rhinol. 37: 403, 1958

Edgerton, M. T., Wolfort, F. G.: The dermal flap canthal lift for lower eyelid support. Plast. Reconstr. Surg. 43: 42, 1969

Erlacher, P.: Hyperneurotisation; muskuläre Neurotisation, freie Muskeltransplantation. Zbl. Chir. 41: 625, 1914

Felix, W.: Spätergebnisse und biologische Beobachtungen bei operierten Fazialisparesen. Langenbecks Arch. Klin. Chir. 298: 940, 1961

Fisch, U.: The surgical treatment of facial hyperkinesia. In: Plastic and Reconstructive Surgery of the Face and Neck, Vol. II, ed. by J. Conley, J. T. Dickinson. Thieme, Stuttgart 1972

Frey, L.: Le syndrome du nerf auriculotemporal. Rev. Neurol. 30: 97, 1923

Gillies, H. D.: Proc. R. Soc. Med. 27: 1372, 1934

Gohrbandt, E.: Quoted in: Ch. Wilberg: Neuartige Operationsmethoden zur Beseitigung der Fazialisparese. Zbl. Chir. 75: 1550, 1950

Hogg, S. P., Kratz, R. C.: Surgical exposure of the facial nerve. Arch. Otolaryng. 67: 560, 1958

Janes, R. M.: Treatment of tumors of the salivary glands. Surg. Clin. North. Am. 23: 1429, 1943

Kornblut, A. D., P. Westphal, A. Miehlke: The effectiveness of a sternomastoid flap in preventing post-parotidectomy occurrence of the Frey-Syndrome. Acta Otolaryng. (Stockholm) 77: 368, 1974

Lathrop. F. D.: Affections of the facial nerve. J. Am. Med. Ass. 152: 19, 1933

Lexer, E.: Die gesamte Wiederherstellungschirurgie. Barth, Leipzig 1931

McLaughlin, C. R.: Surgical support in permanent facial paralysis. Plast. Reconstr. Surg. 11: 302, 1953

Mennig, H.: Plastischer chirurgischer Eingriff bei irreparabler Fazialislähmung. H. N. O. (Berlin) 12: 160, 1964

Miehlke, A.: Probleme der operativen Behandlung des Spasmus facialis. Arch. Ohren-, Nasen-, Kehlkopfheilk. 175: 464, 1959

Miehlke, A.: Surgery of the Facial Nerve. Urban & Schwarzenberg, Munich, Saunders, Philadelphia 1973

Millesi, H., Berger, A. Meissl, G.: Experimentelle Untersuchungen zur Heilung durchtrennter peripherer Nerven. Chir. Plast. (Berlin) 1: 174, 1972

Moser, F.: Zur operativen Behandlung der Parotisgeschwülste. Z. Laryng. Rhinol. 33: 195, 1954

Naumann, H. H.: Parotisgeschwülste und ihre Behandlung. Münch. Med. Wochenschr., 101: 1001, 1959

Nessel, E.: Die Succinyl-Kontraktur an der gelähmten Fazialismuskulatur, ein neues Diagnostikum zur Beurteilung aller Lähmungen. Arch. Klin. Exp. Ohren-, Nasen-, Kehlkopfheilk. 196: 198, 1970

Perzik, S. L.: Diagnosis and management of parotid tumors. Arch. Otolaryng. 67: 319, 1958

Ragnell, A.: A method for dynamic reconstruction in cases of facial paralysis. Plast. Reconstr. Surg. 21: 214, 1958

Rankow, R. M.: An Atlas of Surgery of the Face, Mouth and Neck. Saunders, Philadelphia 1968

Rosenthal, A.: Die bleibende Fazialislähmung und ihre Behandlung. Dtsch. Z. Chir. 223: 261, 1930

Rosenthal, A.: Die Eingriffe bei der Fazialislähmung. In: Allgemeine und spezielle chirurgische Operationslehre, Vol. IV, ed. by N. Guleke, R. Zenker. Springer, Berlin 1930

Sautter, H.: Die Fazialisparese vom augenärztlichen Standpunkt aus. Fortschr. Kiefer- u. Gesichtschir. 2: 127, 1956

Schuchardt, K.: Die Operationen am Gesichtsteil des Kopfes. In: Chirurgische Operationslehre, ed. by Bier, Braun, Kümmell. Barth, Leipzig 1954

Scoville, W. B.: Partial section of proximal seventh nerve trunk for facial spasm. Surg. Gynec. Obstet. 101: 494, 1955

Shambaugh Jr., G. E.: Surgery of the Ear, 2nd edn. Saunders, Philadelphia 1967

Stein, A. E.: Die kosmetische Korrektur der Fazialislähmung durch freie Faszienplastik. Münch. Med. Wochenschr. 25: 1370, 1913

Struppler, A., Scheininger, R.: Elektromyographische Untersuchungen zur Frage der Innervationsübernahme usw. Pflügers Arch. Ges. Physiol. 274: 48, 1961

Index

Numerals beginning with 2/ refer to page numbers in Volume 2